H. Porst · Penile Disorders

Springer

Berlin
Heidelberg
New York
Barcelona
Budapest
Hong Kong
London
Milan
Paris
Santa Clara
Singapore
Tokyo

H. Porst (Ed.)

Penile Disorders

International Symposium on Penile Disorders
Hamburg, Germany, January 26–27, 1996

With 95 Figures and 61 Tables

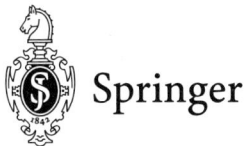 Springer

Prof. Dr. med. Hartmut Porst
Neuer Jungfernstieg 6a
20354 Hamburg
Germany

Acknowledgement

This publication has been supported and made possible by a generous grant from
SCHWARZ PHARMA AG, Alfred-Nobel-Str. 10, D-40789 Monheim.
Federal Republic of Germany

ISBN 3-540-61674-8 Springer-Verlag Berlin Heidelberg New York

Die Deutsche Bibliothek – CIP-Einheitsaufnahme

Penile disorders: with tables / International Symposium on Penile Disorders, Hamburg,
Germany, January 26-27, 1996. H. Porst (ed.).- Berlin; Heidelberg; New York; Barcelona;
Budapest; Hong Kong; London; Milan; Paris; Santa Clara; Singapore; Tokyo: Springer, 1997
    ISBN 3-540-61674-8
NE: Porst, Hartmut [Hrsg.]; International Symposium on Penile Disorders (1996, Hamburg)

© Springer-Verlag Berlin Heidelberg 1997
Printed in Germany

Typesetting: Michael Kusche, Goldener Schnitt, Sinzheim
Bookbinding and Printing: Druckhaus Beltz, Hemsbach

SPIN: 10545599   13/3133-5 4 3 2 1 0   Printed on acid-free paper

Contents

Foreword

This book contains a compilation of papers based on presentations made at the International Symposium on Penile Disorders held in Hamburg, Germany, 26–27 January 1996, under the Chairmanship of Hartmut Porst. This was a unique conference in that it comprehensively addressed various disorders that affect the organ situated at the "center of the male", the penis.

As an important beginning, the sociocultural aspects of the erect phallus were presented by G. Wagner from Copenhagen. The anatomy of the penis and the physiological conditions of erection were then discussed by K.-P. Jünemann from Mannheim, Germany. Previous conferences on the penis had concentrated only on specific areas of disease such as impotence. However, it became readily apparent that at this conference something new for almost every aspect of disease would be discussed, including congenital disorders such as hypospadias and epispadias, sexually transmitted and noninfectious dermatological diseases, and congenital and acquired penile curvatures and penile fractures. An excellent presentation of managing penile cancer by stage related therapeutic decision was presented by S. C. Müller from Bonn, Germany. There is no better person to present a discussion of Peyronie´s disease in 1996 from a historical and management perspective than J. Pryor from London, UK. This same degree of expertise was also demonstrated by I. Saenz de Tejada from Madrid, Spain, regarding priapism. Even the controversial subject of indications and management of penile lengthening and girth enhancement procedures was presented. Beginning late

Friday afternoon, the focus of the conference moved to
erectile difficulties, with an excellent historical perspective
presented by G. Wagner. Epidemiology and a diagnostic
plan for impotence were presented by W. H. Weiske from
Stuttgart, Germany. For me, the highlight of the conference
was a presentation on cavernous tissue neuropharma-
cology by I. Saenz de Tejada. He elegantly put together the
vast amount of molecular information now available to
explain the erectile cycle. Reports on various therapeutic
treatments, including oral drug and hormonal replacement,
topical and intraurethral therapy, vacuum therapy, and
vasoactive drug injection were presented. In fact, the
vasoactive drug injection program was presented in three
separate talks – an overview and two comparative studies.
Finally, the surgical treatment of erectile dysfunction was
presented in three talks directed at venous surgery, penile
revascularization, and penile implants.

This symposium was a heroic endeavor by Hartmut
Porst, who also made two presentations. I must admit that
I was somewhat skeptical that this symposium would be of
any real educational value, however, I am sure that it was
one of the best conferences on penile disorders ever put
together and that the other participants would agree.
Hopefully, with the chapters in this book the authors will
be able to share the experience of a truly excellent international symposium with the readers.

RONALD W. LEWIS, MD
Chief of Urology
Medical College of Georgia

Preface

About 15 years ago at the onset of my qualification in Urology I participated in an international symposium on adrenal diseases in which all aspects of this organ from embryological development to cancer disease were elucidated in order to give a complete survey of this organ to the audience. Indeed the imparted scientific knowledge was very impressive and during my further training period I missed similar symposiums focused on other urological organs and arranged likewise as the aforementioned one. Surely, there is a plenty of international congresses, symposiums and workshops offered to urologists all over the world, but in these meetings ordinarily only special scientific aspects of the respective urological organs are discussed. Therefore these meetings are not able to offer a complete overview on all physiological and pathophysiological conditions of the "organ of interest".

The intention of the subsequent International "Symposium on Penile Disorders" was to present a very actual survey of all important physiologic, pathophysiologic, paediatric, dermatologic and urologic aspects of this organ in one meeting. For this reason international renowned and out-standing experts from all over the world were invited and accepted this invitation being convinced, that this meeting must be a success. Indeed the unexpectedly enormous demand for this symposium indicated the great interest of urologists from all European countries and unfortunately forced us to cancel a lot of registrations due to the limited room capacity.

Both for all the participants and those who did not suc-
ceed or could not participate, this book presents nearly all
contributions with a considerable number of tables and
illustrations. I am deeply indebted to all those, who contri-
buted to the great success of this symposium encouraging
me to edit this volume.

Finally I wish to express my appreciation to my partner
Elfie Meier for her perfect assistance in planning and or-
ganizing this meeting.

Last, but not least I would like to thank all sponsors, first
of all Schwarz Pharma AG for their generous support, both
for the meeting and the publication of this book.

HARTMUT PORST

Contributors

J. Buvat
(EPARP)
49, rue de la Bassée, 59000 Lille, France

S. O. Burman
MSK Institute
3401 N. Central Ave., Chicago, IL 60634, USA

W. L. Furlow
4301 Gulf Shore Blvd. N., 1000, Naples, FL, USA

B. Habermann
Klinikum Marburg
Abt. Dermatologie und Andrologie
Deutschhausstraße 9, 35033 Marburg, Germany

P. W. Heaton
Kingston General Hospital
76 Stuart St., Kingston K7L 2V7, Ontario, Canada

K.-P. Jünemann
Klinikum der Stadt Mannheim
Theodor-Kutzer-Ufer, 68135 Mannheim, Germany

T. P. Kelly
MSD Institute
3401 N. Central Ave., Chicago, IL 60634, USA

W. KRAUSE
Klinikum Marburg
Abt. Dermatologie und Andrologie
Deutschhausstraße 9, 35033 Marburg, Germany

A. LEMAIRE
EPARP
49, rue de la Bassée, 59000 Lille, France

R. LEWIS
Section of Urology
Medical College of Georgia, Augusta, GA 30912-4050, USA

A. MORALES
Kingston General Hospital
76 Stuart St., Kingston K7L 2V, Ontario, Canada

S. C. MÜLLER
Universitätsklinik Bonn, Urologie
Sigmund-Freud-Straße 25, 53127 Bonn, Germany

H. PADMA-NATHAN
University of Southern California
2025 Zonal Ave., Ste GH 5900, Los Angeles, CA 90033, USA

CH. PERSSON-JÜNEMANN
Städtische Kliniken Kassel, Urologische Klinik
Mönchebergstraße 41–43, 34125 Kassel, Germany

E. PESCATORI
Cattedra di Urologia, Policlinico di Modena
Via del Pozzo 71, 41100 Modena, Italy

J. P. PRYOR
Institute of Urology
University College London Medical School
48 Riding House Street, London W1P 7PN, UK

H. PORST
Neuer Jungfernstieg 6a, 20354 Hamburg, Germany

G. SCHOENEICH
Universitätsklinik Bonn, Urologie
Sigmund-Freud-Straße 25, 53127 Bonn, Germany

I. SAENZ DE TEJADA
Departamento de Investigacion
Hospital Ramon y Cajal
Francisco Sanfiz 7, Aravaca Madrid 28023, Spain

G. WAGNER
Department of Medical Physiology
The Panum Institute
University of Copenhagen
Blegdamsvej 3, 2200 Copenhagen, Denmark

W.-H. WEISKE
König-Karl-Straße 38, 70372 Stuttgart, Germany

Anatomy of the Penis and Elementary Physiology of Erection

KLAUS-PETER JÜNEMANN

Knowledge of the anatomical structures and of the physiological and neuropharmacological processes involved in the mechanism of erection is necessary for a pathophysiologic understanding of both erectile dysfunction and the therapeutic approach to be taken. The possibility of pharmacologically inducing erections led, in the first half of the 1980s, to a redefinition of the anatomical and physiological and likewise of the neuropharmacological basis of the mechanism of erection [4, 7, 9, 10, 14, 15, 19–23, 25, 26]; this new concept differed greatly from the shunt theory of erection, proposed by Conti [3] and later by Newman and co-workers [24], that had been prevailing until the early 1980s. According to Conti´s original concept [3], erection was initiated and maintained by an arterial shunt alone, that would divert the blood flow into the cavernous bodies through both the afferent and the efferent penile vasculature as a result of the muscular bolsters described by von Ebner [5]. Thus the cavernous cavities were only a passive reservoir to hold the elevated volume of blood resulting from the intense influx during erection.

It was no longer possible to maintain this theory of mechanism of erection controlled by the regulation of arterial influx alone and with "passive cavernous cavities" following radiologic examinations [4, 23, 26] and subsequent animal experiments [7, 9–11, 19–22]. Our own histomorphologic examinations in canine[1] cavernosal muscles with and without erection have shown that the smooth cavernosal muscles in particular are very important in initiating and maintaining erection [7, 13]. Hemodynamic experiments with pharmacological stimulation confirmed that the mechanism of erection is a complex phenomenon based on arterial dilatation, cavernosal relaxation, and venous restriction [9–11, 19–22].

---

[1] Dogs have a complete septum so that, following the pharmaceutically induced erection of one cavernous body, direct histomorphologic comparisons can be made with the flaccid contralateral cavernous body.

Scanning electron microscopy of the penile anatomy of men and animals has shown for the first time the architecture of the erectile tissue as a three-dimensional image, both during erection and in the flaccid state [7, 13]. These examinations enabled a new concept of the mechanism of erection to be derived, a mechanism in which the relaxation of the smooth cavernosal muscle has a key function. On the basis of today's knowledge, penile erection can be explained as follows:
- Dilatation of the penile arteries and subsequent increase in arterial influx to the penis
- Relaxation of the smooth cavernosal muscles, followed by a decrease in intracorporeal resistance
- Occlusion of the subtunical venous drainage system, resulting in an increase in the resistance to venous outflow

Based on this extended knowledge of the fundamentals of erection, the anatomy and the physiology of penile erection can be described in a new way.

Anatomy

Contrary to the situation in various animal species (cf. above), the two cavernous bodies in man are directly linked with each other by an incomplete septum (Fig. 1). The two cavernous bodies are ensheathed by the rigid tunica albuginea, so the spongy body, which surrounds the urethra and is directly linked with the glans anatomically, is completely separated from the cavernous bodies above it. As shown in Fig. 2, the two cavernous bodies are supplied with blood by the two deep penile arteries, while the neuronal supply is provided by the cavernous nerves. The two dorsal penile arteries and the two dorsal penile nerves are situated between Buck's fascia and the tunica albuginea; they travel laterally on either side of the central deep dorsal vein of the penis into which the circumflex veins empty (Fig. 2). Muscular ligaments (ischiocavernosus muscles and bulbospongiosus muscle) fix the penile base to the symphysis and the abdominal wall.

Blood is supplied to the two cavernous bodies primarily via the paired deep penile arteries with their helicine arterioles. The glans is supplied through the two dorsal penile arteries that have a common origin in the

Fig. 1. Cross-section through the human penis. Note the incomplete septum and the two deep penile arteries (*arrow*). (From [13])

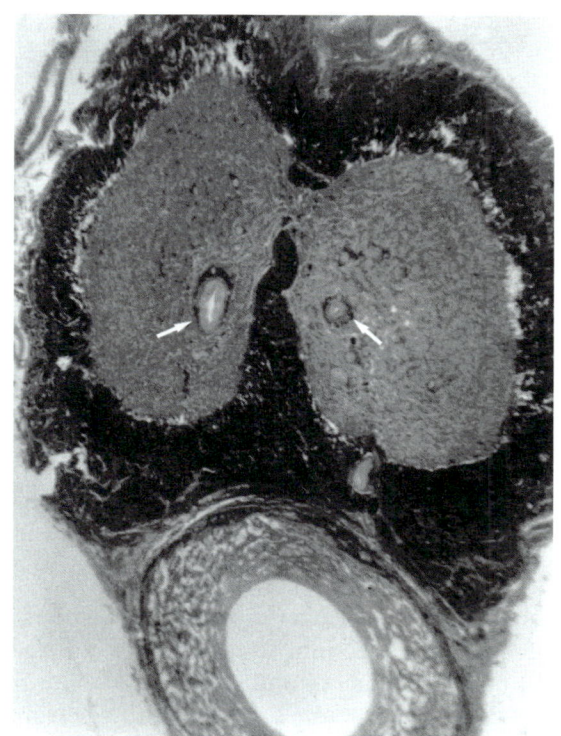

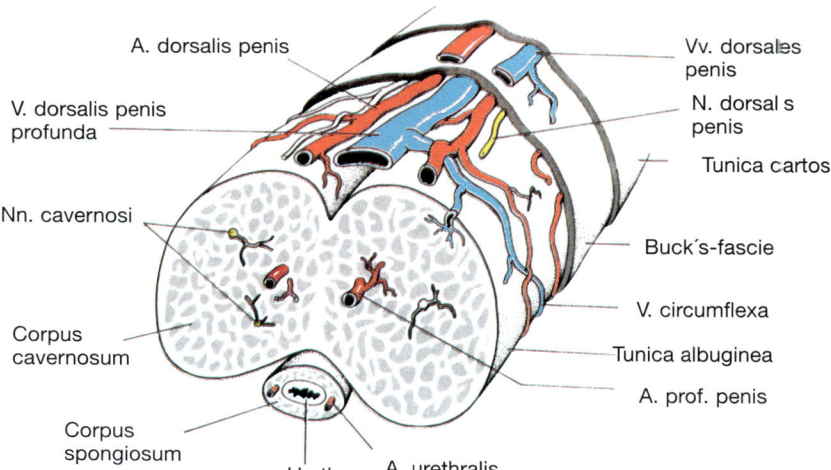

A. dorsalis penis

Vv. dorsales penis

V. dorsalis penis profunda

N. dorsal s penis

Tunica cartos

Nn. cavernosi

Buck´s-fascie

Corpus cavernosum

V. circumflexa

Tunica albuginea

A. prof. penis

Corpus spongiosum

Urethra   A. urethralis

Fig. 2. Serial section through the penis in man. (From [17])

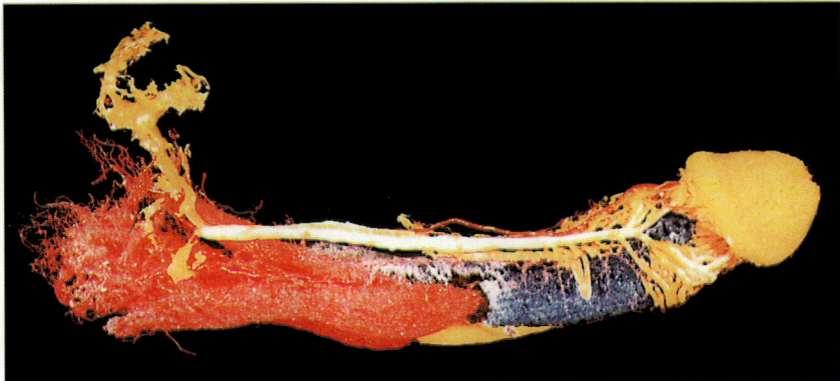

Fig. 3. Corrosion preparation from a 47-year-old man, several segments of which were used for scanning electron microscopy. Red Batson´s solution was injected into both deep penile arteries to visualize the arterial vasculature; the distal part of the cavernous bodies was punctured and perfused with blue Batson´s solution to visualize the venous drainage system. The same solution in yellow was injected through the glans to visualize the communications between the spongy body, the glans, and the outflow through the deep dorsal vein of penis. (From [13])

internal pudendal artery. Only the cavernous bodies give rigidity to the penis during erection. They consist of a three-dimensional network of connective tissue and smooth muscle cells. Apart from the deep cavernous veins at the penile base, the drainage from the cavernous cavities is effected, via the circumflex veins, by a distal, subtunical venous network. This purely descriptive anatomy of the flaccid penis gains in importance increasingly as a result of electron-microscopic scans of the erect and the flaccid penis (Fig. 3). In the flaccid penis, the small arterioles that empty into the sinusoids are constricted and helical (Fig. 4a). It is the helical form of the arterioles that allows the penis to increase in length, a process which leads to an elongation of not only the erectile tissue, but also the vascular structures of the cavernosal muscles. The cavernous cavities are linked by intersinusoidal communications (Fig. 4a). Contrary to Ebner´s [5] description, the electron-microscopic scans were not indicative of the existence of intravascular muscular rims that could be interpreted as bolsters. While scans of the flaccid penis show the arteries to be constricted and the sinusoids to be in a state of maximum contraction, the functional anatomical picture during erection is completely different: elongated arterioles, dilated by a factor of 3–4 (diameter 90–100 μm vs. 20–30 μm) end in markedly distended sinusoids of the cavernous bodies (Fig. 4b). Besides these functionally relevant arterioles,

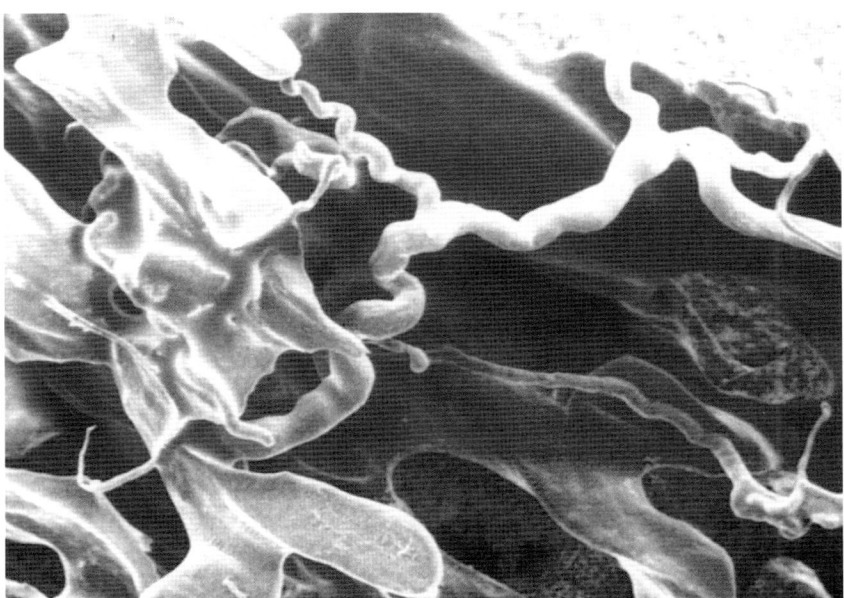

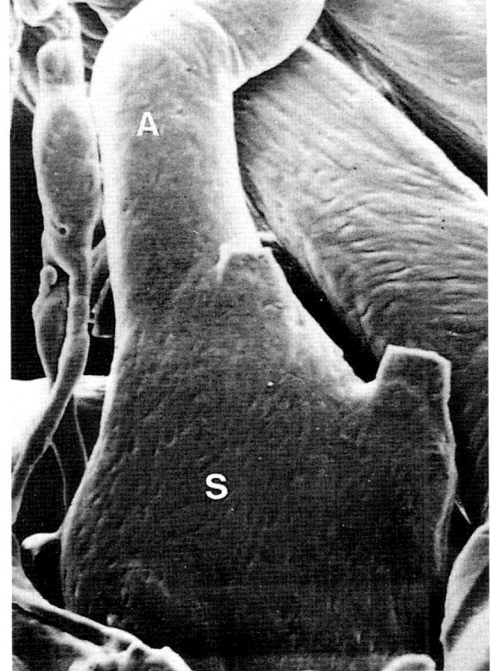

Fig. 4a. Electron-microscopic scan showing part of a human cavernous body in the flaccid state. Note the helical arterioles (20–30 µm) that originate in the deep penile artery and empty into the contracted sinusoids of the cavernous bodies. The sinusoids have multiple intersinusoidal communications. (From [13])
b Visualization of the three-dimensional architecture of the cavernous bodies in a dog during pharmacologically induced erection. During erection, the arterioles (**A**) dilate by a factor of 3–4 (90–100 µm) and transport blood to the markedly distended sinusoids (**S**) of the cavernous bodies. Also note the parallel nutritive capillaries. (From [13])

there are small nutritive capillaries with a maximum diameter of 15 µm. As the intersinusoidal communications between the cavernous cavities are markedly dilated, a free exchange between sinusoids is possible, so that the cavernous bodies become a functional unit (Fig. 5a).

As to the venous vasculature, there is a subtunical venous network between the smooth corporeal muscles and the rigid tunica albuginea in the distal third of the penis. This network, which is clearly visualized in the flaccid penis, comprises several emissary veins, which penetrate the tunica albuginea (Fig. 5a). The cavernous cavities that are covered at right angles to the tunica albuginea by the venous system draining them show maximum contraction (Fig. 5a).

While the subtunical venous plexus is completely visualized when the penis is not erect, the picture differs markedly during erection: due to the specific anatomic situation of the subtunical venous network, the massive relaxation of the smooth corporeal muscles that is accompanied by distention of the sinusoids and their filling with blood (Fig. 5b)

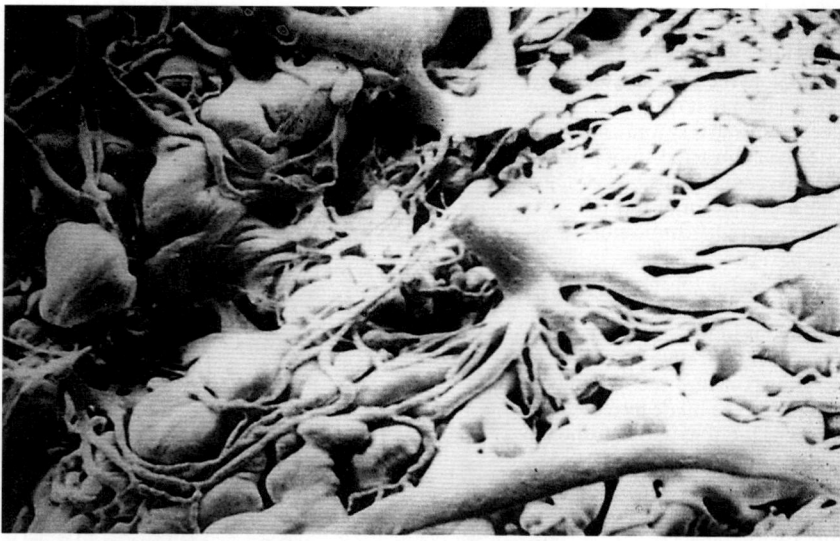

Fig. 5a. Visualization of the subtunical venous drainage system in a dog. Note the multiple small venules (50–120 µm) draining the cavernous cavities, that can be seen on the distended sinusoids. The image further shows some emissary veins, in which the venules end and which in turn empty into a circumflex vein, after they have penetrated the tunica albuginea (removed by etching) (flaccid state).

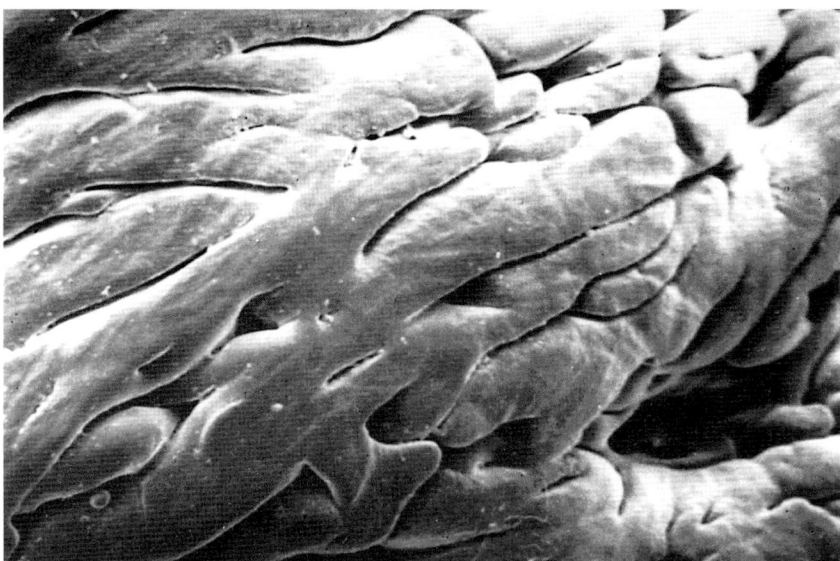

Fig. 5b. Relaxation of the smooth corporeal muscles during erection, on the other hand, leads to a massive distention of the cavernous cavities and subsequent compression of the subtunical intermediary venules, whose courses are longitudinally parallel to the surface; this causes venous restriction in the penis (the venules are not visualized during erection; contralateral cavernous body of the same animal as in 5a). (From [13])

leads to compression of the minor and major intermediary venules (Fig. 5b) and subsequent venous occlusion. Only some emissary veins that penetrate the tunica albuginea stay patent and ensure a continuous exchange of blood in the penis even during full erection.

Based on our examinations using scanning electron microscopy, we can describe the mechanism of erection as follows: In the flaccid penis, while the intracorporeal deep penile arteries and their arterioles, as well as the cavernous cavities, show maximum contraction, the venous drainage system is dilated to the maximum, so that a free outflow of blood through the emissary veins is possible (Fig. 6a). During erection, on the other hand, the arterial bed is dilated so that the blood flow into the maximally relaxed and distended sinusoids of the two cavernous bodies is consecutively increased. The smallest venules between the surface of the cavernous bodies and the tunica albuginea are compressed between the distended sinusoids and the tunica, which results in venous restriction. Only a few emissary veins are patent to ensure the blood exchange

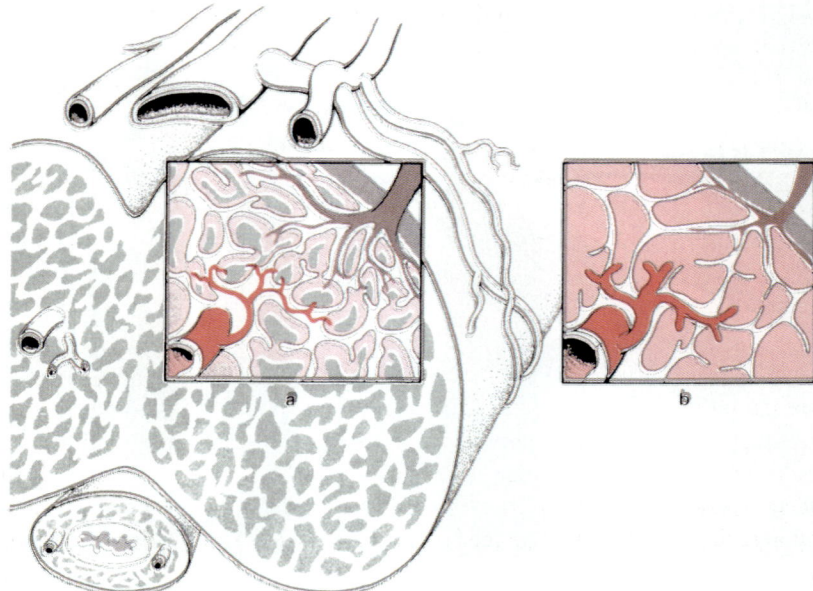

Fig. 6a, b. The mechanism of erection. **a** In a flaccid penis, the penile and intracorporeal arteries are constricted and the corporeal muscles show maximum contraction, while there is free outflow of blood through the emissary veins and the circumflex veins. **b** Arterial dilatation and cavernous relaxation result in a massive influx of blood into the cavernous bodies, with consequential increases in volume and pressure, which in turn lead to venous occlusion of the subtunical venous network (From [17])

even during full erection (Fig. 6b). The mechanism of erection can be comprehensively explained by three phenomena:

1. Arterial dilatation
2. Cavernous relaxation
3. Venous restriction

Physiology

Contrary to the purely descriptive anatomy, the physiological process of penile erection is much more difficult to describe because of essential neuropharmacological physiological processes. However, when the description is limited to purely physiological aspects, a clear picture can be drawn of the mechanism of erection; it can also be demonstrated in patients clinically, for instance, by means of Doppler sonographic examinations.

Two basic kinds of erection can be distinguished:

a) psychogenic erection and

b) reflexogenic erection. The former is mediated, among others, by the sympathetic nerves and is not subject to the patient's will [1, 2]; the latter is of a purely reflexogenic nature and uses primarily spinal pathways [16].

Conducted by the erection center(S2–S4) [8], the stimulating impulses are transmitted by the cavernous nerves that were described by Eckhard as early as 1863 [6]. Animal experiments that we performed [15] showed that penile erection is initiated by the relaxation of the corporeal muscles, receiving parasympathetic impulses via the cavernous nerves, and by arterial dilatation. This leads to an increase in intracorporeal pressure to a level of 20–30 cm H_2O below the systemic blood pressure (Fig. 7). The increase in the intracorporeal blood volume and pressure results in the compression of the subtunical venous plexus between the distended sinusoids and the tunica albuginea. This purely vascular mechanism that is controlled by the parasympathetic nervous system produces maximum tumescence of the cavernous bodies.

Only when, shortly before orgasm, the ischiocavernous muscles compress the tumescent cavernous bodies, does complete rigidity of the cavernous bodies result, with pressures far above those of the systemic blood pressure (> 400 cm H_2O) (Fig. 7). These results correlate with the findings of Lavoisier and co-workers [18]; examining patients, they obtained similar results regarding the reflex contraction of the ischiocavernous muscles and the increase in intracorporeal pressure.

Contrary to earlier assumptions that detumescence was a purely passive mechanism, recent experiments [14] have shown that the stimulation of the sympathetic hypogastric plexus leads to detumescence of the cavernous bodies as a result of the contraction of corporeal smooth muscles and penile arteries (Fig. 7). This mechanism can also be described as an inhibitory mechanism of erection.

In conclusion, it can be stated that full erection with maximum rigidity depends on the parasympathetic as well as the sympathetic and the somatomotor nerve systems being intact. Whereas the initiation and

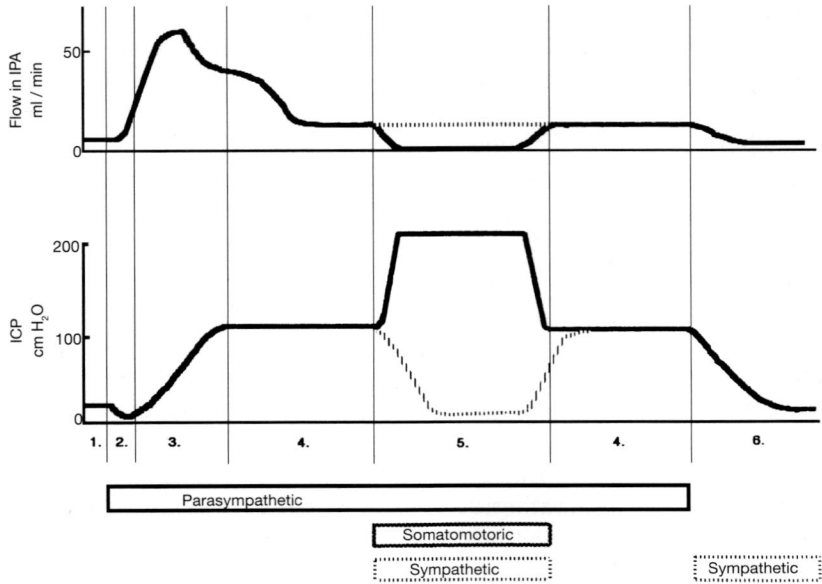

Fig. 7. Hemodynamic physiological examinations in dog and primates. The relation is shown between the arterial blood flow into the penis (*above*) and the behavior of the intracorporeal pressure (*below*). The stimulation of the parasympathetic nerve fibers innervating the penis results in an initial decrease in intracorporeal pressure (relaxation of the smooth corporeal muscles) and then in an influx of arterial blood and an increase in intracorporeal volume and pressure, until maximum tumescence is reached. The stimulation of the somatomotor pudendal nerve leads to complete rigidity of the erection with intracorporeal pressures that are markedly above the systolic pressure. When the somatomotor stimulation is stopped, the pressure falls back to the initial value of parasympathetic stimulation (maximum tumescence). The additive stimulation of the sympathetic nerve fibers of the hypogastric plexus results in a decrease in intracorporeal pressure without the arterial influx being modified, since the smooth corporeal muscles are contracted.(IPA Internal pudendal artery; ICP intracorporeal pressure) (From [15])

maintenance of erection are purely parasympathetic vascular phenomena, maximum rigidity is achieved only when somatomotor impulses cause the ischiocavernous muscles to contract while the penis is tumescent. Detumescence and the decline of erection are a phenomenon that is controlled primarily by the sympathetic system and is induced by the contraction of the smooth muscles; it can be described as an inhibitory mechanism.

References

1. Bors E, Comarr AE (1960) Neurological disturbances in sexual function with special reference to 529 patients with spinal cord injury. Urol Surv 19: 191–222
2. Comarr AE (1970) Sexual function among patients with spinal cord injury. Urol Int 25: 1970
3. Conti G (1952) L'érection du pénis humain et ses bases morphologico-vasculaires. Acta Anat (Basel) 14: 217
4. Ebbehøj J, Uhrenholdt A, Wagner G (1980) Infusion cavernosography in the human in the unstimulated and stimulated situations and its diagnostic value. In: Zorgniotti AW, Rossi G (eds) Vasculogenic Impotence: Proceedings of the 1st International Conference on Corpus Cavernosum Revascularization. Thomas, Springfield, Illinois, USA, p. 191–196
5. Ebner von V (1900) Über klappenartige Vorrichtungen in den Arterien der Schwellkörper. Anat Anz 18: 79
6. Eckhard C (1863) Untersuchungen über die Erektion des Penis beim Hunde. Beitr Anat u Physiol 3: 123
7. Fournier GR Jr, Jünemann K-P, Lue TF, Tanagho EA (1987) Mechanisms of venous occlusion during canine penile erection: An anatomic demonstration. J Urol 137: 163–167
8. Gaskell WH (1986) Preliminary communication to Proceedings of the Physiology Society of London, 1985, on the structure, distribution and function of the nerves which innervate the visceral and vascular systems. J Physiol 7: 1–17
9. Jünemann K-P, Lue TF, Fournier GR jr, Tanagho EA (1986) Hemodynamics of papaverine- and phentolamine-induced penile erection. J Urol (Baltimore) 136: 158
10. Jünemann K-P, Luo JA, Lue TF, Tanagho EA (1986) Further evidence of venous outflow restriction during erection. Brit J Urol 58: 320
11. Jünemann K-P, Lue TF, Abozeid M, Hellstrom WJG, Tanagho EA (1986) Blood gas analysis in drug-induced penile erection. Urol Int (Basel) 41: 207
12. Jünemann K-P, Persson-Jünemann C, Lue TF, Tanagho EA (1988) Neurophysiological aspects of penile erection. In: Proceedings 3rd World Meeting on Impotence. Oct 6–9, Boston, USA, p. 49
13. Jünemann K-P (1988) Physiologie der penilen Erektion. In: Bähren W, Altwein JE (eds.) Impotenz. Diagnostik und Therapie in Klinik und Praxis. Thieme Verlag, Stuttgart, p. 11
14. Jünemann K-P, Persson-Jünemann C, Lue TF, Tanagho EA, Alken P (1989) Neurophysiological aspects of penile erection: The role of the sympathetic nervous system. Brit J Urol 64: 84–92
15. Jünemann K-P, Persson-Jünemann C, Tanagho EA, Alken P (1989) Neurophysiology of penile erection. Urol Res 17: 213–217
16. Jünemann K-P, Persson-Jünemann C, Alken P (1990) Pathophysiology of erectile dysfunction. Sem Urol 2: 80–93
17. Jünemann K-P (1992) Erektionsstörungen. In: Alken P, Walz H (eds) Urologie. VCH-Verlagsgesellschaft, Weinheim, ch. 12, p 305–315
18. Lavoisier P, Proulx J, Courtois F (1989) Bulbocavernosus reflex: Its validity as a diagnostic test of neurogenic impotence. J Urol 141: 311–314

19. Lue TF, Zeineh SJ, Schmidt RA, Tanagho EA (1983) Physiology of penile erection. World J Urol 1: 194
20. Lue TF, Takamura T, Schmidt RA, Palubinskas AJ, Tanagho EA (1983) Hemodynamics of erection in the monkey. J Urol (Baltimore) 130: 1237
21. Lue TF, Zeineh SJ, Schmidt RA, Tanagho EA (1984) Neuroanatomy of penile erection: Its relevance to iatrogenic impotence. J Urol (Baltimore) 131: 273
22. Lue TF, Takamura T, Umraiya M, Schmidt RA, Tanagho EA (1984) Hemodynamics of canine corpora cavernosa during erection. Urology 24: 347
23. Metz P, Wagner G (1981) Penile circumference and erection. Urology 18: 268
24. Newman HF, Northup JD, Devlin J (1964) Mechanism of human penile erection. Invest Urol 1: 350
25. Wagner G, Uhrenholdt A (1980) Blood flow measurement by the clearance method in the human corpus cavernosum in the flaccid and erect states. In: Zorgniotti AW, Rossi G (eds) Vasculogenic Impotence: Proceedings of the 1st International Conference on Corpus Cavernosum Revascularization. Thomas, Springfield, Illinois, USA, p. 41–46
26. Wagner G (1981) Erection. Physiology and endocrinology. In: Wagner G, Green R (eds) Impotence. Physiological, psychological, surgical. Diagnosis and treatment. Plenum, New York, pp. 25–36

Etiology and Management of Hypospadias and Epispadias

Charlotta Persson-Juenemann

In contrast to the majority of adult male patients suffering from erectile disturbances revealing a normal external genitalia, two congenital entities may combine an abnormal anatomic appearance with impossibility of sexual intercourse.

Hypospadias

This is a quite frequent congenital malformation with an overall incidence of about 8.2 in every 1000 male births. Fortunately the less severe forms are the most common, with the glandular and coronal varieties representing 87% of the total. A ventral urethral orifice localized anywhere between the glans penis and perineum is the constituent responsible for the greek name and has been the base for classification. The embryology behind this malformation is a simple developmental arrest, occurring any time between the fifth and twelfth week of gestation, determined by the fact that the urethral folds fail to fuse in the ventral midline. Failure of the urethra to reach the tip of the glans is inevitably accompanied by the absence of the ventral foreskin. Unquestionably a genetic factor exists, most likely based on a multifactorial mode of inheritance. It is important to keep in mind, that if the father has a hypospadia, the risk of having a second son with hypospadias is as high as 26%. In addition the male external genitalia are formed under the influence of testosterone and derivates. Abnormalities of androgen production or utilization can lead to hypospadias.

In order to appraise the malformation correctly, all elements concerned must receive attention, including glans-configuration, amount and distribution of the dorsally hooded foreskin as well as skin tethering or chordee.

Distal Hypospadias.   In the large group of distal hypospadias (glandular, coronal, and subcoronal), the indication for surgical correction is almost always cosmetic. If parents demand an operative intervention it seems feasible for performance around the age of two. In other cases it is reasonable to wait for the child to reach an age to decide for himself. The aim should always be a reconstructed penis appearing normal to the patient and parents. Presently one stage procedures are standard, the operative technique dependent upon the individual anatomic situation and surgeons preference. The MAGPI-procedure focuses on a glanduloplasty after mild distal extension of the meatus employing the Heinecke-

Fig. 1. The individual steps of the MAGPI-procedure in distal hypospadias repair

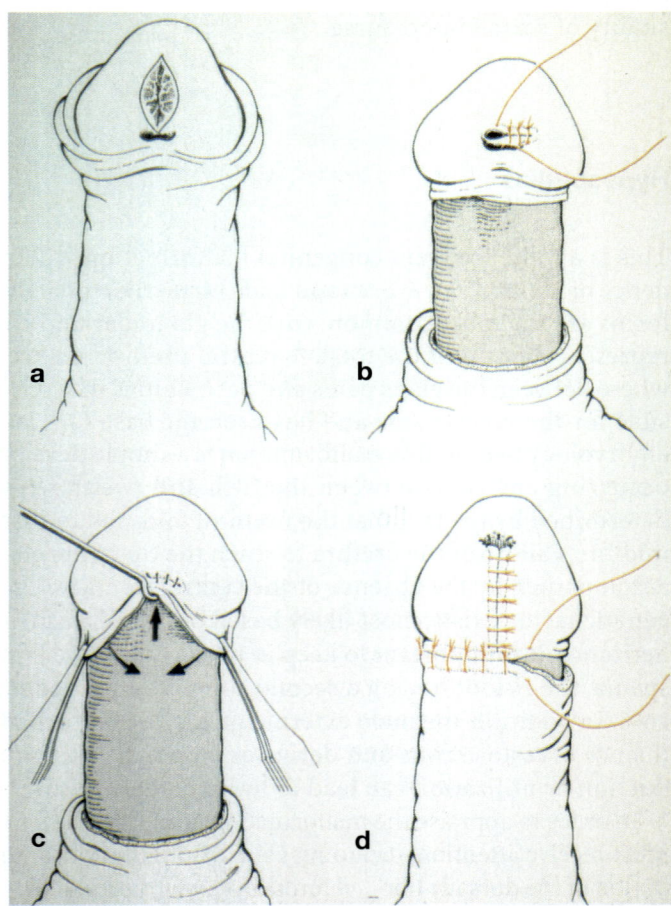

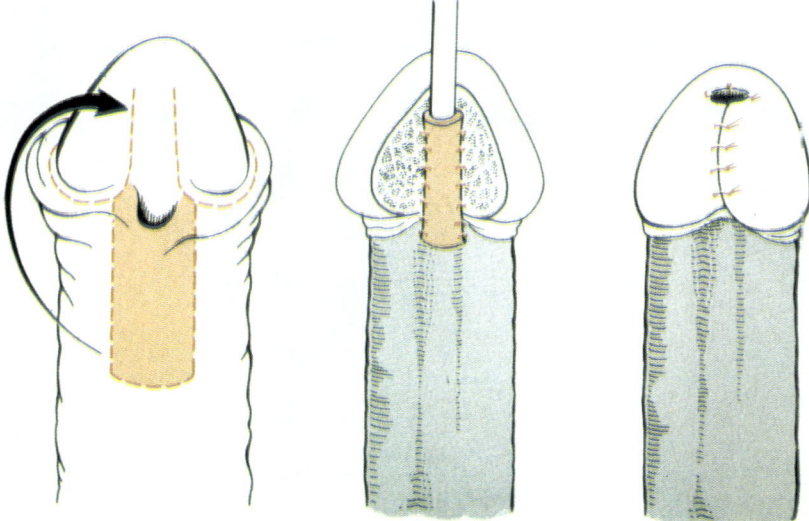

Fig. 2. The meatal-based flap (MATHIEU) in distal hypospadias repair

Mikulicz procedure. Following complete mobilization of the skin, ruling out any chordee under artificial erection, the flat glans wings are completely mobilized then approximated in the midline during distal traction of the urethra with a hook. The result is a meatus located on the tip of a now conical glans [3] (Fig. 1). In cases in which the meatus is patulous or noncompliant or the glans configuration unfavourable, a meatal-based skin flap for distal reconstruction of the urethra is employed (MATHIEU) followed by glans approximation [4] (Fig. 2). Presently the demand for foreskin reconstruction is high in Europe. In many cases this can be incorporated in the MAGPI or MATHIEU repair, or done as the main element of reconstruction as in the VAP-procedure [5] (Fig. 3). This simple operative technique focuses on reapproximation of the separated inner and outer layers of the dorsally localized prepuce in the ventral midline after distal meatotomy.

If intraoperative erection should reveal chordee this demands reclassification of the hypospadias to a more proximal shaft variant after chordectomy. In most cases true chordee is not present in distal hypospadias, the slight bending is most often a result of superficial skin tethering or glandular tilt.

Fig. 3. Approximation of the mobilized and separated layers of the foreskin in the ventral midline judging the feasibility of foreskin reconstruction applying the VAP-procedure

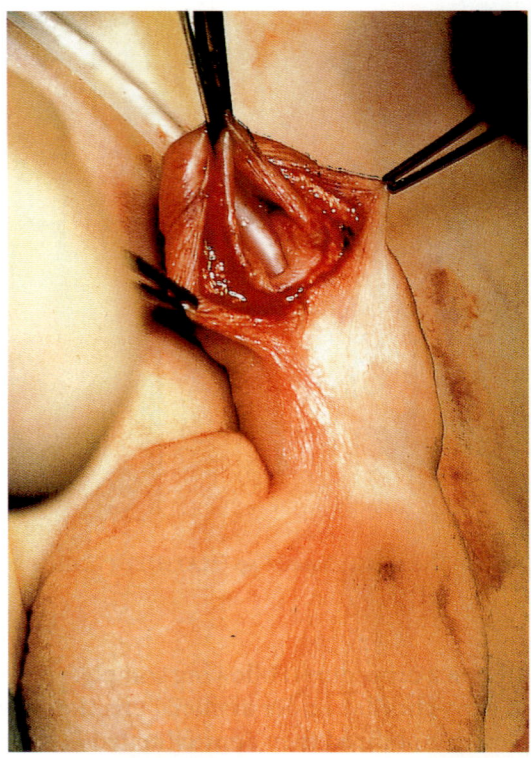

Penile-Shaft Hypospadias.   Numerous operative techniques of urethral reconstruction have been described. In the distal- and midshaft variants one stage procedures are most often possible after exclusion of chordee or concomitant correction. Studies have shown that the preservation of the distal urethral plate incorporating an onlay urethroplasty is, in the cases possible, superior to the employment of a tube reconstruction. In most cases a preputial island onlay pedicle flap (DUCKETT; Fig. 4) harvested transversely from the inner layer of the foreskin enables reconstruction of an up to 8 cm deficient urethra. For skin coverage the outer layer of the prepuce is incised in the dorsal midline and then brought to the ventrum following the glans reapproximation.

Proximal Hypospadias.   In the case of proximal hypospadias (penoscrotal, scrotal, and perineal), the presence of chordee in addition to a most often insufficient urethral plate or demand of transsection to cor-

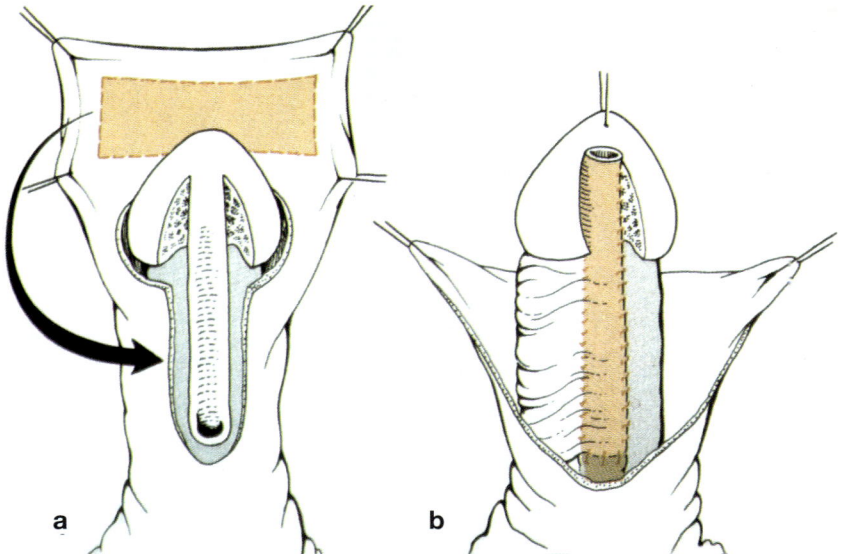

Fig. 4a, b.   Preputial island onlay pedicle flap in penile shaft hypospadias

rect chordee will often make a two-stage procedure mandatory for repair. Tube urethroplasties are necessary, with recent studies demonstrating the superior properties of buccal mucosa in comparison to bladder mucosa. Often the urethral reconstruction will demand a mixed repair combining buccal mucosa with preputial skin.

Male Epispadias

Isolated male epispadias is an exceedingly rare anomaly occurring in approximately 1:118 000 births (Fig. 5). However, in 90% of cases male epispadias are associated with bladder exstrophy, with an incidence of 1:50 000. As in hypospadias the position of the urethral meatus located on the dorsum of the penis determines the classification in balanic, penile or complete penopubic epispadias, the complete form being equivalent with the combined exstrophy-epispadias complex after bladder closure. The typical appearance includes a short and flat penis with a splayed glans (Fig. 6). Sexual intercourse is most often not possible due

Fig. 5.   A very rare case of isolated male epispadias

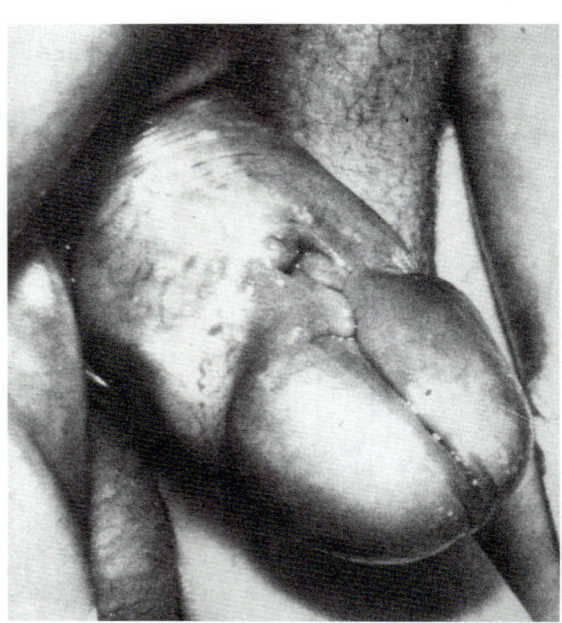

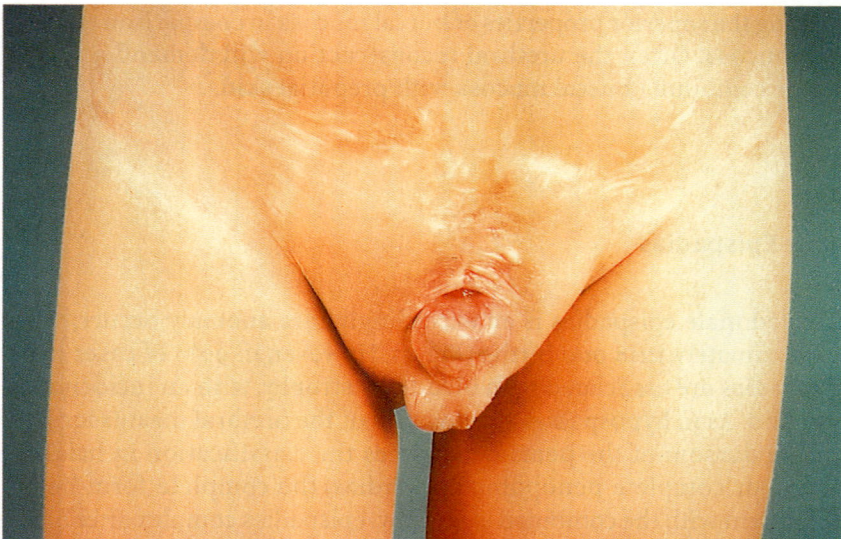

Fig. 6.   The more typical aspect of epispadias. A complete penopubic epispadia equivalent with the combined exstrophy-epispadias complex after bladder closure

to dorsal chordee resulting in an erection directed firmly against the abdominal wall, the cause related to an intrinsic deformity of the corporal bodies. The incontinence rate is high except in the very rare isolated balanic epispadias.

From a practical standpoint the embryology of the exstrophy-epispadias complex is inseparable from that of epispadias alone. Up to date several theories try to explain the embryological defect leading to this malformation, and opposed to hypospadias it is not consistent with simple developmental arrest. MUECKE describes an abnormally large cloacal membrane which could prevent normal mesodermal migration and proper development of the lower abdominal wall structure in combination with an aberrant development of the genital folds resulting in a splayed penis [1]. Others describe a premature dehiscence of the cloacal membrane, the anatomic level of dehiscence accounting for the variability of clinical defects.

The history of operative repair dates back to CANTWELL 1895 and numerous other operative procedures following, revealing considerable

Fig. 7a, b.
The two major steps of the modified CANTWELL procedure

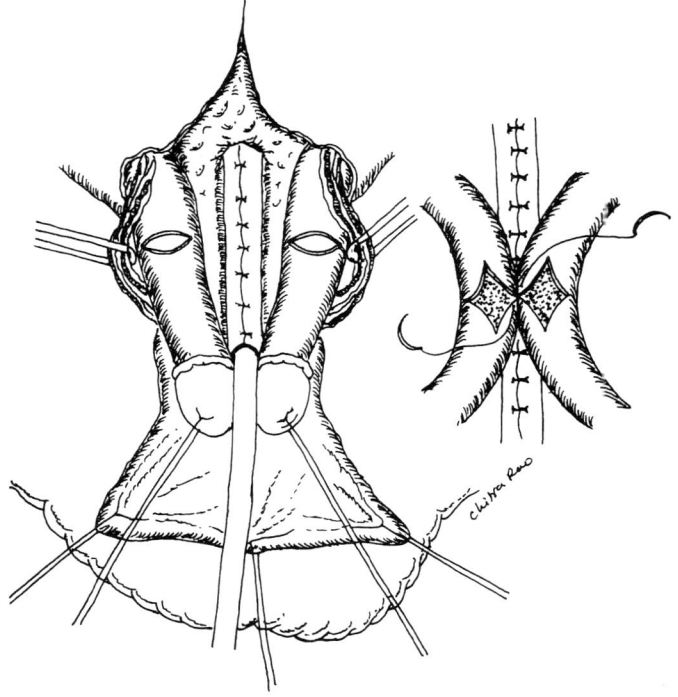

complications in the differently focused attempts to mobilize the urethral plate, provide a urethroplasty ventral to the corpora and overcoming the divergent symphysis pubis in epispadias to enhance penile length as well as rotation of the corporal bodies in attempt to correct the dorsal curvature.

The current reconstructive approach to epispadias is the modified CANTWELL procedure [1] (Fig. 7):

Urethral Reconstruction.   The dorsally located urethral plate is completely mobilized off the corporal bodies. The combination of a highly elastic urethral plate and the rotation underneath the corporal bodies provides sufficient length for a tension free urethroplasty from the prostate up to the tip of the glans. To reconstruct the urethra the urethral plate is tubularized and dorsally sutured with interrupted absorbable sutures providing maximum elasticity.

Corporeal Rotation and Cavernocavernostomy.   To overcome the dorsal curvature a transverse dorsal relaxing incision of the tunica albuginea of both corpora is performed after complete mobilization of the neurovascular bundles which in epispadias have a favourable lateral course. Then the corporeal bodies are rotated and the cavernocavernostomy of the resulted defects performed fixating the bodies in the dorsal midline. The dorsal coverage of the urethral reconstruction has reduced the rate of fistulas.

Glanuloplasty and Skin Coverage.   The urethral plate on the epispadic glans terminates on the dorsum. To achieve a centrally located urethral meatus the urethra must be extended distally toward the ventrum of the glans. Typical for the glans wings is a bulk of irregular tissue on both sides lateral to the urethral plate which has to be exzised aggressively in order to achieve a conical glans configuration. A two-layer closure completes the reconstruction.

Skin closure can be difficult. In most cases the employment of a pedicle flap from the inner layer of the ventral foreskin can achieve coverage of the distal dorsum penis. The proximal dorsal aspect of the penile shaft is effectively covered utilizing a Z-plasty from the midline abdominal incision.

The aim of reconstruction in all congenital malformation of the external genitalia must be a close to normal appearing penis enabling normal function in the sexually active young man. Complications are not rare and must be kept in mind when dealing with minor deviations from the normal.

References

1. Muecke EC (1964) The role of the cloacal membrane in exstrophy: the first success-ful experimental study. J Urol 92: 659
2. Diamond DA, Ransley PG (1995) Male epispadias. J Urol 154: 2150–2155
3. Duckett JW (1981) MAGPI (meatoplasty and glanuloplasty). A procedure for sub-coronal hypospadias. Urol Clin N Amer 8: 513
4. Mathieu P (1932) Traitement en un temps de l´hypospadias balanique et juxtabalani-que. J Chir 39: 481
5. Persson-Juenemann MC, Seemann O, Koehrmann KU, Potempa D, Juenemann KP, Alken P (1993) Correction of distal hypospadias: Ventral adaption of the prepuce and meatal advancement. Urol Int 51: 216–219

Sexually Transmitted and Non-infectious Diseases of the Penile Skin

WALTER KRAUSE AND BARBARA HABERMANN

General Remarks

Anatomical Considerations

The penile skin is very thin and contains only a few terminal hair bulbs, large sebaceous glands and apocrine glands. The cutis is rich of elastic fibers. A subcutis is lacking on the glans, on the shaft it is very thin and contains only little fatty tissue. The prepuce also shows thin epidermis with a small horny layer and an elastic cutis. No hairs are present, however, some sebaceous glands up to 1 mm of diameter may be seen (ectopic sebaceous glands). They may be confused with condylomata.

The blood vessels of the penile skin correspond to those of the corpora cavernosa. The lymph vessels are drained to the inguinal lymph nodes and after this to the iliacal nodes.

Treatment Modalities

Like in other dermatological diseases a topical treatment should be preferred also in those of the penile skin. Moistening skin regions with diffuse secretion must not be treated with fatty ointments or occluded by tight dressings. Alcoholic solutions are not suitable because they frequently produce irritations.

The thin skin permits rapid penetration of exogenous compounds and therapeutic preparations. Thus the concentration of drugs topically applied have to be much lower than in other skin regions. The penetration rate of e.g. topical corticoids in the penile skin is more than 40 times higher than in the forearm. Also toxic reactions are facilitated, e.g. the use of gentian violet is strictly prohibited in the penis, because it is frequently followed by erosive reactions.

Ulcerations must not be treated with antibiotic creams without a correct diagnosis. A syphilitic infection may be suppressed by this treatment, since its typical appearance is masked, but a complete healing is not achieved.

When a disease recurs after primary healing, one should think of sexually transmitted infections. The patient´s attention should be called to this fact and he should be asked to cause his sexual partner(s) to see a dermatologist or a gynecologist.

Psychosomatic and Sociological Considerations

The penis plays a specific role in the emotions of a man. The sexuality and the reproductive function are important aspects of human life. Recurrent penile skin diseases therefore should draw the attention to possible problems in the sexual relationships. Repeated diagnostic investigations in order to clarify persistant symptoms may negatively influence the course of a disease. A patient with a latent neurosis will react with anxiety and stress to diagnostic procedures.

Another psychic symptom related to genital diseases is venerophobia, when the patient is afraid of having acquired a sexually transmitted infection. In these cases, the patients present harmless and long-lasting lesions (ectopic sebaceous glands) and suggest a previous sexual affair to be the cause of these symptoms. A thorough investigation reveals that they are ashamed of their affair and feel themselves guilty.

Diseases of the Penis

Diseases with Disorders of Skin Color, Scaling and Itching

Balanitis simplex

Inflammations of the glans penis, irrespective of their origin, are called balanitis. When the inner sheet of the prepuce is also involved, the term balanoposthitis is used. The term balanitis simplex describes a clinical feature when the region shows more or less reddish color, small papules and anular scaling. The appearances change within a few days, and the patient describes itching and the feeling of dry skin.

The etiology of balanitis may be an infection (bacterial, mycotic), allergy (contact dermatitis), irritation, or unknown in special sensitivity (atopic dermatitis) or a sum of these influences. The clinical feature does allow to draw conclusions to the etiology.

As an example, the case of a patient may be described (Fig. 1), who presented with a diffuse erythema of glans and prepuce without papules or scaling. He washed his penis at least twice a day and always rubbed it to dryness. On request, he reported that one year ago his marriage had been dissolved. His daughter had been treated for depressive symptoms, and during the treatment, the psychoanalyst had suggested a sexual abuse of the daughter by her father as a cause of the depression. The father, our patient, strictly denied such a suspicion, but his wife was not able to trust him and therefore retired from the marital community. Three months ago he started a novel sexual partnership and the "balanitis" appeared some weeks later. This new partnership was also burdened by erectile dysfunction, for this reason the patient already presented to an urologist, who proposed a treatment by intracavernous

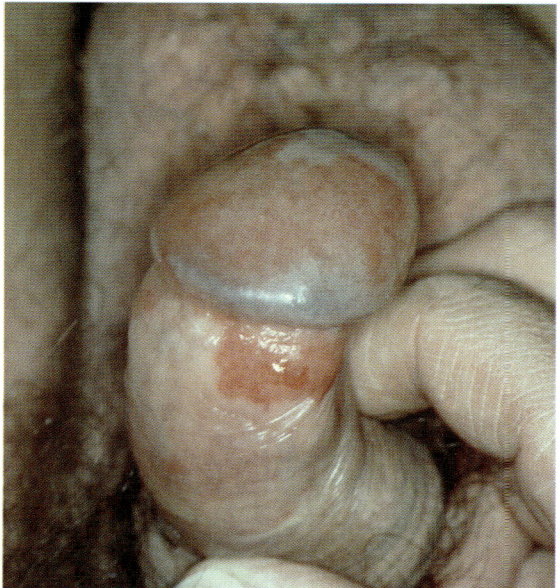

Fig. 1. Balanitis simplex. A patient presented with a diffuse erythema of glans and prepuce without papules or scaling

injections of prostaglandin E$_1$. This balanitis was clearly induced by psychosomatic mechanisms. The patient always tried to clean his penis and to wash away the sexual disgrace. Following counseling with a focus on this problem, the balanitis resolved spontaneously.

Microbiological agents of a balanitis are difficult to discriminate in normal resident flora or pathogenic agents. It is a frequent mistake to consider bacteria or yeasts as the cause of balanitis, only because they grow in culture.

The immunologic factor is often neglected, although a contact dermatitis or a balanitis in atopy is not rare. In contact dermatitis a test with a test patch is required. The most frequent contact allergens in balanitis are scents, latex, ointments.

The following history presents an example of contact dermatitis (Fig. 2). One of our patients presented with small, circinary erosions on glans and the swollen prepuce. The clinical diagnosis was herpes genitalis, however, the herpesvirus could not be isolated. Aciclovir ointment was prescribed, eight days later the erosions and the edema resolved. 2 months later the patient reported new vesicles and erosions, and we decided to begin a continuous treatment with aciclovir orally as

Fig. 2. Balanitis from contact dermatitis. One of our patients presented with small, circinary erosions on glans and the swollen prepuce

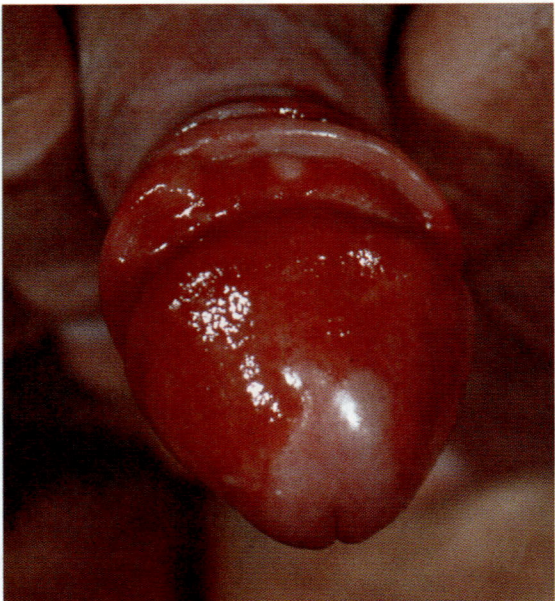

a prophylaxis. However, already 4 weeks after the beginning of this treatment, the patient presented again with an extended ulcerative-erosive balanoposthitis. He was then treated with topical and systemical corticoids. The balanitis slowly regressed, but 8 weeks later there was a severe recurrence. This was again treated with corticoids topically. Following total clearance of the balanitis a patch test was performed. A positive reaction to mactacyd, a desinfectious agent, was found. All other allergens including condoms were negative.

A dermatitis is a frequent cause of balanitis. Hillman et al. (1992) reported on 60 patients, in whom the diagnoses were confirmed by histological investigation. The most frequent pre-biopsy diagnosis, therefore, was fungal balanitis. However, most of the patients showed histological changes typical for dermatitis.

Also Birley et al. (1993) evaluated clinical features and diagnostic investigations in 43 patients with recurrent or unresponsive balanitis. All patients were asked for a history of atopic illness and about their practice of genital washing. All patients were investigated for bacterial and viral culture. In 31 (72%) of the patients a diagnosis of irritant dermatitis was made. In comparison with the remaining patients, they had a greater lifetime incidence of atopic illness and more frequent daily genital washing with soap. For 28 (90%) of these patients, use of emollient creams and restriction of soap washing alone controlled symptoms satisfactorily. The authors concluded that a history of atopic illness and of the practice of penile washing are important aspects in the evaluation of patients with recurrent balanitis.

The treatment of balanitis depends on the etiology. If the cause of the balanitis is an infection, antibiotic or antimycotic creams are applied. The systemical application of antibiotics is not necessary. Allergic or irritative dermatitis may be treated by topical corticosteroids, if it does not alleviate after cessation of the etiologic agent. The use of corticosteroids should not exceed one week, because severe irreversible skin atrophy may follow. In recurrent balanitis of different origins a circumcision should be recommended.

Balanitis Plasmacellularis

A particular feature of balanitis was described in 1952 by Zoon. In his cases he found that the inflammatory cells infiltrating the upper dermis

Fig. 3. Balanitis plasmacellularis. The clinical feature is characterized by a
non-erosive, erythema-
tous, moistly appearent
macule on the glans

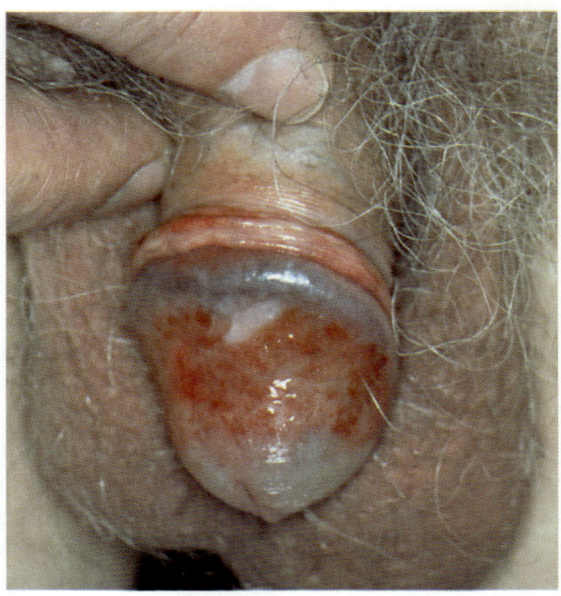

consisted mainly of plasma cells. Therefore he claimed this inflammatory process as "balanitis plasmacellularis". Zoon´s patients claimed a
long-lasting history of the disease (more than 20 years), but none of
them had a history of venereal diseases.

Until now, the etiology of the disease remains unknown. In the literature, allergic reactions, toxic influences, reactions to traumata, or infections with mycobacterium smegmatis were discussed. The clinical feature is characterized by a non-erosive, erythematous, moistly appearent
macule on the glans (Fig. 3). It does not change its size. The typical
plasma cells are easily seen by histological investigation.

In immunotyping, we found in one patient IgG- and IgA- as well as
IgM-positive plasma cells (Fig. 4). Modern techniques, like the polymer-
ase chain reaction (PCR) were not applied to this disease so far.

As a treatment, topical corticosteroids are mostly successful. However,
the disease tends to a recurrence after cessation of treatment. Most
authors confirm a disappearance of the disease following circumcision
(Jolly et al. 1993).

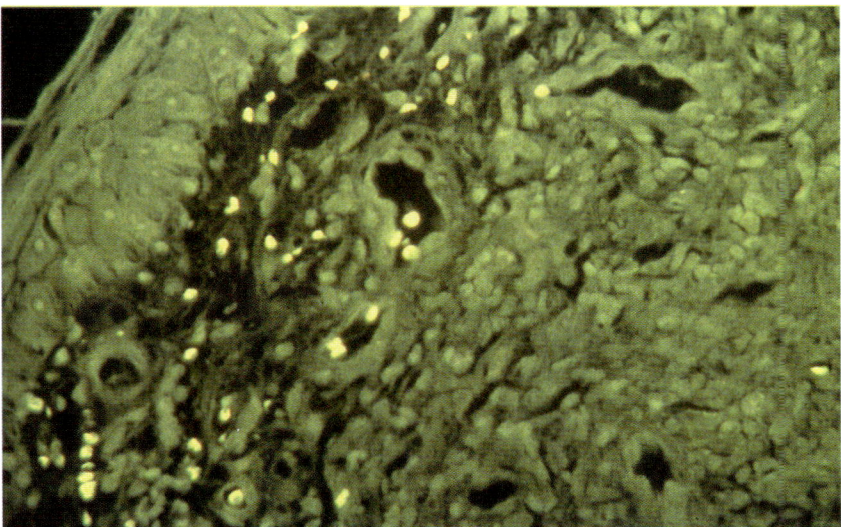

Fig. 4.   Immunotyping in plasma cell balanitis. In one patient IgG- and IgA- as well as IgM-positive plasma cells were found

Lichen Sclerosus et Atrophicus (LSA)

The changes of the glans are diffuse or localized white, blue-white, or yellow-white plaques with atrophic appearance (Fig. 5). The sulcus coronarius and the meatus urethrae may become stenosed. The prepuce is often involved in the disease, and its shrinking leads to a phimosis. It begins as a constricting band, which appears white or blue-white, thus sometimes mimicking a vitiligo (see below).

Histologically, the LSA is characterized by an edema of the cutis and a band-like lymphocytic infiltrate of the lower dermis. Hinchliffe et al. (1994) performed an immunopathological study on LSA cases in boys aged between 3 and 14 years. The infiltrate in LSA patients was totally composed of T cells in all cases. B cells were found only focally in small, discrete aggregates. In 9 of 12 control specimens T-cells were rare and distributed atypically. The authors concluded that immunophenotyping of lymphocyte infiltrates may be helpful in the diagnosis of LSA.

A specific treatment for LSA is not known. A phimosis is usually treated by circumcision. Following this one often observes a remission also involving the glans. Some authors propose a treatment of the ac-

Fig. 5. Lichen sclerosus et atrophicus (LSA): The changes of the glans are diffuse or localized white, blue-white, or yellow-white plaques with atrophic appearance. The sulcus coronarius and the meatus urethrae may become stenosed. The prepuce is often involved in the disease, and its shrinking leads to a phimosis

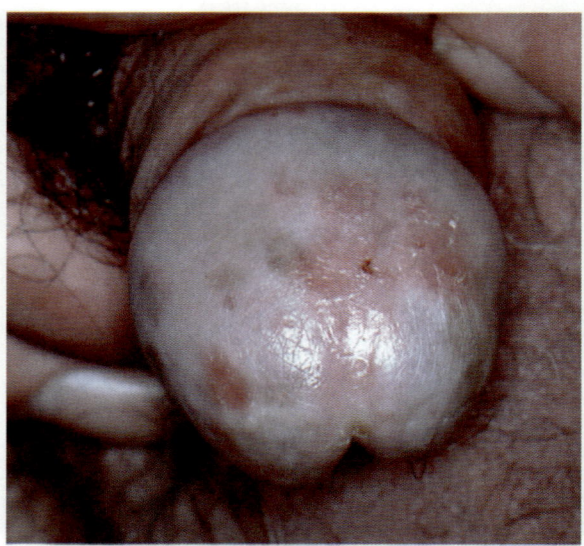

quired phimosis secondary to LSA plastic of the foreskin to avoid circumcision. Although there is no doubt that circumcision in childhood diminishes the risk of balanoposthitis and penis carcinoma in later life, it is not known, whether this will also hold true for LSA (Wiswell 1992).

As a differential diagnosis vitiligo has to be considered. The penile skin shows smaller or larger areas of depigmentation without structural alterations. The lesions tend to spread over the unaffected skin, and spontaneous repigmentation occurs as well. The etiology is unknown. Histologically, there is a normal number of melanocytes, but these are inactive with respect to melanin synthesis. A lymphocytic infiltration accompanies the lesions. High doses of UVA may be useful as a treatment.

Tumorous Diseases

Penile tumors are at least in part the consequence of infections with *human papilloma virus (HPV)*. This DNA-virus is under research in many laboratories. The knowledge of its DNA metabolism, the induction of cellular growth, and other characteristics of the virus has grown to large extent. HPV is highly prevalent in the general population, including a substantial number of cytologically normal men and women. Although HPV detection is often transient in these individuals, it is not known whether the virus is truly eliminated or whether it remains below the threshold of detection in a latent state. Little is known about the interaction between HPV and other risk factors for cancer, but it is possible that variables such as pregnancy, immunosuppression, and use of oral contraceptives may alter the natural history of HPV infection (Morrison 1994).

The role of HPV in the pathogenesis of genital preinvasive carcinoma is highlighted by several studies. HPV-DNA was found in about half of the tumors. Aynaud et al. (1994) studied 1000 male sexual partners of women with genital condyloma or intraepithelial (cervical) neoplasia for penile intraepithelial neoplasia (PIN). Ninety-two patients who presented with lesions suggesting intraepithelial neoplasia underwent biopsy for histologic and virologic studies. In 93% of the specimens penile intraepithelial neoplasia was found. HPV DNA from potentially oncogenic papillomaviruses was detected in 75% of patients with Grade I PIN, in 93% of patients with Grade II PIN, and in all patients with Grade III PIN. The rate of PIN was significantly higher in uncircumcised men than in circumcised men (10% vs. 6%; OR = 1.77; 95% confidence interval, 1.02–3.07). The mean age of patients with Grade III PIN was 7 years higher than the mean age of patients with Grade I PIN, which suggests a progression similar to that of cervical intraepithelial neoplasia.

Condylomata Acuminata

The primary disease caused by HPV is condylomata acuminata. The typical condylomata (warts) are protuberant, papilliferous small-based, reddish tumors of different size (Fig. 6). These lesions predominate in moist and intertriginous areas. Papular lesions, resembling to warts of the fingers, occur on fully keratinized parts of the penile shaft. Flat lesions, which may be invisible to the naked eye, are common on the glans. They often are recognized only after touching the skin with acidic acid, which induces white staining of the thickened horny layer of the warts.

A newly described, distinct entity is the balanoposthitis caused by HPV. Wikstrom et al. (1994) concluded that HPV might be associated with long-lasting balanoposthitis, although the data still are circumstantial for a causative association.

Penile Intraepithelial Neoplasie (PIN)

The clinical features of PIN comprise the *Erythroplasia Queyrat*, an erythematous plaque found on the glans that is round or slightly irregular, measuring 1 to 1.5 cm in diameter. The disease has an overwhelming preponderance in uncircumcised men (Fig. 6).

As a treatment, mostly surgical excision with adequate margins (5 mm) is sufficient. In addition, it is essential to remove deeper tissue layers along with the lesion to document the absence of tumor invasion below the epidermis. The presence of metastases is generally believed to be rare. In addition, circumcision is generally recommended to decrease the risk of local recurrence. Alternative approaches include radiotherapy, the use of topical fluorouracil may be successful, and laser surgery.

Another clinical feature of PIN is *bowenoid papulosis*. The lesions appear as round, reddish to violaceous papules raising on the glans, or, more commonly, the shaft of the penis (Fig. 7). The typical patient is 20 to 35 years old. The majority of the affected patients are circumcised.

Histologically, a lower number of mitotic cells and lesser cellular dysplasia should allow this disorder to be reliably differentiated from carcinoma in situ. In addition, it is a completely benign lesion with no reported development of progression to invasive carcinoma. However, the strong association with the presence of HPV presents a significant risk for the development of cervical neoplasia in the female partner. Observations of partnerships were described. The standard therapy is superficial excision without the removal of additional margins. The

Fig. 6. The clinical features of PIN comprise the *Erythroplasia Queyrat*, an erythematous plaque found on the glans that is round or slightly irregular, measuring 1 to 1.5 cm in diameter

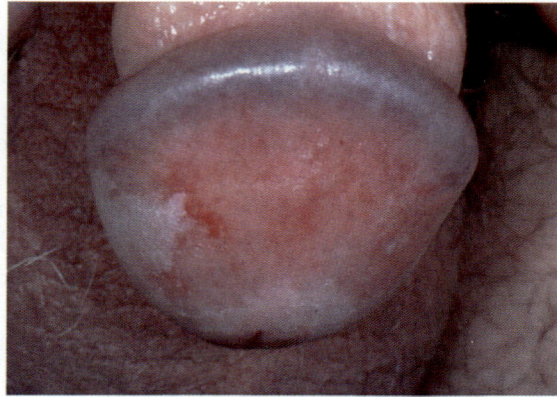

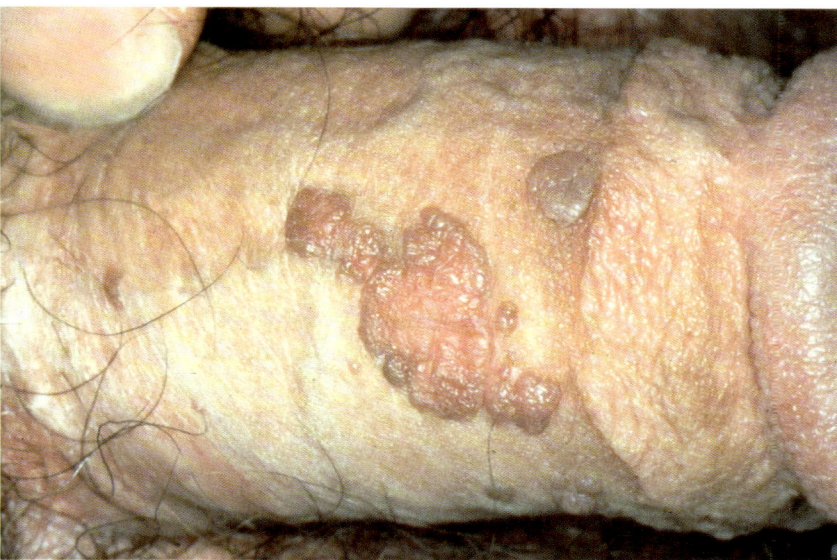

Fig. 7.   Another clinical feature of PIN is *bowenoid papulosis*. The lesions appear as round, reddish to violaceous papules raising on the glans, or, more commonly, the shaft of the penis

recurrence rate may be significant (e.g. 15 of 74 patients, the median follow-up being 5 years).

As a differential diagnosis, *lentigines* have to be separated from PIN. These hyperpigmented macules of different diameters and in different numbers are commonly seen on the glans and the shaft of the penis. They tend to increase in number, size and pigmentation with increasing age until about the 50th year of age. The etiology is unknown, they may be considered as a special type of melanocytic naevi. They are completely benign and may only be removed by excision for cosmetical reasons.

Ulcerative Diseases

Syphilis

Syphilis is caused by *treponema pallidum*. It is nearly exclusively acquired by sexual contacts. The features of the first stage, the chancre, appears usually 3 weeks after infection. Classically, it forms an indurated, punched-out, granular based, nontender ulcer (Fig. 8). The induration and the rolled border confers to the button-like consistency at palpation. The site of predilection is the penis, in particular the coronary sulcus.

In the later stages of the chancre, a firm and nontender enlargement of regional lymph nodes appears. Spontaneaous resolution usually occurs within 4 to 6 weeks. This means a spontaneous healing of the disease in about 60 to 70% of the patients.

The diagnosis is confirmed by the demonstration of

1. treponema and
2. of specific antibodies in blood serum. As the bacteria cannot be grown in culture, the only evidence is given by direct microscopic observation. The surface of a suspicious lesion has to be wiped off with a swab, and this should be pressed on a slide immediately. It is also possible to press the slide directly on the lesion and cover the attached fluid immediately. This procedure inhibits drying which would immobilize the treponemate within a short time. The sample is observed by a phase-contrast microscope (in previous times by a dark-field microscope). Another technique is the staining of dried smears with antibodies specific for treponema pallidum.

The specific antibodies reach a concentration in serum which is measurable by serologic tests within three weeks after inoculation. The test

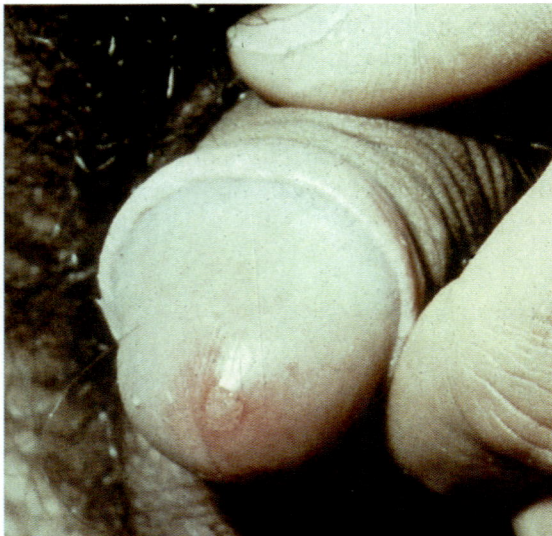

Fig. 8. Syphilitic chancre forms an indurated, punched-out, granular based, nontender ulcer. The induration and the rolled border confers to the button-like consistency at palpation. The site of predilection is the penis, in particular the coronary sulcus

widely used is the treponema pallidum hemagglutination test (TPHA). It will be positive at the time of the occurrence of the chancre. The FTA test allows a discrimination between IgG and IgM antibodies, thus indicating whether an acute infection is present.

The treatment is achieved by penicillin, which is given as a dose of 2.4 million units of benzathine penicillin in a single session. Penicillin-allergic patients should be treated with doxycycline (100 mg orally 2 time a day for 2 weeks).

The disease is cured by this therapy, and it will prevent progression to later stages. Controls of healing are recommended after 3, 6 and 12 months.

Herpes Genitalis

Herpesvirus, a DNA-virus, occurs in two serologically different types. Only type II is capable to infect the penis. The virus is acquired by direct sexual contact. As in herpes labialis, there are recurrent diseases. The phases may follow each other within a few days. In acute phases also the recurrent disease is infectious. There are no exact data on prevalence and infection rates. Today, genital herpes is a risk factor for infections with HIV.

Fig. 9. Herpes genitalis: small clear or purulent vesicles, which quickly erode

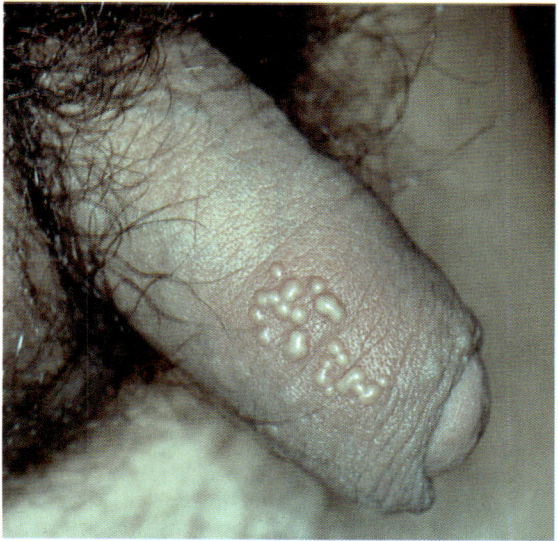

The clinical features comprise of one or more small clear vesicles, which quickly erode (Fig. 9). When the patients present to the physician, mostly the punched-out erosions are the only finding. The lesions are surrounded by inflamed margins; they are painful. Histologically, the vesicle contains isolated, degenerating keratinocytes as round cells.

Mostly, the disease may be diagnosed by clinical investigation. In recurrent disease, the patients themselves are aware of the diagnosis. When necessary, a direct smear from the vesicle or the erosion may be stained with specific herpes antibodies. It is also possible to culture the virus in a tissue culture. The determination of serum antibodies is of no use, for more than half of the adult population are positive for herpes antibodies.

The treatment is achieved with aciclovir or one of the novel derivatives. It should be topically applied to the penis 5 times daily. In recurrent diseases a continuous therapy with aciclovir orally over a period of up to 12 months is able to decrease the number of recurrences.

References

Aynaud O, Ionesco M, Barrasso R (1994) Penile intraepithelial neoplasia. Specific clinical features correlate with histologic and virologic findings. Cancer 74 (6): 1762–1767

Birley HD, Walker MM, Luzzi GA et al. (1993) Clinical features and management of recurrent balanitis; association with atopy and genital washing. Genitourin Med 69 (5): 400–403

Birley HD, Luzzi GA, Walker MM, Ryait B, Taylor-Robinson D (1994) The association of human papillomavirus infection with balanoposthitis: a description of five cases with proposals for treatment. International Journal of STD & AIDS 5 (2): 139–141

Hillman RJ, Walker MM, Harris JR, Taylor-Robinson D (1992) Penile dermatoses: a clinical and histopathological study. Genitourinary Medicine 68 (3): 166–169

Hinchliffe SA, Ciftci AO, Khine MM et al. (1994) Composition of the inflammatory infiltrate in pediatric penile lichen sclerosus et atrophicus (balanitis xerotica obliterans): a prospective, comparative immunophenotyping study. Pediatric Pathology 14 (2): 223–233

Jolly BB, Krishnamurty S, Vaidyanathan S (1993) Zoon´s balanitis. Urol Internat 50 (3): 182–184

Morrison EA (1994) Natural history of cervical infection with human papillomaviruses. [Review] Clinical Infectious Diseases 18 (2): 172–180

Wikstrom A, von Krogh G, Hedblad MA, Syrjanen S (1994) Papillomavirus-associated balanoposthitis. Genitourin Med 70 (3): 175–181

Wiswell TE (1992) Circumcision – an update [Review]. Current Problems in Pediatrics 22 (10): 424–431

Congenital and Acquired Penile Deviations and Penile Fractures

Hartmut Porst

Penile Deviations

Historical Considerations

The scientific description of penile deviations and their surgical repair goes back more than 150 years (Table 1). Thus Mettauer described the existence of ventral penile deviations in cases of hypospadias as early as in 1842, and in 1844 Philip Syng. Physik published details for the first time about the dorsal plication technique for the correction of ventral deviations in hypospadias (references in [3]).

Table 1. History of penile curvatures

Author	Year	Description
J. P. Mettauer	1842	Ventral penile curvature or chordee as a remnant of urethral corpus spongiosum
Philip Syng. Physik	1844	Dorsal plication to correct hypospadias curvature
Sievers	1926	Penile chordee without hypospadias
Reed M. Nesbit	1965	Wedge excision for repair of congenital penile curvature
Pryor/Fitzpatrick	1979	Nesbit´s procedure in Peyronie´s curvatures
Essed/Schroeder	6/1985	Plication of tunica albuginea
Ebbehøj/Metz	7/1985	Plication of tunica albuginea

The entity of congenital penile curvature and its successful repair by means of a special surgical technique was published for the first time by Nesbit in 1965 [35], thanks to whom help became increasingly available for men with penile deviations. Pryor and Fitzpatrick [42] applied the surgical technique described by Nesbit for the first time in cases of acquired penile deviations, with Peyronie´s disease, in which context the study group of J. Pryor presented their long-term results with 359 patients in 1995 [43]. Finally, Essed and Schroeder [14] and Ebbehøj and Metz [9] described a new plication technique for acquired and congenital penile curvatures independently of each other in 1985.

Epidemiology and Etiology

According to research by Ebbehøj and Metz [10], the prevalence of congenital penile deviation in Denmark is about 0.4/1000, although the authors are of the opinion that penile deviations occur considerably more often. By contrast, the prevalence of Peyronie´s disease is estimated as over 1%. More than 90% of patients with Peyronie´s disease develop penile curvature in the further course of the disease, in most cases with a dorsal bending [52].

Nesbit [35] assumes that congenital penile deviations are due to an asymmetry of the corpora cavernosa, the etiology of which remains speculative. Catuogno et al. [6] postulate a fetal androgen deficiency, or a local deficiency of 5 α-reductase as a cause of the different development in length, since dihydrotestosterone (DHT) is responsible for the development of the external genitalia. By the external application of a suspension containing DHT (0.15 mg/cm^2) once daily for 2–3 months, with interruptions, the authors achieved almost complete removal in five of 11 patients (aged 4–21 years) with penile deviations but without simultaneous hypospadias and a 30% improvement in two further patients. Interesting in this context is the fact that during the fetal development a ventral penile curvature is physiological. Therefore, Kaplan and Lamm [21] attribute its persistence beyond the embryo stage to an androgen deficiency or to androgen insensitivity. Devine and Horton [8], based on their own comprehensive experience, classify three types of ventral penile curvature without simultaneous hypospadias: type I, with absence of distal differentiation of the corpus spongiosum (hypoplastic urethra); type II, normal differentiation of the corpus spongiosum, but with fibrous formation of Buck´s and Colle´s fascia; type III, normal differentiation of the corpus spongiosum and solely fibrous formation of Colle´s fascia.

Following the Devine and Horton classification, Perovic [39] distinguishes between four different types of penile deviations and subsequently derives four different surgical procedures on the basis of the underlying etiology (Table 2). Baskin and Duckett [3] come to the con-

Table 2.   Congenital penile curvatures (from [8, 39])

Etiological Concepts

Hypospadias sine Hypospadias (short urethra syndrome)

Congenital ventral deviation		Treatment
1. Cutaneous chordee: (urethra and spong. normal)	Dysgenetic unelastic tissue in tunica dartos and Buck´s fascia	Mobilization
2. Fibrous chordee: (spongiosam abnormal)	Fibrous tissue from Buck´s fascia lateral to spongiosum	Excision
3. Corporocavernosal chordee: (spongiosum normal)	Shortness and/or inelasticity of tunica albuginea	Nesbit procedure
4. Congenital short urethra:	Dysmorphic corpus spongiosum and/or Buck´s fascia	Resection of urethra, chordectomy, dorsal corporoplasty

clusion that congenital penile curvature is attributable to an abnormal differentiation of the skin, of Buck´s or Colle´s fascia, or to a disproportion of the corpus cavernosum, which is due to a discrepancy in the longitudinal growth of the tunica albuginea. The authors also maintain that, normally, the urethral plate is healthy in congenital penile curvature and does not represent an attributable cause of this anomaly.

Material and Methods

From 1988 to 1996, 155 patients with congenital penile curvatures and 153 patients with acquired penile curvatures were personally operated on by the author. Diagnostic screening methods used are shown in Table 3.

Table 3.   Procedures for diagnostic evaluation of penile curvatures

Intracavernous injection of 10–20 µg PGE_1
Duplexsonography of penile arteries
Pharmacocavernosography in nonresponders to 20 µg PGE_1
Uroflowmetry
Retrograde urethrography in dorsal penile curvatures

Irrespective of the underlying etiology, an intracavernous injection of 10–20 µg PGE_1 (Prostavasin, Schwarz Pharma) was carried out in each patient to assess the extent of the penile curvature. The test was combined with simultaneous duplex sonography of the penile arteries in order to verify any circulation deficiencies, in particular in cases of acquired curvature. Patients with semi-erections not sufficient for sexual intercourse underwent pharmacocavernosography to prove or exclude a relevant cavernous insufficiency.

In addition, all patients were submitted to uroflowmetry and evaluation of urine residual volume for assessment of the infravesical situation. In cases with pathological findings, as well as for all patients with dorsal curvatures, in whom mobilization of the corpus spongiosum was required intraoperatively, a retrograde urethrogram was performed preoperatively.

Surgical Technique

The surgical procedure was the same for all penile curvatures and corresponded to the technique described by Nesbit [35]. Depending on the patient´s wishes, the foreskin was either left or circumcised. In cases with preservation of the foreskin, 1.0 cm proximal to the sulcus coronarius the preputial inner layer and Colle´s fascia were incised sharply to Buck´s fascia. In the sleeve technique the penile skin with the adherent Colle´s fascia was prepared down to the penile basis. Subsequently, following the application of a tourniquet and intracavernous insertion of a butterfly cannula, an artificial erection was induced with normal saline solution (Fig. 1a, b).

In cases of ventral deviation, the dorsal nerve-vessel bundle was prepared lateral to medial, without the need for complete detachment in most cases.

In patients with dorsal deviation, complete liberation of the urethra, marked with an indwelling catheter, is mandatory (Fig. 2a, b). Buck´s fascia is then incised at the angle of the curvature and a wedge excision of the tunica albuginea of each corpus cavernosum is performed, the extent of the excision depending on the degree of the curvature. The defect is closed transversely with a running Vicryl or PDS suture, which is additionally secured by interrupted sutures. The result of the surgery

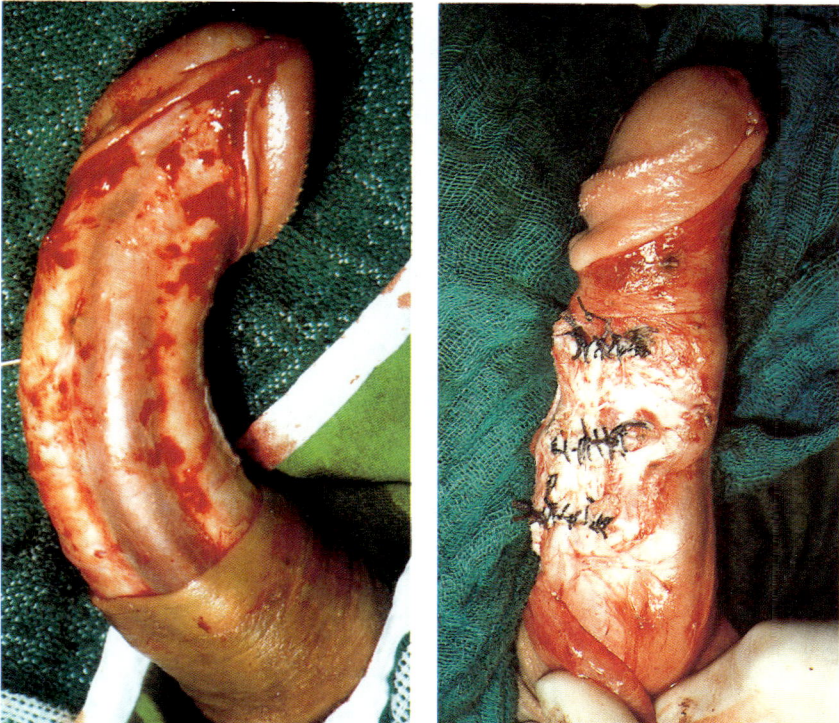

Fig. 1a, b.   Severe kongenital left-lateral deviation requiring three wedge excisions for complete straightening

is verified by an artificial erection and, if required, a second wedge is excised from the tunica or a plication suture is applied using prolene. Buck´s fascia is reapproximated using catgut 4/0 interrupted sutures (Fig. 3a). After reapproximation of the skin with 4/0 Catgut sutures a light circular compression bandage is applied to the penis and the penis is fixed to the abdominal wall with adhesive tape (Fig. 3b).

Urine drainage is ensured in dorsal deviations for 3–4 days by means of a suprapubic cystostomy, following intraoperative removal of the catheter. In all other cases, urine drainage is carried out for 1 day by means of a 14-Ch. indwelling catheter.

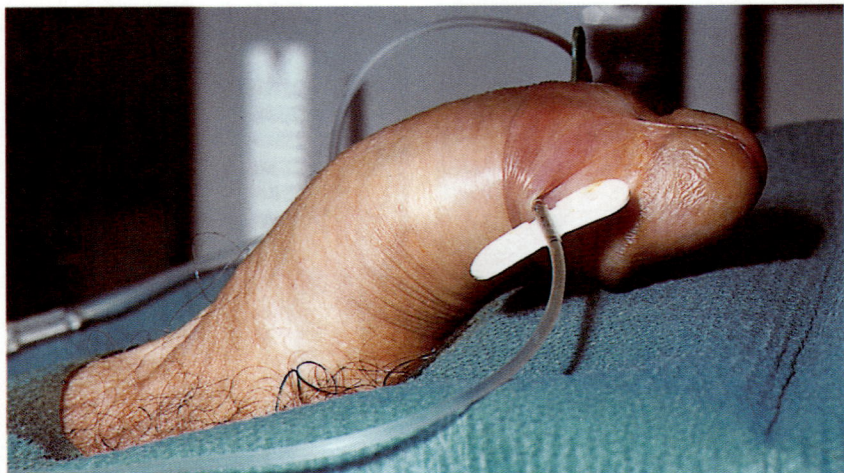

Fig. 2a

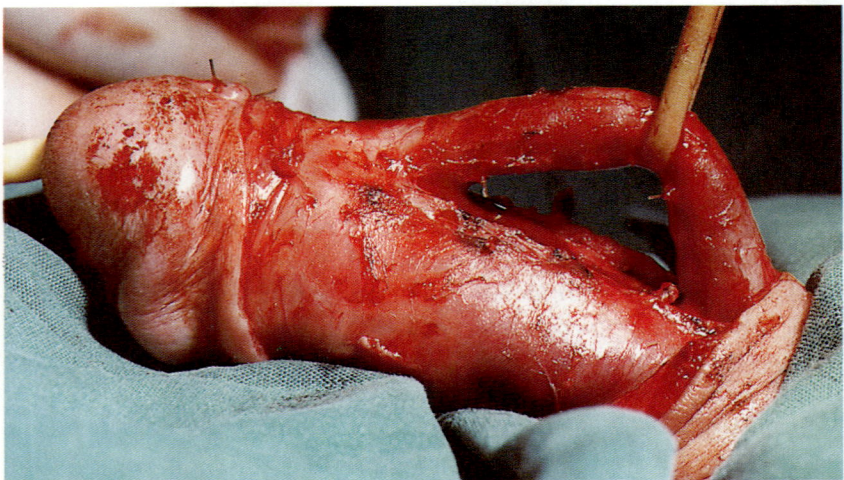

Fig. 2b.   In dorsal deviations complete mobilization of the urethra is mandatory to ensure complete correction

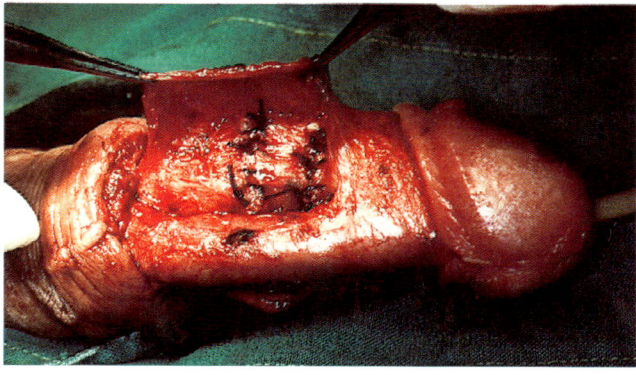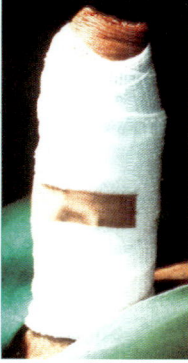

Fig. 3a, b.   After closure of the tunical wedge excisions, the sutures are covered with the preserved Buck's fascia. A moderate compressing bandage is applied for 24 h and urine drainage is secured with a 14 Ch Foley catheter

Results

Congenital Penile Deviations

Of the 155 patients with congenital penile curvatures who underwent surgery, 110 (71%) were available for follow-up. Average age was 21 years (15–31) and average follow-up 34 months (6–78). The distribution of penile deviations was as follows:

Ventral: 63%   (69/110)   mean angle of curvature 70°   (40°–95°)
Left-lateral: 27%   (30/110)   mean angle of curvature 53°   (40°–90°)
Right-lateral: 4%   (4/110)   mean angle of curvature 45°   (40°–60°)
Dorsal: 6%   (7/110)   mean angle of curvature 75°   (70°–90°)

Details of preoperative and postoperative sexual performance are summarized in Table 4. It is interesting that 23% had not yet attempted coitus and a further 36% were unable to successfully penetrate the vagina due to the degree of the curvature. A further 35% reported problems with vaginal penetration. Among couples for whom coitus was possible, 31% of the sexual partners complained of painful sensations during intercourse attributable to the curvature. Postoperatively, 80% indicated that coitus was normal, while a further 9% had still not performed sexual intercourse. With respect to the evaluation of the final results, 89% indicated that they were very satisfied or satisfied with the outcome of the

Table 4. Sexual performance in congenital penile curvatures in 110 patients

Problem	Preoperative (%)	Postoperative (%)
No attempt at coitus	23	9
Unsuccessful coitus (due to bending)	36	2
Unsuccessful coitus (due to erectile failure)	6	4
Coitus successful but with problems	35	5
Normal coitus possible	1	80
Coitus painful for sexual partner	31	Not stated

Table 5. Results of corporoplasty for congenital penile curvatures in 110 patients followed up via telephone interview or questionnaire 1988–1995

Very satisfied/ or satisfied	Fairly satisfied	Dissatisfied	Repeated consent to operation
89% (98/110)	10% 11/110	1% 1/110	98% 108/110

operation, 10% were satisfied to a limited degree, 1% were not satisfied, and 98% would again agree to an operation in light of the result of their surgery (Table 5).

Direct postoperative complications arose in 1.9% (3/155) of cases in terms of wound infections and in 1.3% (2/155) due do partial necrosis of the foreskin, with the results that these patients required subsequent circumcision. A further two patients developed hematoma, with the result that the postoperative course of healing was somewhat delayed. In terms of *late complications*, recurrent deviations of > 20° were indicated in 5.4% of cases (6/110), numbness in 0.9% (1/110), and shortening of the penis in 1.8% (2/110).

Acquired Penile Deviations

Of the 153 patients with acquired penile deviations, an average follow-up of 39 months (6–86) was possible with 118 (77%). The average age was 53.4 years (17–70 years). A total of 86% (132/153) of the curvatures were the result of Peyronie´s disease, 8% (12/153) were caused by scar formation following self-injection therapy into the cavernous bodies, and 6% (9/153) were attributable to penile fractures.

The distribution of the acquired deviations was as follows:

Dorsal: 79%   (93/118)   mean angle of curvature 82°
Left-lateral: 16%   (19/118)   mean angle of curvature 65°
Right-lateral: 2%   (2/118)   mean angle of curvature 80°
Ventral: 3%   (4/118)   mean angle of curvature 75°

With regard to the preoperative and postoperative sexual performance of the patients, 58% indicated that preoperative coitus was no longer possible, a further 38% complained of difficulties but were able to achieve penetration, and 4% indicated that coitus was normal; 45% of all patients presented additional erectile dysfunction preoperatively. Postoperatively, coitus was still not possible for 18%, and a further 16% reported difficulties in performing sexual intercourse (Table 6).

Table 6.   Sexual performance of 118 patients with acquired penile curvatures

	Preoperative (%)	Postoperative (%)
Coitus not possible	58	18
Coitus possible, but with problems	38	16
Normal coitus	4	66
Additional erectile dysfunction	45	34

The patients assessed the postoperative result as follows: very satisfied/satisfied, 77% (91/118); satisfied with limitations 10% (12/118); dissatisfied 13% (15/118).

Assessment of the postoperative results with regard to the preoperative erectile capacity shows that 90% of the patients with preoperatively

Table 7. Results of corporoplasty in 118 patients with acquired penile curvatures

	Subjective evaluation	(%)
Patients with erectile dysfunction, n = 53 (45%)	Very satisfied/satisfied	61
	Fairly satisfied	16
	Dissatisfied	23
Patients with normal erectile function, n = 65 (55%)	Very satisfied/satisfied	89
	Fairly satisfied	5
	Dissatisfied	5

normal erectile capacity were satisfied with the postoperative results, whereas the satisfaction rate was only 61% in those patients with preoperatively impaired erectile function (Table 7).

Direct postoperative complications occurred in 4% (6/153) with severe skin gangrene in a case of poorly controlled diabetes, which made plastic skin surgery necessary, one preputial necrosis with subsequent circumcision, two cases of peripheral bleeding of the wound edges with the need for suture, and two cases of bleeding from the suprapubic cystostomy requiring premature removal without subsequent complications.

Late complications were reported as follows: shortening of the penis by 1–2 cm, 35%; shortening of the penis > 2 cm, 7%; only 6% of the patients complained that penile shortening was associated with functional impairment during sexual intercourse. Recurrence of deviations > 20°, 12%; 20°–50°, 3%; > 50°, 4%.

Discussion

Our comprehensive personal experience with corporoplasty using the surgical technique originally described by Nesbit has shown that this is a very reliable procedure, both with congenital and with acquired penile curvatures. The satisfaction-rate of 89% in our own patient group with congenital curvatures was within the percentage scales reported in the literature, which ranged between 81 and 96% in larger patient series (Table 8). The rate of satisfaction with the postoperative outcome

Table 8.   Results of surgical therapy of congenital penile curvatures

Author	No of patients	Mean follow-up	Technique	Satisfaction rate (%)
Poulsen [41]	163	6 months–5 years	Nesbit: 138	82
			Ebbehøj: 25	60
Ebbehøj [10]	140	6 months–10 years	Ebbehøj plic.	94
Kelami [22]	100	1–10 years	Nesbit	96
Ralph/Pryor [44]	88	10 months	Nesbit	94
Popken [40]	55	1–10 years	Nesbit	90
Klevmark [23]	58	24 months	Plication	81
Porst	110	34 months	Nesbit	89

was less favorable in acquired penile deviations. While this was 77% in the present series, the figures in the literature ranged between 35 and 89% (Table 9).

The reason for these discrepancies between congenital and acquired penile curvatures in the assessment of postoperative results is the substantial age difference between the two groups, with an average of more than 30 years (see personal series). On the one hand, the probability of simultaneous erectile dysfunction increases with age; on the other hand, it is a well-known fact that in the course of Peyronie´s disease the incidence of erectile problems increases. In particular, the occurrence of so-

Table 9.   Results of surgical therapy of acquired penile curvatures

Author	No of patients	Mean follow-up	Technique	Satisfaction rate (%)
Ralph/Pryor [43]	359	21 months	Nesbit	82[a]
Klevmark [23]	57	20 months	Plication	82
Schubert [48]	54	> 3 years	Plication	89
Nooter [38]	33	42 months	Plication	64
Mufti [33]	30	31 months	Nesbit/plication	63
Knopf [24]	23	39 months	Schroeder/Essed	35
Porst	118	39 months	Nesbit	77

[a] Bending up to 30°.

called cavernous insufficiency, i.e. a disorder of the veno-occlusive mechanism (also described as cavernous leak), is frequently reported in cases of Peyronie´s disease [5, 20, 27, 28]. Especially plaque-associated texture problems of the tunica albuginea, with a reduction of the elastic fibers and, as a result, a clearly reduced compliance of the tunica, seem to be responsible for simultaneous cavernous insufficiency [1, 19].

Moreover, arterial circulation disorders play a part among the predominantly older patients with Peyronie´s disease and associated deviations. Therefore, various authors have pointed out the importance of preoperative vascular assessment by means of penile duplex sonography [5, 20, 45]. In this respect, the present series also demonstrated that 45% of all patients with acquired penile deviations also had simultaneous erectile disorders, and that the percentage of 61% who were satisfied with the outcome of the operation was less than those without simultaneous erectile dysfunction (90%).

For this reason, most authors have come to the conclusion that in patients with simultaneous erectile dysfunction, plastic surgery alone should be carried out only in exceptional cases, and that this patient group is better treated with the implantation of a hydraulic penile prothesis [5, 43, 52], which corresponds to the personal approach.

Based on the above comments, an exact preoperative diagnostic screening of the cavernosal function as well as of the penile circulation by means of pharmacotesting with PGE, and duplex sonography, as well as pharmacocavernosography in nonresponders to 20 µg PGE_1, is essential. An important point in the assessment of the postoperative results is the degree of penile shortening. It obviously plays no part at all in the surgical repair of congenital curvatures but has indeed an importance with regard to curvatures due to Peyronie´s disease, since this disorder already leads to penile shortening preoperative, due to the fibrous transformation processes which take place and which cause patients to complain. For this reason, plaque surgery at an early stage, with simultaneous grafting by means of dermal grafts or Goretex or Durapatch, has been propagated as an alternative to corporoplasty alone. However, the long-term results with these patients have shown that a high percentage suffer from postoperative erectile disorders as a consequence of graft-associated cavernous insufficiency, and few authors prefer this procedure [16, 27]. Apart from that, both the comprehensive series of Ralph et al. [43] and the present series show that functionally important shortening of more than 2 cm occurs only in 5–7%. For this reason, it may be stated that corporoplasty with sustained erectile function continues to be the procedure of choice and is clearly superior to any plaque excision procedures with simultaneous grafting.

Another topic in the consideration of postoperative results, in congenital as well as acquired penile curvatures, is the percentage of recurrent deviations and the question of whether the plication techniques as described by Essed and Schroeder [14] or Ebbehøj and Metz [9], which are considerably easier from the technical point of view, could provide comparable results.

With regard to the frequency of recurrence of deviations, it has been demonstrated that the incidence is considerably higher in educational clinics with several surgeons, as is the overall incidence of postoperative complications [15, 24, 40, 50]. Therefore, in the interest of the patient, corporoplasty should not be regarded as a training operation.

While some authors have also published very good results with plication techniques, with satisfaction rates of up to 81–94% [9, 13, 23, 48], others have shown substantially less favorable postoperative results, with satisfaction rates of 35–64% [24, 33, 38, 41]. In particular, Poulson and Kirkeby [41] and Fritz et al. [15] were able to show, in a direct comparison, that the original Nesbit procedure provides very good postoperative results in 82%, which was substantially better than the plication technique with 60%.

I abandoned the plication technique years ago in favor of the Nesbit procedure, due to the considerably more frequent recurrences of deviations. Undoubtedly, the suture material used plays a not negligible part in the incidence of recurrent deviations.

There is general agreement that with the use of the plication technique only nonabsorbable suture material should be used, whereby an inverted suture technique with concealment of the knots is mandatory; otherwise, the palpable knots could later lead to painful sensations or cause the formation of fistulas [13].

For wedge excisions, as described in Nesbit's original method, my own experience has shown that slowly absorbed material such as Vicryl, Dexon, or PDS is sufficient. Finally, with congenital penile deviations, which mostly involve young patients, physical growth should be complete at the time of surgery; my experience has shown that if the operation is carried out during puberty, between the ages of 13 and 16, the incidence of recurrent deviations will be substantially higher.

Penile Fractures

Etiology and Symptomatology

A review of the literature of the past 10 years shows that publications with series of more than ten patients are still rare, even today [2, 11, 12, 29, 34, 49]. A survey of 393 penile fractures (Fig. 4) reported by a total of 25 authors shows that the overwhelming majority of penile fractures occurred during forced masturbation (43%), while only 28% occurred during actual sexual intercourse; 11% of all fractures actually occurred at night, unnoticed during sleep, when the male rolled over his erect penis during a nocturnal penile erection. Finally, 16% of penile fractures were encountered as a result of direct trauma to the penis (blow or push). The classical penile fracture is characterized by a loud cracking sound, like the tear of a bow string, accompanied by penile pain and rapid loss of erection and onset of penile hematoma and represents a dramatic event for both the affected man and his sexual partner.

A survey of 169 penile fractures (23 references), in which the authors also considered urethral injuries, shows that an average of 11% (0–38%) of all cases of penile fractures were combined with simultaneous rup-

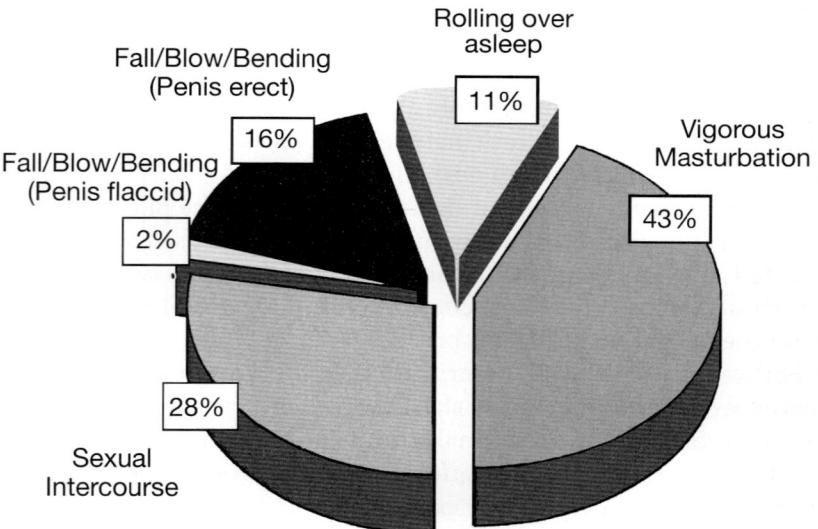

Fig. 4. Etiology of penile fracture based on a worldwide survey of 25 references including 393 cases

ture of the urethra. A typical feature of a simultaneous rupture of the urethra is the emergence of blood from the urethral orifice and initial macrohematuria during micturition. In some cases, hematuria may be pronounced, depending on the severity of urethral damage.

Besides these classic symptoms of the acute, clinically apparent penile fracture there are more frequently encountered penile fractures which, in my own experience of the past 15 years, are for a while clinically latent. They are not noticed by the patient until later, when palpable scar formation with detectable induration of the penis occurs; it is often accompanied by penile deviation and only this prompts the patient to consult a physician. These primarily latent penile fractures do not cause apparent hematoma but, when the patient´s history is taken, are remembered as a slip during coitus, with a short cracking sound, sometimes accompanied by a short pricking pain with subsequent subsidence of erection and early termination of sexual intercourse. Depending on the extent of the lesion of the tunica a notch or deviation of the penis may occur days or weeks later, with the result that the originally responsible rupture of the tunica later gives the impression of classical Peyronie´s disease. Such men also frequently present with a certain degree of erectile dysfunction. In the author´s own experience of more than 1500 patients with penile disorders per year, about 30–40 men present with a history of such clinically latent penile fractures.

Diagnostic Assessment

The classical acute penile fracture manifests as a large penile hematoma. It must be differentiated from rupture of a dorsal or circumflex vein as well as of a dorsal artery [31, 37]. These likewise lead to a hematoma, but they occur substantially less often than penile fracture.

The diagnosis of penile fractures may indeed represent a "first-look diagnosis," but the severity and location of the tunica rupture requires additional imaging procedures to provide better insight. In this context, the first step is cavernosography, which is recommended by a number of authors and the diagnostic value of which corresponds to the personal experiences (Fig. 5a, b). Several authors [7, 34] have also reported on localization of the rupture by means of sonography, although this diagnostic method has not gained general acceptance. If there is any suspi-

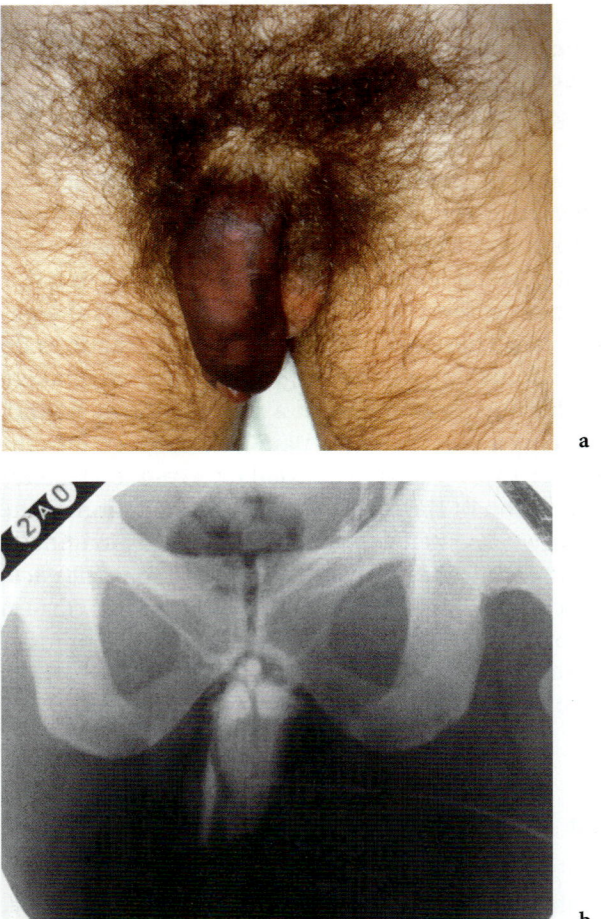

Fig. 5a, b.   Penile fracture with extravasation of contrast medium during cavernosography. In this case surgical intervention with closure of the rupture should be obligatory. (From Porst, H. Erektile Impotenz, Enke-Verlag Stuttgart, 1987)

cion of a concomitant rupture of the urethra, a retrograde urethrogram is mandatory, whereby the use of catheterization in these cases should be absolutely avoided due to the potential risk of converting a partial rupture into a complete rupture. If possible, a urine culture should be taken preoperatively, enabling antibiotic treatment according to the bacteria found in case of the presence of urinary tract infection.

Therapy

There is uniform agreement in the literature that for acute penile fractures surgical intervention is mandatory [2, 7, 11, 12, 26, 29, 34]; this con-
curs with my own approach. However, some cases are problematical, and
the consultation is delayed for some days. In these cases, a decision must
be made on an individual basis, depending on the symptoms and the
local findings, as to whether an operative or a conservative approach
should be adopted. In my experience, the extent of the hematoma is a
landmark indicator.

In most publications, a subcoronary approach with the sleeve technique is recommended [2, 7, 12, 34, 36, 46]. Other authors prefer a longitudinal or transverse incision of the penile skin above the rupture site
to the subcoronary technique [11, 26, 29, 46]. In individual cases, an
infrapubic or high scrotal incision with eversion of the penis is also
described, as recommended by Lue for penile venous surgery [30, 34]. I
generally prefer a subcoronary approach, but for individual cases with
fracture close to the penile base or with simultaneous rupture of the
suspensory ligament I choose an infrapubic incision.

After evacuation of the hematoma, which may be a very time-consum-
ing procedure in penile fractures that occurred some days earlier, the
tunica rupture is exposed and any simultaneously present intracavernous hematoma is likewise evacuated. The tunica is then closed off with
interrupted sutures or with a running suture, and practically all cited
authors use absorbable suture material (Dexon, Vicryl, PDS). Most authors maintain urine drainage for several days. In the author's opinion,
preference should always be given to a suprapubic cystostomy. In the
event of simultaneous rupture of the urethra, a tissue-sparing trimming
of the urethral wound edges should be carried out, with subsequent
suture of 5/-o Chrome Catgut or Dexon. Antibiotic prophylaxis is recommended by all authors.

Results and Late Complications

With immediate surgical repair it was possible to preserve potency in
97% of 169 cases (23 references); this is a convincing argument in favor
of surgical treatment for penile fractures. By contrast, Volz and Brode-

rick [51] describe an impotence-rate of 100% in six cases of conservative treatment of penile fractures. This does not, however, correspond to the author's own observations, whereby three of four patients with penile fractures who presented at the clinic with a delay of 36–72 hours after the fracture event and were therefore treated conservatively, remained potent. Further late complications of penile fractures treated either surgically or conservatively are penile curvatures or indurations, which indeed resemble genuine Peyronie's disease [2, 11, 12, 29].

Very rare late consequences of penile fractures with simultaneous rupture of the urethra were described in the form of cavernoso-urethral fistulas [18, 32] or the occurrence of a urethral stricture [17].

With latent penile fractures an erectile dysfunction may often occur in addition to the formation of penile induration or penile deviation. In these cases, according to the author's experience, intracavernous stimulation therapy with PGE$_1$ (Prostavasin) 6–10 times has at intervals of 8–14 days proved to be effective; in most cases a clear improvement of this temporary cavernous insufficiency has been achieved. Functionally relevant penile curvature as a sequela of penile fracture must be treated by corporoplasty.

References

1. Akkus E, Carrier S, Rehman J, Baba K, Nunes L, Morgan D, Padma-Nathan H, Lue TF (1994) Structural alterations in the tunica albuginea: relevance to Peyronie's disease and impotence. Int J Impotence Res 6 Suppl 1: D206
2. Asgari MA, Hosseini SY, Safarinejad MR, Samdzadeh B, Bardideh AR (1996) Penile fractures: Evaluation, therapeutic approaches and long-term results. J Urol 155: 148–149
3. Baskin LS, Duckett JW (1994) Dorsal tunica albuginea plication for hypospadias curvature. J Urol 151: 1668–1671
4. Benson G (1993) Editorial comment: Peyronie's disease. J Urol 149: 1326
5. Broderick GA, Wessels H, Wein AJ (1994) Peyronie's disease: a functional and anatomic assessment with duplex doppler ultrasound. Int J Impotence Res 4 Suppl 2: A112
6. Catuogno C, Lanza T, Ventrice GA, Scalfari A, Lanza P (1994) Medical therapy of congenital curving of the penis without hypospadias. Int J Impotence Res 6 Suppl 1: D225
7. Cendron M, Whitmore KE, Carpiniello V, Kurzweil SJ, Hanno PM, Snyder HM, Duckett JW (1990) Traumatic rupture of the corpus cavernosum: evaluation and management. J Urol 144: 987–991
8. Devine CH, Horton CE (1973) Chordee without hypospadias. J Urol 110: 264–271
9. Ebbehøj J, Metz P (1985) New operation for Krummerik (penile curvature). Urology 26: 76–78
10. Ebbehøj J, Metz P (1987) Congenital penile angulation. Brit J Urol 60: 264–266

11. El-Sherif AE, Dauleh M, Allowneh N, Vijayan P (1991) Management of fracture of the penis in Quatar. Brit J Urol 68: 622–625
12. Ercole CJ, Sneiders A, Gordon BE, Gleich WP, Motilla P, Corica A (1991) Preservation of sexual potency following surgical repair of traumatic corpus cavernosum rupture. J Urol 145/4 Suppl: 403A
13. Erpenbach K, Rothe H, Derschum W (1991) The penile plication procedure: an alternative method for straightening penile deviation. J Urol 146: 1276–1278
14. Essed E, Schroeder FH (1985) New surgical treatment for Peyronie´s disease. Urology 25: 582–587
15. Fritz T, Müller SC, Bürger RA, Hohenfellner R (1990) Operative Korrektur von Penisdeviationen: Erfahrungen mit der Methode nach Nesbit und dem modifizierten Verfahren nach Schröder und Essed. Akt Urol 21: 126–131
16. Grein U, Noll F (1993) Schwellkörperinsuffizienz nach Dermalgraft-Corporoplastik. Urologe A 32 Suppl 2: S18
17. Gross M, Arnold TL, Peters P (1977) Fracture of the penis with associated laceration of the urethra. J Urol 117: 726–727
18. Hargreaves DG, Plail RO (1994) Fracture of the penis causing a corporo-urethral fistula. Brit J Urol 73: 97
19. Iacono F, Barra S, de Rosa G, Boscaino A, Lotti T (1993) Microstructural disorders of tunica albuginea in patients affected by Peyronie´s disease with or without erection dysfunction. J Urol 150: 1806–1809
20. Jordan GH, Angermeier KW (1993) Preoperative evaluation of erectile function with dynamic infusion cavernosometry/cavernosography in patients undergoing surgery for Peyronie´s disease: correlation with postoperative results. J Urol 150: 1138–1142
21. Kaplan GWD, Lamm DL (1975) Embryogenesis of chordee. J Urol 114: 769–772
22. Kelami A (1987) Congenital penile deviation and its treatment with the Nesbit-Kelami-technique. Brit J Urol 60: 261–263
23. Klevmark B, Andersen M, Schultz A, Talseth T (1994) Congenital and acquired curvature of the penis treated surgically by plication of the tunica albuginea. Brit J Urol 74: 501–506
24. Knopf HJ, Engelmann UH, Haupt G, Senge T (1991) Operative Korrektur der angeborenen und erworbenen Penisdeviation. Akt Urol 22: 371–375
25. Koga S, Saito Y, Arakaki Y, Nakamura N, Matsuoka M, Saita M, Yoshikawa M, Ohyama C (1993) Sonography in fracture of the penis. Brit J Urol 72: 228–229
26. Krauß B (1983): Penisfraktur. Pathologie-Diagnostik-Therapie. Akt Urol 14: 141–144
27. Lakin BL, Carter MF (1991) Venogenic impotence following dermal graft repair for Peyronie´s disease. J Urol 146: 849–851
28. Lopez JA, Jarow JP (1993) Penile vascular evaluation of men with Peyronie´s disease. J Urol 149: 53–55
29. Mansi MK, Emran M, El-Mahrouky A, El-Mateet MS (1993) Experience with penile fractures in Egypt: long-term results of immediate surgical repair. J Trauma 35: 67–70
30. Mellinger BC, Douenias R (1992) New surgical approach for operative management of penile fracture and penetrating trauma. Urology 39: 429–432
31. Mostafa H (1967) Rupture of the dorsal artery of the penis as a result of sexual intercourse. J Urol 97: 314
32. Motiwala HG (1993) Urethrocavernous fistula following sexual intercourse. J Urol 149: 371

33. Mufti GR, Aitchison M, Bramwell SP, Paterson PJ, Scott R (1990) Corporeal plication for surgical correction of Peyronie´s disease. J Urol 144: 281–283
34. Nane J, Esen T, Tellaloglu S, Selhanoglu M, Akinci M (1991) Penile fractures: emergency surgery for perseveration of penile functions. Andrologia 23: 309–311
35. Nesbit RM (1965) Congenital curvature of the phallus: report of three cases with description of corrective operations. J Urol 93: 230–233
36. Nicolaisen GS, Melamud A, Williams RD, McAninch JW (1983) Rupture of the corpus cavernosum: surgical management. J Urol 130: 917–919
37. Nicoly ER, Costabile RA, Moul JW (1992) Rupture of the deep dorsal vein of the penis during sexual intercourse. J Urol 147: 150–152
38. Nooter RJ, Bosch JLHR, Schroeder FH (1994) Peyronie´s disease and congenital penile curvature: long-term results of operative treatment with the plication procedure. Brit J Urol 74: 497–500
39. Perovic S (1992) Hypospadias sine hypospadias. World J Urology 10: 85–89
40. Popken G, Wetterauer U, Hakenberg O, Katzenwadel A, Kreutzig T (1994) Long-term results of surgical correction of congenital deviation. Int J Impotence Res 6 Suppl 1: D158
41. Poulsen J, Kirkeby HJ (1992) Treatment of penile curvature – a retrospective investigation of 163 patients. Int J Impotence Res 4 Suppl 2: A150
42. Pryor JP, Fitzpatrick JM (1979) A new approach to the correction of the penile deformity in Peyronie´s disease. J Urol 122: 622–623
43. Ralph DJ, Al-Akraa M, Pryor JP (1995) The Nesbit operation for Peyronie´s disease: 16 year experience. J Urol 154: 1362–1363
44. Ralph D, Al-Akraa M, Coker C, Pryor J (1994) Surgery for congenital curvature of the penis. Int J Impotence Res 6 Suppl 1: D159
45. Ralph DJ, Hill PD, Kellet MJ, Pryor JP (1992) Erectile dysfunction in Peyronie´s disease. Int J Impotence Res 4 Suppl 2: A113
46. Ruckle HC, Hadley HR, Liu PD (1992) Fracture of penis. Urology 40: 33–35
47. Sarramon JP, Escourrou G (1991) The diagnosis and management of Peyronie´s disease. Int J Impotence Res 3: 69–83
48. Schubert J, Kümmerling St (1992) Induratio penis plastica. Untersuchungen zum Staging, Erektionsverhalten und operativen Möglichkeiten. Akt Urol 23: 242–247
49. Tan LB, Chiang CP, Huang CH, Chou YH, Wang CJ (1991) Traumatic rupture of the corpus cavernosum. Brit J Urol 68: 627–628
50. Theiß M, Grups JW, Heckl W, Bergmann M, Frohmüller H (1990) Langzeitergebnisse und histologische Untersuchungen nach operativer Korrektur der kongenitalen Penisdeviation. Urologe A 29: 342–344
51. Volz LR, Broderick GA (1994) Conservative management of penile fracture may cause cavernous-venous occlusive disease and permanent erectile dysfunction. J Urol 151 5 Suppl: 358A
52. Weidner W (1993) Internationale Konferenz über Induratio penis plastica (IPP) 17.– 19. März, Washington Bethesda. Akt Urol 24: 372–374

Penile Cancer: Stage-Related Therapy

Georg Schoeneich and Stephan C. Müller

Incidence

Squamous cell carcinoma (SCC) of the penis is a rare disease in well-developed countries, but remains a significant health problem in some areas of the world where infantile circumcision and good genital hygiene are not routinely practiced. In Central Europe and in the USA, its age-adjusted annual incidence is 0.9/100 000 men. In Israel, reflecting the rate of circumcision, its rate is 0.1/100 000 men. This is in contrast to certain areas of Asia, Africa, India, and the Third World, where SCC of the penis is prevalent and one of the most frequently diagnosed malignant tumors in men (Table 1) [1–5].

Table 1. Geographic incidence of squamous cell carcinoma (SCC)

Geographic area	Incidence (% of male cancers)
Europe/USA	1.0
Vietnam	11.5
Thailand	6.6
Uganda	12.0
Brazil	17.0
Mexico	10.0
Puerto Rico	20.0

Etiology

SCC of the penis is associated with absence of circumcision or poor genital hygiene. Smegma has been implicated in the carcinogenesis of penile cancer. Phimosis is found in as many as 75% of the patients with SCC of the penis and is the most common coexisting abnormality in men with this neoplasm [6–8]. However ten cases of penile cancer after neonatal circumcision have been reported, which implies the need for caution even after circumcision [9]. On the other hand, there is an increasing evidence and prevalence for a viral role in the development of at least some cases of penile cancer. Desoxyribonucleic acid (DNA) sequences of human papilloma-viruses (HPV) were found in the majority of benign or malignant penile lesions: HPV-6, -11, -42, -43 in condylomata acuminata; HPV-16 in intraepithelial neoplasia (M. Bowen); HPV-16, -18 in penile and zervix carcinoma [10–15]. An increasing incidence and prevalence of penile lesions in men whose female partners have cervical carcinoma or intraepithelial neoplasia have also been reported [16]. Similar to skin cancer, ultraviolet radiation also appears to have carcinogenic potential for SCC of the penis: oral 8-methoxypsoralen and ultraviolet A phototherapy (PUVA) or ultraviolet B in men with psoriasis greatly increase the incidence of penile and/or scrotal SCC [17].

Clinical Presentations

The spectrum of clinical presentation varies, ranging from itching or burning under the foreskin, erythema and ulceration or induration of the glans and prepuce, to obvious extensive carcinoma of the glans or penile shaft. Chronic irritation beneath a phimotic foreskin typically precedes recognition of the tumor. Primary SCC of the penis may occur at any anatomic location of the penis (Table 2) [8, 18, 19]. Depending on the history of the patient, the length of delay in diagnosis, and the tumor size, superficial inguinal lymph nodes may be palpable at presentation (metastases/inflammatory lymphadenopathy).

Table 2. Primary sites of origin of penile cancer

Site	Percentage
Glans penis	48
Prepuce	21
Prepuce, glans, shaft	14
Glans and prepuce	9
Coronal sulcus	6
Shaft	2

Differential Diagnosis

By far the most common cancer of the penis is squamous cell carcinoma, which accounts for more than 95% of cases [20], but abnormal penile growths must include the discussion of both benign or malignant tumors. Some penile lesions are strictly benign. Some are premalignant or at least possess the potential for malignancy. Metastatic spread to the penis from another origin has to be evaluated and distinguished from primary SCC of the penis. With the increasing incidence of the acquired immundeficiency syndrome (AIDS), it has been estimated that 20% of patients with AIDS-related Kaposi´s sarcoma will have involvement of the genitourinary tract, and in 3% the initial lesion is located on the penis [21, 22]. An overview of common benign, premalignant, carcinoma in situ (CIS), and other malignant penile lesions is listed in Table 3 and shown in Figs. 1–3.

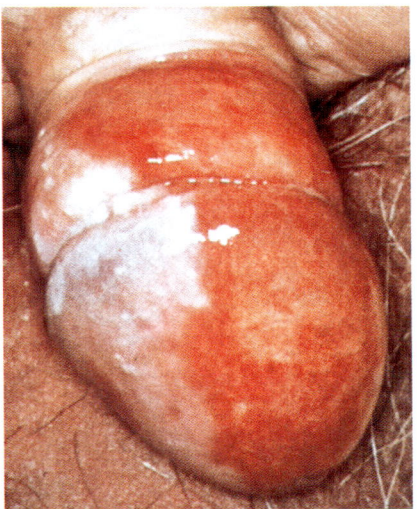 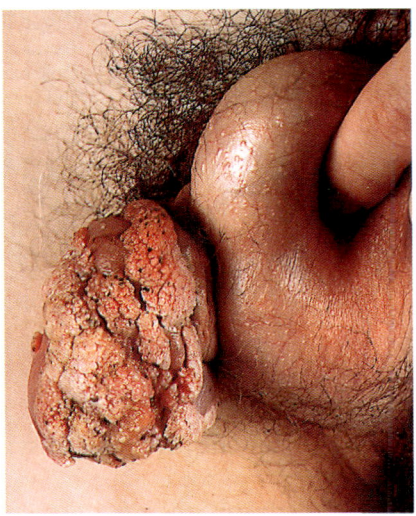

Fig. 1. Chronic balanitis at the glans penis and sulcus coronarius (benign). (From [7])

Fig. 2. Giant condyloma acuminatum of the penis, Buschke-Löwenstein-tumor (premalignant)

Fig. 3. Squamous cell carcinoma of the glans penis (pT1, pNo, Mo, WHO grade I)

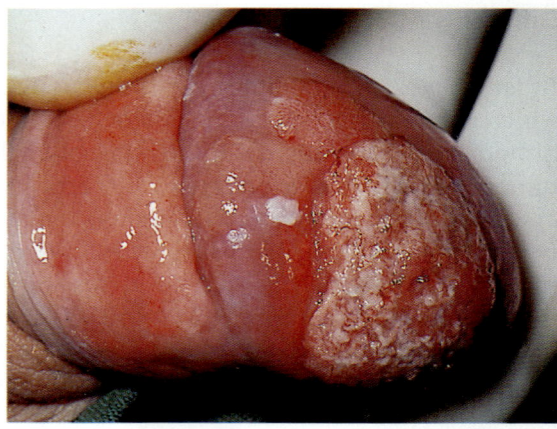

Table 3. Differential diagnosis of penile lesions

Lesion	Status
Angioma, fibroma, myoma	Benign
Condylomata acuminata	Benign
Cutaneous horn	Premalignant
Buschke Löwenstein tumor	Premalignant
Balanitis xerotica obliterans	Premalignant
Leukoplakia	Premalignant
Erythroplasia of Queyrat	CIS
Bowen´s disease	CIS
Kaposi´s sarcoma	Malignant
Malignant melanoma	Malignant

CIS, carcinoma in situ

Diagnosis

The time from the first signs or symptoms to the patient´s presentation in a doctor´s office is usually long. Penile lesions that do not respond to a short trial of conservative treatment require biopsy immediately. No reason appears to justify not doing so.

Examination

Primary Tumor (T).   The assessment of the primary tumor should include size and location and whether the tumor involves the corporal bodies. In addition to palpation ultrasonography, cavernosography and/or magnetic resonance imaging (MR) of the penis may be helpful [23–25]. Identifying carcinoma of the penis, knowledge about histologic grade, and depth of invasion is mandatory before initiation of any therapy.

Lymph Nodes (N).   As the prognosis depends on the degree of lymphatic spread, both groins have to be palpated for inguinal lymphadenopathy. Palpable inguinal lymph nodes are common at the time of presentation in men with penile cancer. Differentiation between inflammatory lymphadenopathy secondary to infection or metastatic involvement cannot be made by palpation. Lymph node biopsy or inguinal lymphadenectomy is recommended, because computed tomography (CT) and MRI of the small pelvis and/or pedal lymphangiography have poor diagnostic value. Because of the failure of noninvasive techniques to evaluate the inguinal lymph nodes, alternatives such as "sentinal node" biopsy [26], aspiration biopsy [27], or "modified lymphadenectomy" [28] have been reported.

Distant Metastases (M).   Distant metastases may be excluded by chest radiography, CT, or MRI and bone scan together with the physical examination.

Tumor Marker – Squamous Cell Carcinoma Antigen.   Squamous cell carcinoma antigen is a recommended marker for the carcinoma of the cervix [29, 30]. More than 90% of penile cancers are squamous cell carcinomas. The squamous cell carcinoma antigen, with a specificity of 95% and sensitivity of about 70–80%, correlates with the tumor volume, stage, and metastases. The marker decreases under therapy, and an increasing marker profile has been reported under progress and/or relapse [31, 32]. Squamous cell carcinoma antigen could be a useful tumor marker for the follow-up of men with squamous cell carcinoma of the penis.

Biopsy.   An initial biopsy is mandatory for histological confirmation of penile cancer. Biopsy can be performed as a separate procedure or as frozen section prior to a planned excisional operation.

Classification

TNM Classification

The two main classifications for staging SCC are the Jackson classification [33] and the UICC-TNM [34]. The Jackson system was used as a retrospective classification, based on the findings at surgery and therefore with a limited clinical use. The new TNM classification is the more useful system, as it classifies the primary lesion according to whether the corpora are invaded or not, which correlates best with the presence or absence of inguinal lymph node metastases, and a differentiation is made whether single or multiple nodes are involved. The TNM classification should be used to make all future publications and studies comparable (Table 4).

Table 4.   Penile cancer, TNM classification (1993)

T0	No evidence of primary tumor
Tis	Carcinoma in situ (CIS)
Ta	Non invasive verrucous carcinoma
T1	Tumor infiltration of subepithelial soft tissue layers
T2	Tumor infiltration of the corpora cavernosa or spongiosa
T3	Tumor infiltration of the urethra
T4	Tumor invading adjacent structures
N0	No evidence of regional node involvement
N1	Involvement of a single superficial inguinal node
N2	Involvement of multiple unilateral or bilateral superficial nodes
N3	Involvement of the deep inguinal or pelvic nodes
M0	No evidence of distant metastases
M1	Distant metastases present

Therapy of the Primary Lesion in Carcinoma of the Penis

Tis, Ta, T1 Tumors

Organ-Preserving Surgical Therapy.   Surgical therapy of SCC of the penis is strictly stage related, and we recommend organ preservation for Tis, Ta, and T1 tumors. Circumcision, local excision, or Nd:YAG/CO_2 laser coagulation after tumor excision are the treatment modalities of choice. Stage Ta or CIS tumor, located at the distal prepuce, can be cured by circumcision alone if the surgeon ensures a wide safety margin (2 cm) free of tumor [35–37]. Proximal preputial tumors have a higher incidence of local recurrence after circumcision so the patient has to be followed very closely [4, 38]. An indication for Nd:YAG laser coagulation is superficial penile carcinoma of the prepuce or glans penis stage Tis, Ta, and T1 [39–41]. Rothenberger and Hofstetter reported a 7-year disease-specific survival rate of 95% ($n = 23$) [42]. Three of four men had a local recurrence and were successfully treated with a second laser coagulation; partial penectomy was performed in one of the four patients [42]. For the sake of completeness, mention should be made of Mohs micrographic surgery, an alternative for organ-preserving surgical therapy of penile cancer [43]. The author reported a 5-year disease-specific survival rate of 86% in stage I and 62% in stage II, respectively (Jackson classification) [44].

Organ-Preserving Nonsurgical Therapy.   Organ preservation can also be achieved by radiation therapy of superficial penile cancer. Gebraulet and Lambin reported 109 men who were treated with interstitial brachytherapy with iridium-192; the 5- and 10-year disease-specific survival rate was 74% and 52%, respectively [45]. With regard to surgery of the primary lesion alone, radiation therapy has an increased incidence of side effects and/or complications, such as urethral/meatal strictures, superficial skin necrosis, and/or deep penile necrosis, which are sometimes hard to differentiate from relapse or local recurrence [46, 47]. Because recurrence may develop years after radiation therapy, close follow-up is important. Local recurrence in the penis has to be treated by partial or total penectomy.

Partial and Total Penectomy – T2, T3/4 Tumors

T2 carcinomas of the penis involving the glans or distal shaft should be treated with partial penectomy excising 2 cm of normal, histologically proven tissue proximal to the margin of the tumor. A stump 2–3 cm in length is needed to allow directable micturition in an upright position and some coital function as well. If the penile stump appears too short (< 2 cm), we recommend a total penectomy. To avoid total penectomy, augmentation of the phallic length is reported by dividing the suspensory ligament of the penis and mobilizing lateral skin flaps to the prepubic area [48]. T2 carcinomas of the proximal shaft are better treated by total penectomy to ensure a tumor-free margin of at least 2 cm. Penile cancers > T2 have to be treated by total penectomy. A perineal urethrostomy allows micturition in a sitting position.

Management of Regional Lymph Nodes

Penile cancer metastasizes primarily to the inguinal lymph nodes. The prepuce and skin of the penis drain into the superficial nodes located medial to the femoral vein. A bilateral involvement due to the superficial lymphatics decussate has been reported [49–51]. The corpora and glans drain into the deep inguinal and/or iliac nodes. The management and cure of patients with penile cancer depend on the tumor stage, grade, and an accurate knowledge of the regional node status, but the optimal evaluation or management of ilioinguinal lymph nodes is still controversial. Controversy exists, for example, about whether we can predict the likelihood of lymph node metastases from the clinical presentation, stage, or tumor grade. On the other hand, discussion is ongoing on whether staging-lymphadenectomy for men with nonpalpable lymph nodes should be recommended or whether early versus delayed lymphadenectomy should be performed in men with palpable lymph nodes.

Palpable inguinal nodes are common at the time of presentation (26–64% of patients) [4, 52–54], but palpable nodes are not metastatic in 40% (false positive), and normal nodes can contain metastases in 10–15% (false negative) [37]. Unilateral palpable lymph nodes are more likely positive than bilateral palpable nodes, which are enlarged secondary to infection rather than metastatic involvement.

The best guide to the likelihood of inguinal lymph node involvement is the clinical stage of the primary tumor: superficially invasive tumors or tumors confined to the glans penis have a mean incidence of 9% (range, 4%–42); men with tumours invading the corpus cavernosum or extending to the shaft have a mean incidence of 47% (range, 21%–66%) [4, 38, 51, 52, 55, 56]. The differentiation of tumor grade might also be very helpful in evaluating the likelihood of nodal metastases: in patients with well-differentiated primary tumors, the mean incidence of nodal metastases is only 14%, with moderately differentiated tumors 72%, and with poorly differentiated tumors 96% [51, 52].

When both stage and grade are combined, it is understandable that patients with well-differentiated T1 tumors rarely have metastases compared to men with poorly differentiated tumors greater than stage T1. Horenblas et al. [57] evaluated the various prognostic factors of survival in 118 patients with SCC and reported a statistical significance between T category, N category, and grade of differentiation: the 5-year disease-specific survival rates for stages T1, T2, and T3 disease were 94%, 59%, and 52%, respectively. The 5-year disease-specific survival rates according to the N category were 93%, 57%, 50%, and 17% for stages N0, N1, N2, and N3, respectively. WHO grade III carcinomas showed a significant difference in 5-year survival compared to WHO grade I tumors (47% and 79%, respectively). There was no significance between WHO grades II and III.

Clinically Nonpalpable Lymph Nodes

Nonpalpable ilioinguinal lymph nodes may contain metastases in up to 15%. The available methods to detect the true node status are completely inaccurate. Cabanas [26] proposed the "sentinel node biopsy," because he observed by lymphangiograms that penile carcinomas drain first into the "sentinel node" located near the junction of the superficial epigastric and greater saphenous vein (Fig. 4). But there are reports of later development of inguinal metastases in patients with negative bilateral sentinel node biopsies [38,58,59]. Pettaway et al. [60] observed that 25% of their patients had inguinal metastases after negative sentinel biospy, and because of this high false-negative rate sentinel node biopsy is of no use for staging penile cancer and cannot longer be recommended.

But what is the best management of men with invasive penile cancer and clinically negative inguinal nodes? The fact is that watchful management of these patients until metastases are present leads to a poor outcome and that survival is dependent on the extent of inguinal metastases.

Therefore, discovery of lymph node metastases at the earliest moment is advantageous, and the option of staging versus delayed lymph node dissection (LND) for patients with clinically negative nodes has to be discussed. Staging ilioinguinal LND is performed at the initial surgery of the primary tumor or within 4–6 weeks postoperatively. Delayed LND is defined as dissection of secondary palpable, suspect groin adenopa-

Fig. 4. Sentinel lymph node in the groin: located lateromedial to the junction of the vena epigastrica superficialis *(V.e.s)*, vena saphena magna *(V.s.m.)*, and vena saphena accessoria *(V.s.a.)* (From [7])

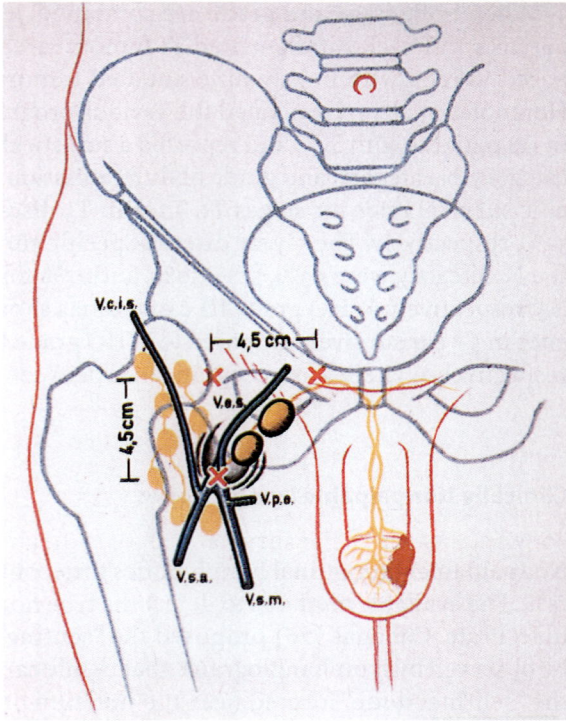

thy. Justification of early LND is based on several reports about a better survival rate compared to the delayed LND: 5-year survival rates of 57%–100% among men with invasive cancer and nonpalpable lymph nodes undergoing early LND versus 8%–24% for those after delayed LND [3, 38, 51, 61]. The rationale for delayed LND is associated with a significant morbidity after bilateral groin dissection [38, 51, 63]. Ravi [63] reported 231 inguinal and 174 ilioinguinal LND on 234 patients with penile carcinoma. The morbidity of inguinal LND included wound infection in 18%, skin edge necrosis in 61%, and seroma formation in 5%. The morbidity of ilioinguinal LND included wound infection in 14%, skin edge necrosis in 64%, and seroma formation in 29%. The routine use of a myocutaneous flap for primary reconstruction of the groin following ilioinguinal LND resulted a 100% primary wound healing and decreased postoperative morbidity. Alternatively, we recommend the use of an omentum majus flap to cover the groin before skin closure.

Clinically Palpable Lymph Nodes

Palpable nodes are common at the time of presentation. Differentiation between metastatic spread or inflammatory reactions cannot be made clinically. A short trial of antibiotic therapy is recommended. Doubtful inguinal nodes are to be reevaluated 4–6 weeks after treatment of the primary tumor with adequate antimicrobial therapy. If nodes persist and are still palpable or suspected, early inguinal LND is indicated on the most likely site.

Positive Lymph Nodes

Regardless of whether early or delayed LND is performed, the presence of positive nodes is a poor prognostic indicator. When the deep inguinal nodes are affected, the survival is poor. When the pelvic nodes are involved, the results are fatal [3, 8, 38, 51, 54, 55, 64].

Ideal Indications for Lymph Nodes Dissection

Horenblas et al. [65] found a clear relationship among T category, grade, and the probability of node invasion. Patients with T1–2 WHO GI–II presented significantly less often with lymphatic invasion. In these cases, the authors recommended surveillance of the regional lymph nodes in patients who present with unsuspected lymph nodes. Patients with stage T2 WHO GIII, stage T3, or operable T4 tumors should undergo staging LND because of a high probability of clinically occult lymph node invasion. Further, they recommended contralateral/and pelvic node dissection when two or more positive lymph nodes were found in the dissected groin specimen. Primary pelvic node dissection should be performed in men who present initially with biopsy-proven positive inguinal nodes.

Abi-Aad and deKernion [66] defined their indications for LND as follows: patients with SCC of the penis not invading into the corpora and clinically nonsuspect lymph nodes should be followed very carefully at 2- to 3-month intervals after surgery of the primary tumor. Patients with persistent node enlargement after tumor control and antibiotic therapy should undergo early LND first, and if positive nodes are found, bilateral deep dissection should be performed. Bilateral LND (inguinal and pelvic) is recommended in patients with penile cancer invading the corpora with clinically negative or positive nodes.

In a retrospective study of 64 patients with infiltrating penile cancer, treated with partial or total penectomy, we evaluated the advantage or disadvantage of LND, divided into early or delayed dissection: 33 patients were treated without LND, early LND was performed 16 times, and delayed LND 15 times. In the group without LND, no evidence of diseases (NED) was observed in 30% of the patients and death from disease (DOD) in 40% (follow-up, 155 months). A total of 31 patients were treated with LND, and NED was observed in 30% and DOD in 61% (follow-up, 88 months). In early ($n = 16$) and delayed ($n = 15$) LND, we observed NED in 31% and DOD in 56% in the early group and NED in 27% and DOD in 67% in the delayed group. In summary, we found that positive lymph nodes during LND are prognostic of a fatal outcome and that there was no therapeutic advantage of early LND.

In conclusion, it should be noted that there is no unique treatment protocol for the management of lymph node involvement in patients with SCC of the penis. Each study group recommends its own treatment, based on retrospective studies and follow-up. If different staging systems are used (TNM vs. Jackson), the results cannot be compared.

At our department, we recommend the following indications: according to the literature, the 5-year disease-specific survival rate of patients with Tis, T1 WHO GI carcinomas with clinically nonpalpable lymph nodes is up to 100% after primary surgery [51, 65]; we recommend watchful waiting and close follow-up in these patients. Staging bilateral LND should be performed in penile cancer stage T1–T4 WHO II–III with nonpalpable lymph nodes. If clinically positive lymph nodes are still palpable at the time of presentation after antibiotic therapy and in relation to the extent of lymph node involvement, the advantage of LND is poor for curative intent. The indication for dissection should be discussed strongly, considering the high morbidity and poor benefit of the LND in disseminated penile cancer.

Role of Chemotherapy in Penile Cancer

The value of chemotherapy is still uncertain. Good results under curative intent were only reported concerning therapy of CIS with 5-fluorouracil [67]. Partial remission with some reproducible results were reported with cisplatin in combination with 5-fluorouracil, methotrexate, and bleomycin in patients with penile cancer and lymph node metastases [67–69]. A neoadjuvant (inductive) polychemotherapy with vincristin, bleomycin, and methotrexate was reported by Pizzocarro et al. [70] for patients with large, fixed inguinal lymph node involvement. Prior to surgery, a complete remission of inguinal lymph node involvement was achieved in eight out of 11 patients. After salvage LND, four out of eight patients were NED up to 2–6 years.

New Treatment Options

According to the medical therapy of patients with squamous carcinoma of the skin, the combination with interferon alpha 2a and retinoid (vitamin A derivate) could be a possible way to treat patients with SCC of the penis in future [71, 72]. Because of the higher prevalence of human papillomavirus DNA in patients with SCC of the penis, Mitropoulos et al. [73] reported their organ preserving investigation in which they treated patients with noninvasive penile carcinoma primarily with a combination of interferon alpha 2b and cisplatin. They observed that this primary treatment combination induced responses in 75% of their patients. A larger number of patients and a longer follow-up will be required for both studies to confirm these preliminary results.

Quality of Life

Surgical treatment of SCC of the penis is associated with a high degree of psychological trauma. The cosmetic results and the loss of sexual activity are reasons to refuse therapy for some patients. Opjordsmoen and Fossa [74] evaluated the long-term psychological well-being of patients after successful physical treatment for penile cancer. Seven of 30 men (23%) reported that, if asked again, they would choose treatment with a lower long-term survival to increase the chance of remaining sexually potent. The authors concluded that, before treatment of penile cancer, the physician should discuss the expected outcome and consequences of the different treatment options with the patient and that psychological treatment might be helpful in certain cases.

References

1. Persky L (1977) Epidemiology of cancer of the penis. Recent Results Cancer Res 60: 97–109
2. Paymaster JC, Gangadharan P (1967) Cancer of the penis in India. J Urol 97: 110–113
3. Ornellas AA, Seixas AL, Marota A (1994) Surgical treatment of invasive squamous cell carcinoma of the penis: retrospective analysis of 350 cases. J Urol 151: 1244–1249
4. Narayana AS, Olney LE, Loening SA (1982) Carcinoma of the penis: analysis of 219 cases. Cancer 49: 2185–2187
5. Hellberg GJ, Valentin J, Eklund T, Nilsson St (1987) Penile cancer: is there an epidemiological role for smoking and sexual behaviour? Br Med J 295: 1306–1308
6. Buddington WT, Kickham CJE, Smith WE (1963) An assessment of malignant disease of the penis. J Urol 89: 442–445
7. Brühl P (1987) Das Peniskarzinom. Urologe B 27: 3–7
8. Fraley EE, Zhang G, Sazama R (1985) Cancer of the penis: prognosis and treatment plans. Cancer 55: 1618–1620
9. Peterson RO (1986) Penis. In: Lippincott JB (ed) Urologic pathology. Saunders, Philadelphia, p 691
10. Gissmann L, DeVilliers EM, Hausen H (1982) Analysis of human genital warts (condylomata acuminata) and other genital tumors for human papilloma virus type 6 DNA. Int J Cancer 29: 143–146
11. Gissmann L, Wolnik L, Ikenberg H, Koldovsky U, Schnürich HG, Hausen H (1983) Human papilloma virus types 6 and 11 sequences in genital and laryngeal papillomas and some cervical cancers. Proc Natl Acad Sct USA 80: 560–563
12. Ikenberg H, Gissmann L, Gross G, Grussendorf-Cohnen EI, Hausen H (1983) Human Papilloma virus type 16 related DNA in genital Bowen's disease and in Bowenoid papulosis. Int J Cancer 32: 563–565
13. McCane DJ, Kalache A, Ashdown K, Andrade L, Menezes F, Smith P, Doll R (1986) Human papilloma viruses types 16 and 18 in carcinoma of the penis from Brazil. Int J Cancer 37: 55–59
14. Strohmeyer T (1993) Das Peniskarzinom: ätiologische Bedeutung der Papillomviren. Hautarzt 44: 113–134

15. Cupp MR, Malek RS, Goellner JR, Smith TF, Espy MJ (1995) The detection of human papillomvirus desoxyribonucleic acid in intraepithelial, in situ, verrucous and invasive carcinoma of the penis. J Urol 154 (3): 1024–1029

16. Barasso R, de Brux J, Croissant O (1987) High prevalence of papillomvirus-associated penile intraepithelial neoplasia in sexual partners of women with cervical intraepithelial neoplasia. N Engl J Med 317: 916–918

17. Stern RS and Members of the Photochemotherapy Follow up Study (1990) Genital tumors among men with psoriasis exposed to psoralens and ultraviolet A radiation (PUVA) and ultraviolet B radiation. N Engl J Med 322: 1093–1096

18. Burgers JK, Badalement RA, Drago JS (1992) Penile cancer: clinical presentaticn, diagnosis and staging. Urol Clin North Am 19: 247–256

19. Maiche AG, Pyrhönen S (1990) Clinical staging of cancer of the penis: by size, by location or depth of infiltration. Eur Urol 18: 16–22

20. Chesney TM, Murphy WM (1989) Diseases of the penis and scrotum. In: Murphy WM (ed) Urologic pathology. Saunders, Philadelphia, p 392

21. Casado M, Jimenez F, Borbujo J (1988) Spontaneous healing of Kaposi's angiosarcoma of the penis. J Urol 139: 1313–1314

22. Lowe FC, Lattimer DG, Metroka CE (1989) Kaposi's sarcoma of the penis in patients with acquired immundeficiency syndrome. J Urol 142: 1475–1478

23. Vapnek JM, Hricak H, Caroll PR (1992) Recent advances in imaging studies for staging of penile and urethral carcinoma. Urol Clin N Am 19: 257–266

24. Raghavaiah NV (1978) Corpus cavernosogram in the evaluation of carcinoma of the penis. J Urol 120: 423–425

25. Horenblas S, Kröger R, Gallee MPW, Newling DWW, van Tinteren H (1994) Ultrasound in squamous cell carcinoma of the penis: a useful addition to clinical staging? Urology 43: 702–707

26. Cabanas RM (1977) An approach for treatment of penile carcinoma. Cancer 39: 456–466

27. Luciani L, Piscioli F, Scappini P, Pusiol T (1984) Value and role of percutaneous regional node aspiration cytology in the management of penile cancer. Eur Urol 10: 294–302

28. Catalona WJ (1988) Modified inguinal lymphadenectomy for carcinoma of the penis with preservation of saphenous veins: technique and preliminary results. J Urol 140: 306–309

29. Kato HT, Torigoe T (1977) Radioimmunassay for tumor antigen of human cervical squamous cell carcinoma. Cancer 40: 1621–1628

30. Meier W, Eiermann W, Stieber P, Fateh-Moghadam A, Hepp H (1989) Erfahrungen mit dem SCC Antigen, einem neuen Tumormarker für Karzinome der Cervix uteri. Geburtsh Frauenheilk 49: 625–629

31. Wishonow KI, Johnson DE, Fritsche H (1990) Squamous cell carcinoma antigen (TA-4) in penile carcinoma. Urology 36/4: 315–317

32. Wiese M, Jansen D, Schlichter A (1995) unpublished data

33. Jackson SM (1966) The treatment of carcinoma of the penis. Br J Surg 53: 33–35

34. International Union Against Cancer (1993) TNM-Atlas, 3rd edn. Springer, Berlin Heidelberg New York, pp 234–240

35. Bissada NK (1992) Conservative exstirpative treatment of carcinoma of the penis. Urol Clin North Am 19: 283–290

36. Brühl P (1992) Penistumoren. In: Krück F, Kaufmann W (eds) Therapiehandbuch. Urban and Schwarzenberg, Munich, pp 1–4
37. deKernion JB, Tynberg P, Pesky L, Fegen JP (1973) Carcinoma of the penis. Cancer 32: 1256–1262
38. McDougal WS, Kirchner FK jr, Edwards RH, Killon LT (1986) Treatment of carcinoma of the penis: the case of primary lymphadenectomy. J Urol 136: 38–41
39. Kriegmaier M, Rothenberger KH, Spitzenpfeil E, Schmeller N, Hofstetter A (1990) Neodymium-YAG laser treatment for carcinoma of the penis. J Urol 143: 351A
40. Schoeneich G, Vogel J, Miersch WD (1993) Carcinoma of the penis: the possibility of organ preservation by ND: YAG laser treatment. Onkology 16: 94–99
41. Malloy JJ, Wein AJ, Carpinielo VL (1988) Carcinoma of the penis treated with neodymium YAG-laser. Urology 31: 25–29
42. Rothenberger KH, Hofstetter A (1994) Lasertherapie des Peniskarzinoms. Urologe A 33: 291–294
43. Mohs FE, Snow SN, Messing EM, Kulgitsch ME (1985) Microscopically controlled surgery in the treatment of carcinoma of the penis. J Urol 133: 961–966
44. Mohs FE, Snow SN, Larson PO (1992) Mohs micrographic surgery for penile tumors. Urol Clin North Am 19: 291–304
45. Gebraulet A, Lambin P (1992) Radiation therapy of cancer of the penis: indications, advantages and pitfalls. Urol Clin North Am 19: 325–332
46. Haile K, Delclos L (1980) The place of radiation therapy in the treatment of carcinoma of the distal end of the penis. Cancer 45: 1980–1984
47. Salaverria JC, Hope-Stone HF, Paris MD (1979) Conservative treatment of carcinoma of the penis. Br J Urol 52: 32–35
48. Das S (1992) Penile amputations for the management of primary carcinoma of the penis. Urol Clin North Am 19: 277–482
49. Daseler GH, Anson BH, Reiman AF (1948) Radical excision of the inguinal and iliac lymph glands: a study based upon 450 anatomical dissections and supportive clinical observations. Surg Gynecol Obstet 87: 679–684
50. Dewire D, Lepor H (1992) Anatomic considerations of the penis and its lymphatic drainage. Urol Clin North Am 19: 211–219
51. Fraley EE, Zhang G, Manivel C, Niehans G (1989) The role of ilioinguinal lymphadenectomy and significance of histological differentiation in treatment of carcinoma of the penis. J Urol 142: 1478–1482
52. Solsona E, Oborra I, Ricos JV (1992) Corpus cavernosum invasion and tumor grade in the prediction of lymph node condition in penile carcinoma. Eur Urol 22: 115–118
53. Horenblas S, van Tinteren H, Delemarre JFM (1991) Squamous cell carcinoma of the penis: accuracy of tumor, nodes and metastases classification system, and role of lymphography, computerized tomography scan and fine needle aspiration cytology. J Urol 146: 1279–1283
54. Srinivas V, Morse MF, Herr HW (1987) Penile cancer: relation of extent of nodal metastases to survival. J Urol 137: 880–882
55. Young MJ, Reda DJ, Waters WB (1991) Penile carcinoma: a twenty-five-year experience. Urology 38: 528–532
56. Pettaway CA, Stewart D, Vuitch F (1991) Penile squamous carcinoma: DNA flow cytometry versus histopathology for prognosis. J Urol 145: 367A (abstr 618)

57. Horenblas S, van Tinteren H (1994) Squamous cell carcinoma of the penis: IV. Prognostic factors of survival: analysis of tumor, nodes and metastases classification system. J Urol 151: 1239–1243
58. Perinetti E, Crane DB, Catalona WJ (1980) Unreliability of sentinel lymph node biopsy for staging penile cancer. J Urol 124: 734–736
59. Wespes E, Simon J, Schulman CC (1989) Cabanas approach: Is sentinel node biopsy reliable for staging penile carcinoma? Urology 28: 279–282
60. Pettaway CA, Pisters LL, Dinney CPN, Jularbal FE, Swanson DA, von Eschenbach AC, Ayala A (1995) Sentinel lymph node dissection for penile carcinoma: the M.D. Anderson cancer center experience. J Urol 154: 1999–2003
61. Johnson DE, Lo RK (1984) Management of regional lymph nodes in penile carcinoma. Five-year results following therapeutic groin dissection. Urology 24: 308–311
62. Ornellas AA, Seixas ALC, de Moraes JR (1991) Analysis of 200 lymphadenectomies in patients with penile carcinoma. J Urol 146: 330–332
63. Ravi R (1993) Morbidity following groin dissection for penile carcinoma. Br J Urol 72: 941–945
64. Ravi R (1993) Correlation between the extent of nodal involvement and survival following groin dissection for carcinoma of the penis. Br J Urol 72: 817–819
65. Horenblas S, van Tinteren H, Delemare JF, Moonen LM, Lustig V, van Waardenburg EW (1993) Squamous cell carcinoma of the penis. III. Treatment of regional lymph nodes. J Urol 149: 492–497
66. Abi-Aad AS, deKernion JB (1992) Controversies in ilioinguinal lymphadenectomy for cancer of the penis. Urol Clin North Am 19: 319–324
67. Roth St, Rathert P (1990) Chemotherapie des Peniskarzinoms. Urologe A 30: 10–16
68. Kattan J, Culine S, Droz JP, Fadel E, Court B. Perrin JL, Wibault P, Haie-Meder C (1993) Penile cancer chemotherapy: 12-years' experience at Institut Gustave-Roussy. Urology 42: 559–562
69. Eisenberger MA (1992) Chemotherapy of carcinoma of the penis and urethra. Urol Clin North Am 19: 333–338
70. Pizzocarro G, Piva L (1992) Primary chemotherapy and surgery for fixed inguinal metastases from squamous cell carcinoma of the penis. J Urol 147: 369A
71. Ubrig B, Roth ST (1995) Peniskarzinom – Neues zu Ätiologie, Prognose und Therapie. Akt Urol 26: 281–389
72. Lippmann SM, Parkinson DR, Itri LM, Weber RS, Schantz StP, Ota DM (1992) 13-cis retinoic acid and interferon alpha-2a: effective combination therapy for advanced squamous cell carcinoma of the skin. J Nat Cancer Inst 84: 235–241
73. Mitropoulos D, Dimopoulos MA, Kiroudi-Voulgari A, Zervas A, Dimopoulos C, Logothetis CF (1994) Neoadjuvant cisplatin and interferon-alpha 2B in the treatment and organ preservation of penile carcinoma. J Urol 152: 1124–1126
74. Opjordsmoen S, Fossa SD (1994) Quality of life in patients treated for penile cancer. A follow up study. Br J Urol 74: 652–657

The Management of Peyronie´s Disease

John P. Pryor

The Management of Peyronie´s Disease

In 1743 Francois de la Peyronie successfully treated patients with induratio penis plastica with the waters of Barrage. He was not the first to describe the condition, Vesalius and Fallopius had both treated the same patient in the 16th Century, but his treatment was more successful than any subsequent reports.

The aetiology and pathophysiology of the condition are ill understood but it is characterised by a plaque of fibrous tissue that is inevitably present when the patient is first seen. The symptoms are variable and usually consist of penile discomfort and deformity on erection. Many patients require no more than reassurance that the problem is not due to malignancy and that the condition is no more than a nuisance that interferes with sexual activity. Medical treatment should be tried in the first instance and surgery is reserved for those patients in whom the disease process has stabilized – usually after one year.

In this review I will concern myself with current management options and will be particularly concerned with the changes that have occurred during the past ten years.

Conservative Management

New Options for Conservative Treatment

The early stages of Peyronie´s disease are characterized by an acute inflammatory reaction in the sub tunical region which leads to collagen formation [1]. This process is reversible in the early stages but in other patients it may lead to the formation of mature fibrous tissue, sometimes with calcification and ossification. The inflammatory excidate consists of T lymphocytes and macrophages which activate the cytokine network to initiate fibrogenesis. The release of cytokine transforming growth factor β (TGF-β) from platelets and activated macrophages has been shown to be important in regulating the inflammatory immune responses and tissue repair [2]. A high concentration of TGF-β causes macrophage deactivation and T lymphocyte suppression, thus decreasing the inflammatory response and reducing fibrogenesis.

Tamoxifen has been shown to increase the secretion of TGF-β from human fibroblasts in vitro and it should inhibit the inflammatory response [3]. It has also been used in the treatment of desmoid tumours [4, 5]. It was therefore used in Peyronie's disease with encouraging results [6]. Thirty-six men were treated with tamoxifen, 20 mg twice daily for 3 months. There was some improvement in 20 (55%) of the 36 patients and there was no deterioration in any patient. There was a significantly greater improvement with patients in the earlier stages of the disease (i.e. less than 4 months since the onset). A small biopsy was taken from the plaque in 12 men with painful Peyronie's disease. An excellent response to tamoxifen was found in 6 of the 8 men in whom an acute inflammatory infiltrate was observed but no improvement occurred in those without an inflammatory response. It is desirable to conduct a double-blind trial to further assess the benefits of tamoxifen but this has not proved to be possible. At the present time I think that it is worthwhile trying tamoxifen for 6 weeks in any patient with painful Peyronie's disease.

Colchicine may decrease collagen synthesis and induce collagenase and was found to be useful in fibromatosis [7]. In a series of 24 men with Peyronie's disease, it was found to produce an improvement in plaque size in 12 and an improvement in pain in 7 of the 9 patients where it was present [8]. Gelbert et al. [9] injected **collagenase** directly into the Peyronie's plaque and in a prospective double-blind randomised controlled trial in 49 men, found a significant benefit over placebo ($P \leq 0.007$). However there was little improvement in the erectile deformity and the better results were obtained in those with lesser degrees of bend. Levine et al. [10] injected the **calcium channel blocking agent verapamil** into the plaque-calcium channel blockers alter the metabolism of fibroblasts to inhibit collagen formation. In a study of 14 men, 12 completed the six month course of treatment and the pain improved in 10 of the 11 men in whom it was present and the deformity improved in 5 (42%). The improvement in pain always has to be observed against the natural history of the disease.

Duncan et al. [11] showed that **interferons** α, β **and** γ are all capable during in vitro culture of inhibiting fibroblast proliferation and collagen production as well as increasing the production of collagenase by Peyronie's tissue. Benson [12] reported favourable clinical results but in contrast Wegner [13] found an improvement in only 1 of 25 patients.

Existing Options of Conservative Treatment

The new methods of treatment all attempt to interfere with fibroblast activity and might be expected to be useful during the early stages of disease. Their efficacy has to be seen against the natural history of the disease and the knowledge that discomfort on erection rarely persists beyond 6 months. **Vitamin E** is the traditional treatment of choice for Peyronie's disease. It is easy to take, cheap, free of side effects and better than placebo for treating the pain [14]. **Paraminobenzoate (Potaba)** is more expensive, unpleasant to take, has more side effects and needs to be taken for 12 months [15]. This permits the disease to stabilize and patients with persisting symptoms may then be candidates for surgery. Beneficial results of low dosage **radiotherapy** are still being reported [16, 17] but it is probably best avoided in men under the age of 60 years. It has also been reported as the cause of extensive penile fibrosis [18].

Surgical Management of Peyronie's Disease

Plaque Excision and Dermal Graft

The surgical management of Peyronie's disease was unsuccessful until Horton and Devine [19] in the United States and Byström et al. [20] in Scandinavia described the operation of plaque excision and dermal graft replacement of the defect in the tunica albuginea. Byström et al. reported that despite good results the late results were disappointing with only 6 of 17 men having a good result after 10 years [20]. Personal experience

Fig. 1.   The plaque of fibrous tissue extends into the erectile tissue and inevitably its excision is accompanied by some loss of erectile tissue

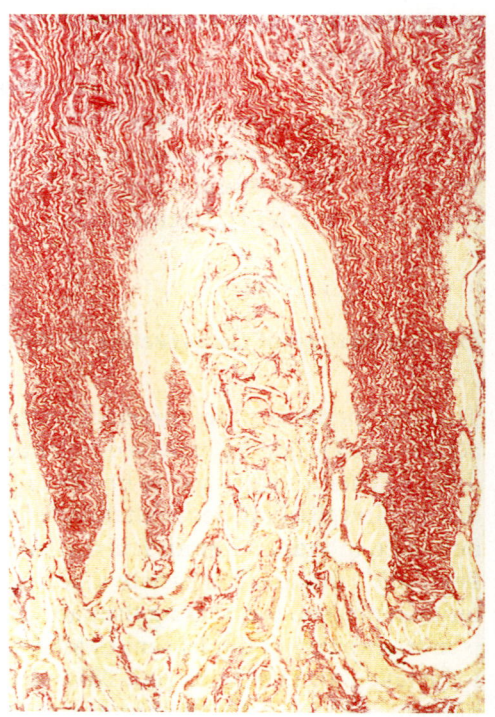

[21] and a subsequent review of the literature [22] confirmed that many patients had poor results with this operation and was the rationale for using the Nesbit procedure in Peyronie´s disease [21].

Austoni [23] has recently reported a large series of 418 men on whom he performed plaque excision and a dermal graft operation. He found that 17% of patients required further surgery for curvature and that 20% of patients had significant impairment of erection. Erectile dysfunction following plaque excision is due to a combination of factors ranging from damage to the underlying erectile tissue adherent to the plaque (Fig. 1), loss of compliance of the dermal graft, new venous channels forming to give veno occlusive dysfunction [24] and a deterioration of the underlying aetiological factors. It is now recognized that the histological changes of Peyronie´s disease are not confined to the plaque but may also be seen in the normal tunica albuginea excised during the Nesbit procedure [25, 26].

The Nesbit Procedure

Reed Nesbit [27] described the correction of erectile deformities due to congenital abnormalities by shortening the opposite side of the penis using plication or the excision of an ellipse of tunica albuginea. The technique has been applied to Peyronie´s disease with success and in 359 men operated upon between 1977 and 1992, 295 (82%) had good results and were able to have intercourse [28]. Operative treatment is only performed when the disease has stabilized – usually at least a year after its onset – and the deformity makes intercourse difficult or impossible.

The operation is usually performed through a circumglandular incision – circumcising the man if necessary in order to prevent a secondary phimosis. An artificial erection is induced by injecting saline from a rapid transfusion apparatus and no tourniquet is used as it sometimes makes for inaccurate assessment of the bend. It is also essential to observe the bend at the time of full erection otherwise the deformity may be underestimated. The site of maximum bend is marked with a stay suture. Buck´s fascia is incised longitudinally (Fig. 2) and dissected medially to bare the tunica albuginea. This technique permits elevation of the corpus spongiosus ventrally, the dorsal vascular bundle and the

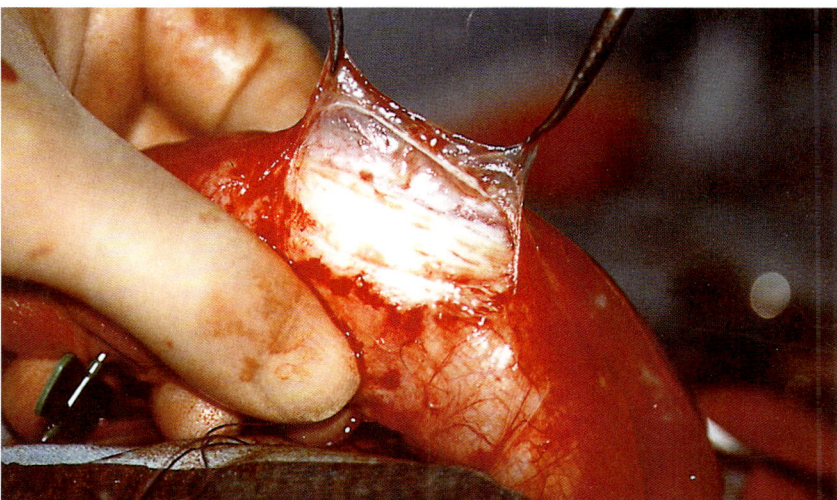

Fig. 2.   Buck´s fascia is incised longitudinally to bare the tunica albuginea. This technique permits elevation of the nerve fibres, corpus spongiosum or dorsal vascular bundle without injury

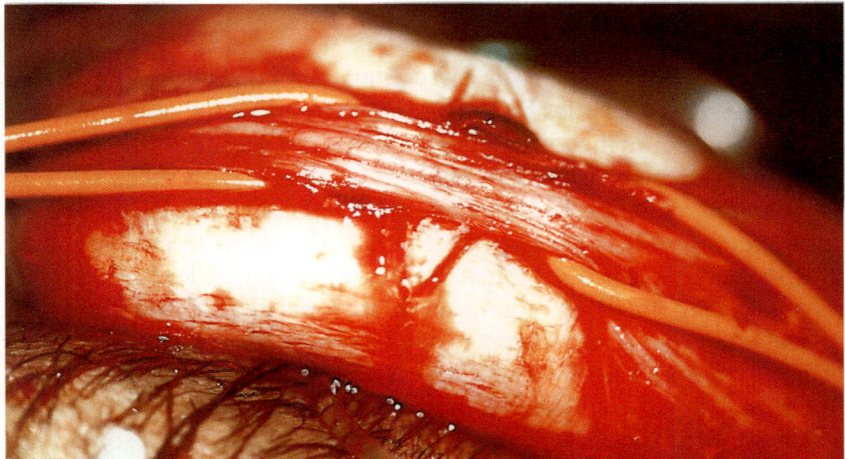

Fig. 3.   The dorsal vascular bundle has been isolated with strings and the Nesbit ellipse outlined with the scalpel

Fig. 4.   Alliss forceps have been applied to the tunica albuginea opposite the stay suture showing the position of maximum deformity. An artificial erection has been induced by an infusion through the butterfly needle and the erection is observed

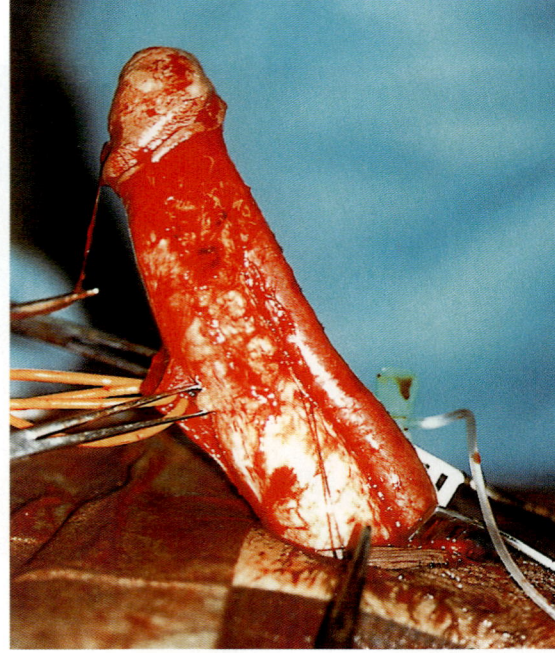

nerves without appreciable damage. The Nesbit ellipse (Fig. 3) is marked out opposite the site of maximum deformity and for every 10° of bend, the ellipse is 1 mm wide. In a retrospective study it was found that the mean width of the ellipse was 7 mm and the angle of deformity was 68°.

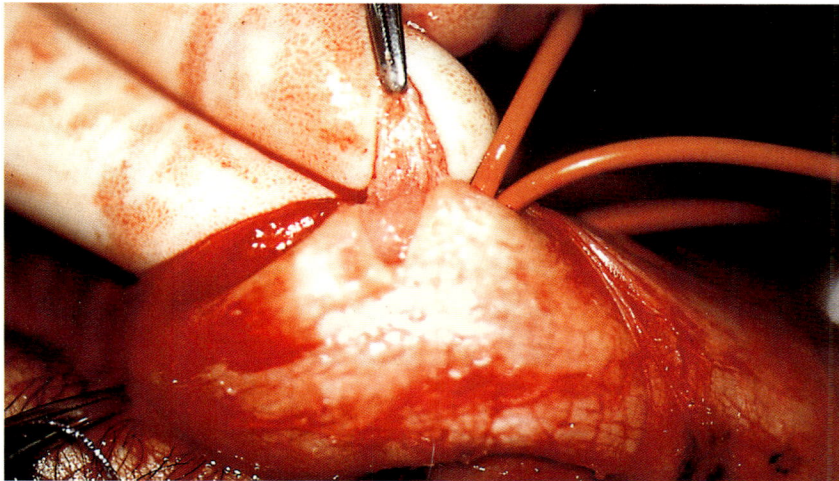

Fig. 5.   The ellipse is excised with little damage to the underlying corpus cavernosus

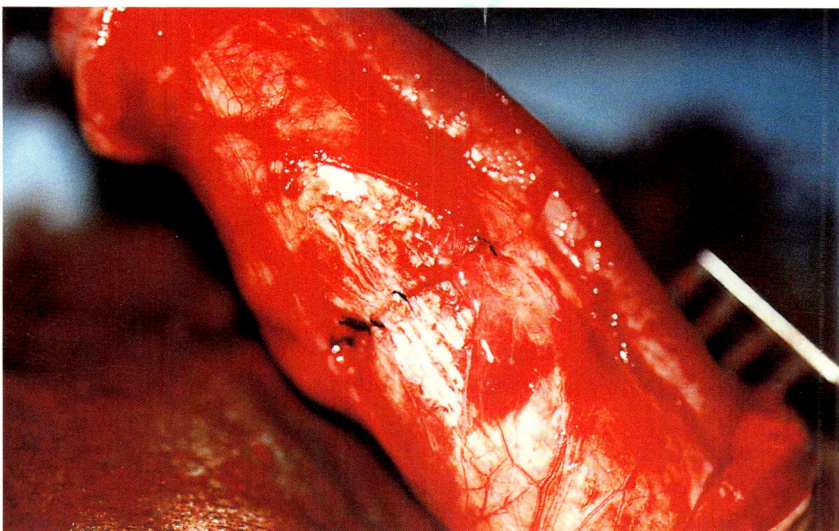

Fig. 6.   Closure of the tunica albuginea

Fig. 7. Artificial erection induced to check that the penis has been straightened

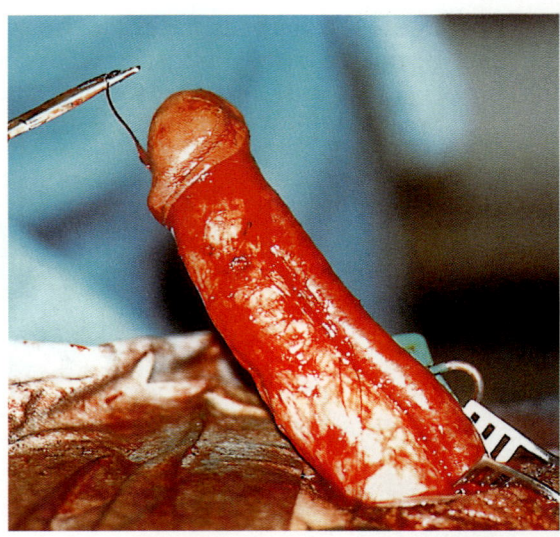

Table 1. Nesbit procedure for Peyronie´s disease

| | 1977 – 1992 | | 1977 – 1984 | | 1985 – 1992 | |
	(*n*)	(%)	(*n*)	(%)	(*n*)	(%)
Number of men	359		174		185	
Excellent result	237	66	101	58	136	73
Satisfactory result	58	16	27	16	31	17
Poor result	64	18	46	26	18	10

When in doubt it is possible to apply two Alliss forceps to the tunica albuginea (when the penis is flaccid) and then inflate the penis to check the correction (Fig. 4). The ellipse is excised (Fig. 5) with minimum disturbance to the underlying muscle of the corpus cavernosus and the defect closed with 0-PDS sutures with the knots on the inside (Fig. 6). Vicryl sutures are a frequent cause for failure of the procedure. Finally an artificial erection is induced to check that the penis has been straightened (Fig. 7).

The overall results of the Nesbit technique are very satisfactory (Table 1). Some of the poor initial results in the period 1977–1983 have been eliminated by preoperative assessment with intracavernous drugs, either alone or combined with colour doppler ultrasound examination

[29]. A literature review confirmed the favourable results [22] as have more recent studies [30, 31].

Alternatives to the Nesbit Procedure

There are a variety of corporoplasties which may be regarded as variants of the Nesbit procedure and these usually give good results [32, 33]. Some authors favour a simple plication technique [34, 35] but the problem with this procedure is that the correction is dependent upon the strength of the suture material and this probably accounts for the unfavourable results of some authors [31] and the late failure in others (as high as 24% in one series [34]).

The alleged drawback of the Nesbit procedure is penile shortening. In Peyronie's disease the penis is shortened by scar tissue and the operation straightens the penis by shortening the unaffected side. In reality the shortening is rarely troublesome and was only more than 2 cm in 17 of 359 men and intercourse was possible in 15 of these [28]. The past five years has seen attempts to lengthen the penis by incising the plaque [36, 37, 38, 39, 40, 41, 42, 43, 44] (Table 2). This is done in the shape of an "I" and the defect should be covered with a substance that does not contract. Dorsal penile, or saphenous, vein would seem to be the simplest but, in the uncircumcised man, the pedicle dermal graft of Krishnamurti [42] is a good alternative. These procedures would seem to have a role to play in those men with an already shortened penis but longer term follow-up is still required.

Table 2. Plaque incision and graft replacement of the tunica albuginea in the surgical treatment of Peyronie's disease

First author	Year	Number of men	Graft technique
Sampaio	1992	7	Dura
Brock	1993	18	Vein
Faerber	1993	9	Dacron
Moriel	1994	10	Vein
Ganabathi	1995	16	Goretex
Gelbert	1995	30	Temporalis fascia
Krishnamurti	1995	17	Pedicled dermal flap
Rigaud	1995	5	Dermal graft
Kim	1995	7	Laser & vein

Implantation of a Penile Prosthesis

Finally, in those older men where there is an appreciable element of vasculogenic impotence it is sensible to implant a penile prosthesis. These have always given excellent results provided that the men have a realistic expectation from the operation. The plaque may cause some narrowing of the corpus cavernosal space but this seldom makes for difficulties. A malleable prosthesis usually corrects the deformity but with an inflatable prosthesis it may be necessary to incise the plaque. Operative moulding of the penis [45] over a prosthesis may look and sound horrible but gives a good result in correcting any deformity.

Conclusion

Many patients require no more than reassurance but in the early stages it is worthwhile trying drugs, such as tamoxifen, which interfere with the laying down of fibrous tissue. Surgery is reserved for those men with a persistent deformity that makes coitus difficult. The Nesbit procedure gives good results but in those men with a short penis it is worth considering plaque incision and inserting a vein graft. A penile prosthesis is inserted when there is a marked vasculogenic deficit.

References

1. Ralph DJ, Mirakian R, Pryor JP, Bottazzo GF (1996) The immunological features of Peyronie´s disease. J Urol 155: 159–162
2. Wahl SM, McCartney-Francis N, Mergenhagen SE (1989) Inflammatory and immunomodulatory roles of TGF-β. Immunol Today 10: 258–261
3. Colletta AA, Wakefield LM, Howell FV et al. (1990) Anti-oestrogens induce the secretion of active transforming growth factor beta from human fetal fibroblasts. Br J Cancer 62: 405–409
4. Kinzbrunner B, Ritter S, Domingo J, Rosenthal CJ (1983) Remission of rapidly growing desmoid tumours after tamoxifen therapy. Cancer 52: 2201–2204
5. Waddel WR, Gerner RE, Reich MP (1983) Nonsteroid antiinflammatory drugs and tamoxifen for desmoid tumours and carcinoma of the stomach. J Surg Oncol 22: 197–211

6. Ralph DJ, Brooks MD, Bottazzo GF, Pryor JP (1992) The treatment of Peyronie's disease with tamoxifen. Br J Urol 70: 648–651
7. Dominguez-Malagon HR, Alfeiran-Ruiz A, Chavanna-Xicotencatl P (1992) Clinical and cellular effects of colchicine in fibromatosis. Cancer 69: 2478–2483
8. Akkus E, Carner S, Rehman J, Breza J, Kadioughu A, Lue TF (1994) Is colchicine effective in Peyronie's disease: a pilot study. Urology 44: 291–295
9. Gelbert MK, Jones K, Raich P, Dovey F (1993) Collagenase versus placebo in the treatment of Peyronie's disease: a double blind study. J Urol 149: 56–58
10. Levine LA, Merrick PF, Lee RC (1994) Intralesional verapamil injection for the treatment of Peyronie's disease. J Urol 151: 1522–1524
11. Duncan MR, Berman B, Nseyo UO (1991) Resolution of the proliferation and biosynthetic activities of cultured human Peyronie's disease fibroblasts by interferon-alpha, -beta and -gamma. Scan J Urol Nephrol 25: 89–94
12. Benson RC Jr, Knoll LD, Furlow WL (1991) Interferon-α2b in the treatment of Peyronie's disease (abstract). J Urol 145 (Suppl): 1342
13. Wegner HEH, Andresen R, Knipsel HH, Miller K (1995) Treatment of Peyronie's disease with local interferon-α2b. Eur Urol 28: 236–240
14. Pryor JP, Farell CF (1983) Controlled clinical trial of Vitamin E in Peyronie's disease. Prog Reprod Biol 9: 41–45
15. Shah PJR, Green NA, Adib RS et al. (1983) A multicentre double-blind controlled clinical trial of potassium paraaminobenzoate (Potaba) in Peyronie's disease. Prog Reprod Biol 9: 47–60
16. Rodrigues CI, Njo KH, Karim AB (1995) Results of radiotherapy and vitamin E in the treatment of Peyronie's disease. Int J Radiat Oncol Biol Phys 31: 571–576
17. Viljoen IM, Goedhals L, Dom MJ (1993) Peyronie's disease: a perspective on the disease and the long term results of radiotherapy. S Af Med J 83: 19–20
18. Hall SJ, Basile G, Bertero EB, Movenas A, Goldstein A (1995) Extensive corporeal fibrosis after penile irradiation. J Urol 153: 372–377
19. Devine CJ, Horton CE (1974) Surgical treatment of Peyronie's disease with a dermal graft. J Urol 111: 44
20. Byström J, Alfthan O, Gustafson H, Johansson B (1972) Early and late results after excision and dermo-fat grafting for Peyronie's disease. Prog Reprod Biol 9:78–84
21. Pryor JP, Fitzpatrick JM (1979) A new approach to the correction of the penile deformity in Peyronie's disease. J Urol 122: 622–623
22. Pryor JP (1987) Peyronie's disease. In: Hendry WF (ed) Recent Advances in Urology, Volume 4. Churchill Livingston, London, pp 245–261
23. Austoni E, Colombo F, Mantovani F, Patelli E, Fenice O (1995) Chirurgia radicale e conservazione dell'erezione nella malattia di La Peyronie. Arch It Urol 67: 359–364
24. Dalkin BL, Carter MF (1991) Venogenic impotence following dermal graft repair for Peyronie's disease. J Urol 146: 849–851
25. Iacono F, Barra S, De Rosa G, Boscaino A, Lotti T (1993) Microstructural disorders of tunica albuginea in patients affected by Peyronie's disease with or without erectile dysfunction. J Urol 150: 1806–1809
26. Anafarta K, Beduk Y, Uluoglu O, Aydas K, Baltaci S (1994) The Significance of histopathological changes of the normal tunica albuginea in Peyronie's disease. Int Urol Nephrol 26: 71–77
27. Nesbit RH (1965) Congenital curvature of the phallus: report of three cases with description of corrective operation. J Urol 93: 230

28. Ralph DJ, Al-Akraa M, Pryor JP (1995) The Nesbit operation for Peyronie's disease: 16-year experience. J Urol 154: 1362–1363
29. Ralph DJ, Hughes T, Lees WR, Pryor JP ((1992) Pre-operative assessment of Peyronie's disease using colour doppler sonography. Br J Urol 69: 629–632
30. Sulaiman MN, Gingell JC (1994) Nesbit's procedure for penile curvature. J Androl Suppl: 545–565
31. Poulsen J, Kirkeby HJ (1995) Treatment of penile curvature – a retrospective study of 175 patients operated upon with plication of the tunica albuginea or with the Nesbit procedure. Br J Urol 75: 370–374
32. Saissine AM, Wespes E, Schulman CC (1994) Modified corporoplasty for penile curvature: 10 years experience. Urology 44: 419–421
33. Yachia D (1990) Modified corporoplasty for the treatment of penile curvature. J Urol 143: 80–82
34. Nooter RI, Bosch JLHR, Schröder FH (1994) Peyronie's disease and penile curvature: long-term results of operative treatment with the plication procedure. Br J Urol 74: 497–500
35. Klevmark B, Andersen M, Schultz A, Talseth T (1994) Congenital and acquired curvature of the penis treated surgically by the tunica albuginea. Br J Urol 74: 501–506
36. Sampaio JS, Passarinho A, Olivera AG et al. (1992) Surgical correction of severe Peyronie's disease without plaque excision. Eur Urol 22: 130–133
37. Brock G, Kadioglu A, Lue TF (1993) Peyronie's disease: a modified treatment. Urol 42: 300–304
38. Faerber GJ, Konnak JW (1993) Results of combined Nesbit penile plication with plaque incision and placement of dacron patch in patients with severe Peyronie's disease. J Urol 149: 1319–1320
39. Moriel EZ, Grinwald A, Rajfer J (1994) Vein grafting of tunical incisions combined with contralateral plication treatment of penile curvature. Urol 43: 697–701
40. Ganabathi K, Dinochowski R, Zimmera PE, Leach GE (1995) Peyronie's disease: surgical treatment based on penile rigidity. J Urol 153: 662–666
41. Gelbert MK (1995) Relaxing incisions in the correction of penile deformity due to Peyronie's disease. J Urol 154: 1457–1460
42. Krishnamurti S (1995) Penile dermal flap for defect reconstruction in Peyronie's disease: operative technique and four years' experience in 17 patients. Int J Impotence Res 7: 195–208
43. Rigaud G, Berger RE (1995) Corrective procedures for penile shortening due to Peyronie's disease. J Urol 153: 368–370
44. Kim ED, McVany KT (1995) Long term follow-up of treatment of Peyronie's disease with plaque incision, carbon dioxide laser plaque ablation and placement of a deep dorsal vein patch graft. J Urol 153: 1543–1546
45. Wilson SK, Delk JR (1994) A new treatment for Peyronie's disease: modelling the penis over an inflatable prosthesis. J Urol 152: 1121–1123

Priapism – New Aetiologic Insights and Medical Consequences

Iñigo Saenz de Tejada

Introduction

Priapism is a pathological state in which the penis is in continuous erection. Priapism may occur at all ages, from the newborn to the elderly and it can even occur in impotent patients. During priapism the erection state is limited to the cavernous bodies, not affecting the corpus spongiosum or the glans [1, 2].

Since the introduction of the intracavernosal injection of vasoactive drugs in the medical practice, the incidence of priapism has increased enormously, passing from being a very rare entity, to be relatively frequent. Veno-occlusive priapism constitutes an urologic emergency, therefore it is important to know the pathophysiology, the diagnosis and the treatment of this entity that, if not identified and treated adequately, can cause complete impotence.

Classification, Aetiology and Pathophysiology

Priapism may be classified in veno-occlusive (ischemic, low-flow) and arterial (non-ischemic, high-flow) (Table 1).

Veno-occlusive Priapism

This is the most common form of priapism and the one that entails a greater potential of causing permanent alteration of erectile function [1]. In veno-occlusive priapism a partial or complete obstruction of corpora cavernosa drainage exists [4, 5]. Once the corporeal bodies are

Table 1.   Classification and features of priapism

	Veno-occlusive	Arterial
Blood flow	low (ischemic)	high (nonischemic)
pathophysiology	Obstruction of corporeal outflow	arterio-lacunar fistula
relative frequency	high	low
Aetiology	Multiple: Vasodilators (I.C.) Psychotropic drugs Antihypertensives Hematologic disturbances	Trauma: perineal or penile
Treatment		
Onset	urgent	deferred
Purpose	increase corporeal outflow	decrease arterial inflow
Method	drainage I.C. vasoconstrictors shunts	selective percutaneous embolisation of bleeding artery

maximally expanded, obstruction to the blood out-flow prevents arterial inflow and, therefore, an ischemic state in the corpora cavernosa is established.

Initial impairment of venous outflow may be due to an extravascular or intravascular obstruction of drainage venules. Priapism initiated by an extravascular compression may end up having an intravascular component added, due to blood clotting in the drainage venules as a consequence of blood stasis. In the same way, priapism initiated by an intravascular obstruction may eventually have an extravascular component due to the development of oedema in the trabecular tissue [6].

Once the ischemic state has been established, and with the passing of time, pO_2 and pH of the trapped blood decrease, reaching levels close to anoxia (pO_2 0–10 mm Hg) and severe acidosis (pH ~ 6.6) [1]. Porst and col. [7] took cavernous blood samples from patients with prolonged erection/priapism of variable duration, demonstrating that 3–4 hours after the establishment of ischemia, the acidosis is severe, while the hypoxia is only partial (pO_2 ~ 50 mm Hg) (Fig. 1). The hypoxia as well as the acidosis cause depression of the contractility of the trabecular

Fig. 1. Cavernosal blood gases in various patients at different duration of prolonged erection/priapism following administration of intracavernosal vasoactive drugs. Soon after the onset of ischemia, acidosis is severe while severe hypoxia occurs many hours later. Data from reference 7

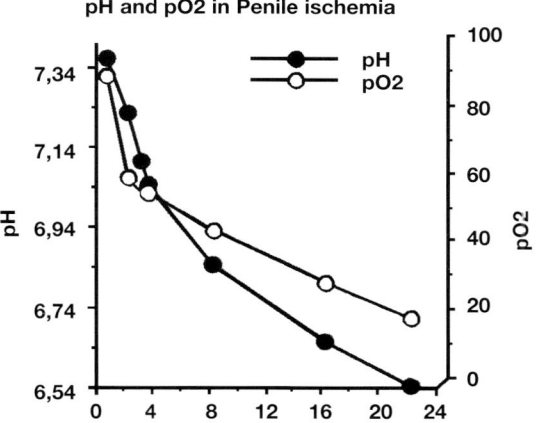

smooth muscle preventing the de-activation of the veno-occlusive mechanism, necessary for the drainage of blood from the cavernous bodies [8]. Nevertheless, in flaccidity, the cavernous tissue is exposed to venous blood (pO_2 ~ 35 mm Hg) so the effects of low oxygen on the contractility are probably not very significant until severe hypoxia is established (pO_2 < 25 mm Hg), late in the evolution of priapism [7]. On the contrary, acidosis is an early event after the initiation of ischemia and its deleterious effects on the smooth muscle contractility precede those of hypoxia.

Nitric oxide and prostacyclin (PGI_2) are potent inhibitors of platelet aggregation, as well as of adhesion and activation of inflammatory cells. Synthesis of both substances in the cavernous body depends on the oxygen concentration and during hypoxia (pO_2 < 25 mm Hg) their synthesis is practically blocked [9, 10]. The absence of nitric oxide and PGI_2 favours platelet aggregation and thrombi formation inside the venules as well as the infiltration of the trabecular tissue by inflammatory cells. Typically, these findings occur late after the onset of ischemia (~ 24 hours), coinciding with the establishment of severe hypoxia.

The prolonged ischemic state may lead to cellular death and subsequent fibrosis during the repair process of the tissue. These structural changes may lead to severe erectile dysfunction. Spycher and Hauri [11], studied the ultrastructure of cavernosal tissue biopsies during priapism and they established precisely the correlation between duration of priapism and severity of structural alterations.

Oxygenation with reperfusion of ischemic corpora cavernosa, after the treatment of priapism, may also have deleterious effects for the cavernosal tissue. Re-oxygenation of a tissue exposed to hypoxia or ischemia is associated with the generation of reactive oxygen species (ROS) which may contribute to tissue damage (Fig. 2). Under normal conditions cells have several anti-oxidant mechanisms, including catalase, superoxide dismutase, and glutathion peroxidase (Fig. 2). The concentration of these enzymes decreases during hypoxia or ischemia, making the tissues less capable of dealing with ROS generated during re-perfusion. It has been shown, for example, that the hypoxic cavernous body, at re-oxygenation, forms ROS that interfere with the synthesis of prostaglandins [12].

There are multiple causes that can lead to veno-occlusive priapism [13–22]. Intracavernosal injection of vasoactive drugs has become the most frequent cause of this type of priapism [1, 2]. Various other drugs, administered by oral or parenteral route have been associated with priapism. Psychotropic agents (antipsychotics and antidepressants) and antihypertensive drugs are among the most common [14–16]. Pharmacological priapism is, probably, initiated by the extravascular occlusion of the drainage veins as a consequence of the persistent relaxation of the trabecular smooth muscle.

Priapism due to intravascular obstruction is less frequent, except in those countries in which there are large populations with haemoglobin disease, such as sickle cell anaemia [19, 20]. Although the initiating event of sickle cell disease is not precisely known, stacking of sickled red cells in the corpus cavernosum veins is considered to be the cause of the venous drainage obstruction. Hypoxia and acidosis, secondary to

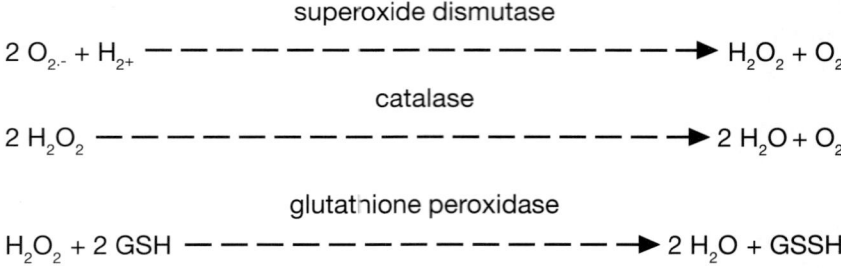

$$2\ O_{2^{.-}} + H_{2^+} \xrightarrow{\text{superoxide dismutase}} H_2O_2 + O_2$$

$$2\ H_2O_2 \xrightarrow{\text{catalase}} 2\ H_2O + O_2$$

$$H_2O_2 + 2\ GSH \xrightarrow{\text{glutathione peroxidase}} 2\ H_2O + GSSH$$

Fig. 2. Reactive oxygen species and endogenous antioxidant systems

ischemia, increase the number of sickled cells, complicating the obstructive situation [19, 20]. Hematological malignancies with hypercellularity, especially leukaemia, and parenteral hyper-alimentation are other causes that may lead to priapism due to intravascular obstruction [1, 2, 21, 22]. Priapism associated with the local extension of solid tumors can be ascribed to extravascular compression as well as to intravascular obstruction of the veins that drain the cavernous bodies.

Arterial Priapism

Arterial flow to the lacunar spaces is regulated by the resistance vessels, the helicine arteries. These arteries are contracted in the flaccid penis, restricting the blood flow to the lacunar spaces, creating a large pressure gradient between the cavernous artery and the lacunar spaces [24]. In arterial priapism, this control mechanism is altered when the cavernous artery, or one of its branches, is lacerated, forming an arterio-lacunar fistula [25, 26]. This fistula establishes a state of high flow and pressure in the cavernous bodies that escapes the physiological regulation of the resistance arteries. In the area adjacent to the arterio-lacunar fistula a turbulent blood flow is produced, creating mechanical forces ("sheer stress") on the endothelial cells lining the lacunar spaces [24–26]. The combination of this stimulus and the increase in oxygenation by high flow, probably favours the synthesis and release of nitric oxide by the endothelium, leading to the vasodilatation of the rest of the corpus cavernosum [9]. The recent observation that methylene blue, an inhibitor of the guanylate-cyclase, causes temporal detumescence in arterial priapism [26], gives support to the concept of the participation of the nitric oxide/cGMP pathway in the maintenance of the erection.

In arterial priapism the penis remains in a state of tumescence but the rigidity is only partial (60–75%). This is due, probably, to incomplete activation of the veno-occlusive mechanism, since the neurogenic mechanisms that relax trabecular smooth muscle are not activated. This is what allows the maintenance of the high flow state (high inflow and high outflow) in the cavernous bodies.

It is not clear what is the effect of the high flow state on the erectile tissue over weeks, or months, as can be seen in some patients with arterial priapism. Spycher and Hauri [11] showed the presence of moderate oedema in the trabecular tissue in patients with high flow priapism lasting from days to months. However, structural alterations in this type of priapism are much less severe than those observed in veno-occlusive priapism lasting more than 24 hours. This form of priapism is always associated to a perineal or penile trauma with laceration of the cavernous artery or one of its branches [24–28]. The result is the formation of an arterio-lacunar fistula. Although priapism associated with intracavernosal injection is usually of the veno-occlusive type, there have been cases of laceration of the wall of the artery by the needle inserted in the cavernous body, resulting in an arterial priapism [24, 25]. This may happen in patients in auto-injection program as well as during cavernosometry. Another iatrogenic cause of arterial priapism was described during penile revascularization surgery by the anastomosis of the inferior epigastric artery to the tunica albuginea. It is also important to be aware that the surgical treatment of veno-occlusive priapism by means of caverno-spongiosal or caverno-saphenous shunts, can be complicated with the laceration of the cavernosal artery or its branches, converting a veno-occlusive priapism into an arterial priapism. Awareness of this possible complication will avoid unnecessarily re-operations on a patient, thinking that his ischemic priapism has not been resolved.

Clinical Presentation

Veno-occlusive Priapism

The patient attends the Emergency room with a painful erection of several hours of duration. Except in the cases associated with intracavernosal injection, the patient typically noted for the first time the prolonged erection upon awakening, in the middle of the night, or after maintaining sexual activity. This temporal relationship with sexual or nocturnal erections suggests that in many cases the primary alteration that leads to priapism is the interference with the physiological mechanisms that regulate the detumescence of the erect penis [1, 2, 4]. The penis tends to present a full and rigid erection and palpation may be very painful. Only the cavernous bodies participate in the priapistic erection: the glans is small and the ventral surface of the penis is flat, not showing the bulging that produces the spongy body in a normal erection.

It is important to establish if the patient is taking any drugs, if he has some kind of haemoglobin disease, and which was the previous erection standard. In some cases the patients refer an history of easily obtaining multiple erections, prolonged erections (as a rule less than 2–3 hours) that eventually resolve spontaneously, or episodes in which the penis has maintained the rigidity during an extended period of time after the ejaculation [5].

Arterial Priapism

The patient always has a history of penile or perineal trauma, which may have occurred some hours or some days before the development of priapism. This is probably because trauma occurs in the flaccid (penile arteries constricted) penis and it is not until there is complete vasodilatation, for example in REM-associated erections, that the arteriolacunar fistula is opened. The appearance of priapism after several days may be explained by the trauma to the arterial wall which after several days is resolved by necrosis of an area which eventually falls apart, making a hole into the artery wall. When the trauma is penetrating, typically by needle, priapism is usually established immediately [24, 25].

Although some patients express some degree of discomfort associated with the erection, this form of priapism tends to be painless and, indeed, it is not associated with the severe ischemic pain that accompanies veno-occlusive priapism. On examination, the penis has incomplete rigidity (60–75%), it is not painful to palpation, and shows an elastic consistency. The blood within the corpora can be emptied by applying external pressure and upon release of pressure the corpora are refilled.

Diagnosis and Treatment

Priapism is a medical emergency and, therefore, the patient must be attended to immediately. The first objective is to define whether it is an ischemic priapism or not, since the therapeutic management of veno-occlusive and arterial priapism differs radically. Figure 3 summarizes the steps that must be followed in the diagnosis and treatment of priapism.

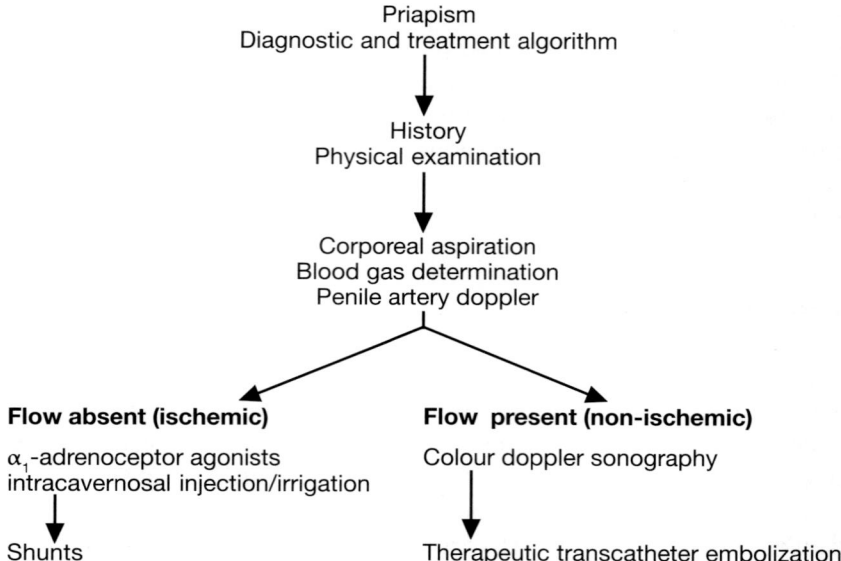

Fig. 3. Diagnosis and treatment of priapism

The main objective of the treatment of priapism is to apply therapeutic measures for the return of the erect penis to the flaccid state, while maintaining as much as possible, and this is of critical importance, its erectile capacity.

The clinical data and the symptoms that the patient refers are, as a rule, enough to suspect one or the other type of priapism. The treatment with drugs known to be associated with priapism (antihypertensive drugs, psychiatric drugs, parenteral feeding) must be interrupted. In the evaluation, the first step is to determine the presence of arterial flow to the cavernous bodies. This can be done through the use of the Doppler and through the measurement of pO_2, pCO_2 and pH in the blood of the cavernous bodies [24, 25].

Veno-occlusive Priapism

The presentation of a patient with a painful priapism, with absent or minimal arterial flow or with ischemic cavernous gasometry (hypoxia, acidosis) establishes the diagnosis of veno-occlusive priapism. It must be emphasized that during the erection the pO_2 in the blood of the cavernous bodies is of arterial type (pO_2 ~ 100 mm Hg). Therefore, the gasometry of the cavernous body should be interpreted through its comparison with the arterial gasometry [1]. If the arterial pO_2 is 100 mm Hg and that of the cavernous body is 60 mm Hg, it is indicative that of ischemia. As it was indicated before, the accumulation of CO_2, together with the reduction of pH, are considerable as early as 3–4 hours since the onset of erection, and should guide us to the diagnosis.

The drainage of the blood of the cavernous bodies in a priapism of short duration (4 to 8 hours) does not usually require anaesthesia, since the penile pain is usually not severe and emptying the ischemic blood, at that stage, does not require much manipulation. Nevertheless, sometimes it is convenient to apply local anaesthesia in the subcoronal sulcus which permits the insertion of big gauge needles. For more painful priapism, of longer duration, blockade of the dorsal nerve as well as of nervous branches to the skin around the base of the penis (sensory blockade of the penis) can be performed. In agitated patients, with severe pain, it is advisable the use of spinal, epidural, or even general anaesthesia. Big gauge needles (of 19G to 14G) should be used. Usually, in pharmacological priapism, with a duration of 4 to 8 hours, drainage may be done through the balano-preputial region with a 19G needle. The cavernous blood aspiration should be made slowly at the same time that compression or massage of the penis is exercised. If the drainage causes complete detumescence of the penis, the draining needle is closed waiting approximately 10 minutes to see if the erection returns or if penis stays flaccid. If the erection reappears, intracavernosal injection of adrenergic agonists should be applied. During this treatment it is advisable to monitor arterial blood pressure and heart rate. An alpha-1 selective adrenergic agonist, as phenylephrine or etilefrine, is probably the drug of choice for this treatment [6, 29]. The alpha-1 selective adrenergic agonist, methoxamine, has also been used successfully. Alpha-adrenergic selectivity avoids the possible complications associated with the stimulation of beta-adrenergic receptors by non-selective agonists (such as epinephrine or norepinephrine). Death, due to hypertensive crisis, has been reported after the use of metaraminol.

Phenylephrine can be prepared in two different ways, depending if it is for injection or for irrigation. For injection a solution of 1 mg of phenylephrine for each ml of saline is used, with doses of 0.2–0.5 ml (of 200 to 500 µg of phenylephrine for injection) that can be repeated several times. A total dose of 1.5–2.0 mg should not be to exceed over a period of 1 hour. For irrigation, 10 mg of phenylephrine are mixed in 1 liter of saline, resulting in a concentration of 10 µg/ml of phenylephrine. The irrigation is made with 20–30 ml of this solution, with each irrigation 200–300 µg of phenylephrine in the cavernous body.

The etilefrine is administered diluted in saline (1 mg/ml), it can be administered among 500 and 1000 µg every time. This injection can be repeated each 15 to 20 minutes until a total dose of 4 mg is reached.

Methoxamine is prepared diluting a vial of 20 mg in 5 ml of saline injecting 1 to 2 ml of this solution (4–8 mg of methoxamine) the dose can be repeated without surpassing a dose of 30 mg in total.

If, after the administration of anyone of these adrenergic agonists, a hypertensive crisis develops (systolic blood pressure > 200 mm Hg) the calcium antagonist nifedipine (10 mg) should be administered via sublingual route.

When the blood of the corpus cavernosum has increased considerably its viscosity due to a prolonged ischemic period of time, the drainage of the cavernous bodies can be difficult. In this case the cavernous body can be irrigated, with 20–30 ml of normal saline, to remove the ischemic blood. Once the cavernous bodies have emptied partially and the presence of red blood (oxygenated) is observed, the drainage and the detumescence of the penis may be completed through the irrigation with phenylephrine. If priapism has a duration superior to 24 hours and the cavernosal blood gasses demonstrate severe ischemia, the trabecular edema, the thrombosis of the drainage veins, and the profound depression of the contractility of the trabecular smooth muscle make, in many instances, the irrigation with alpha adrenergic agonists unsuccessful. In this case shunts connecting the cavernous bodies with a low resistance system (glans, spongy body, or saphenous vein) need to be performed. The objective of these shunts is to increase outflow (drainage) of the lacunar spaces which then allows inflow with the entrance of oxygenated blood.

As mentioned before, reperfusion/oxygenation of the ischemic cavernosal bodies causes the release of oxygen reacting metabolites with deleterious effects to the cavernosal tissue. No clinical trials have been conducted to prove the benefit of antioxidant drugs in the preservation of the erectile tissue. Its utilisation, nevertheless, seems to be rational and advisable, particularly in cases of priapism of long duration. Before the drainage of the corpora is accomplished, antioxidant drugs may be administered, like vitamin E (tocopherol) by intramuscular route (200–400 mg), or vitamin C (ascorbic acid), available in vials for intravenous use.

In the treatment of veno-occlusive priapism, after the irrigation or the shunt surgery, compressive bandages should not be applied in the penis in order to maintain the flaccidity of the penis [30]. These bandages may further reduce the arterial flow to a tissue that has been already submitted to severe ischemia, which may lead to a total or partial necrosis of the penis.

Treatment of the Recurrent Prolonged Erection

A few patients may present spontaneous prolonged erection episodes with a duration of up to 3 hours. This clinical entity may be considered a pre-priapism, the difference with priapism is that spontaneous detumescence of the penis takes place [5]. Typically, these patients awake from their sleep with an uncomfortable erection in the middle of the night or in the morning. Some patients have these episodes all nights, which interferes severely with their sleep pattern, leading patients to a state of extreme weakness, irritability and sometimes depression. Paradoxically, many of these patients exhibit low sexual interest or desire. These individuals have a high risk of developing priapism when they undergo treatment with antihypertensive or psychotropic drugs. The patients that finally develop priapism, after the resolution of the episode, frequently treated with shunts, may have worsening of the clinical picture [5]. The prolonged erections become more frequent and of greater intensity (more difficult to reach detumescence), with some patients developing multiple episodes of veno-occlusive priapism. The pathophysiology of prolonged erections and of recurrent priapism in these patients is not well understood. It is known, however, that most patients respond to adrenergic agonists, which indicate the presence of alpha-adrenergic receptors. During cavernosometry, when the muscle is contracted, obstruction to out-flow is not detected, eliminating the possibility of a mechanical obstruction of the drainage from the cavernous bodies [5]. However, these patients seem to have difficulty in the maintenance of constrictor tone of the trabecular muscle. It is not known if this is due to a deficiency in the autocrine and paracrine mechanisms

Fig. 4. Measurement of sleep associated erectile activity with Rigiscan in a patient with prolonged recurrent erections. In the upper tracing an intense erectile activity is measured. The lower tracing, from the same patient, was recorded after the patient was treated with phenylpropanolamine (225 mg) at bed time

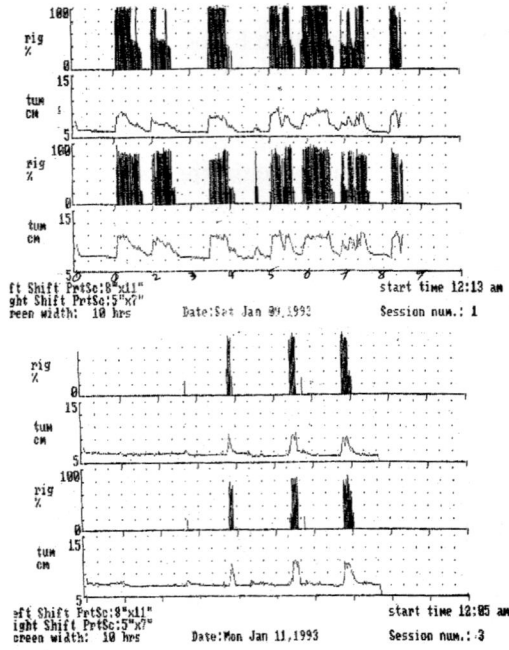

that regulate contraction of penile smooth muscle or to a lack of inhibition of the effectors for relaxation.

Some patients achieve detumescence of the prolonged erection, walking or through the physical exercise, possibly by an increase in the sympathetic activity. The treatment with adrenergic agonists by oral route, as phenylpropanolamine (75–150 mg at bedtime) reduces in some of these patients the frequency and the intensity of the prolonged erections, which permits some patients to sleep all night long [5] (Fig. 4). This treatment has the drawback of producing palpitations and insomnia in some patients. Also, it is convenient to instruct these patients in the intracavernosal self-injection of phenylephrine (200–300 μg) since an early treatment can avoid the development of priapism. Anti-androgens also have been used with success in cases of intolerance or contraindication of this treatment. The mechanism behind this treatment is unclear, as is the role of androgens in erection. The recent observation in animals that reduced levels of androgens decreases the activity of nitric oxide synthase (NOS), could explain the reduced erectile activity, provided that such androgen-NOS relationship holds true in humans.

Arterial Priapism

In this form of priapism the patient always recalls a history of trauma, has a painless erection, there is good arterial flow in the Doppler examination, and the cavernous blood gases demonstrate typical values of arterial blood [24, 25]. Due to the lack of ischemic compromise of the cavernous bodies, the treatment can be deferred. This leads to the question as to the need to treat these patients and when to do so. In general, it is probably reasonable to wait 7–10 day, as some of these priapisms resolve spontaneously. If it does not resolve, several reasons favour treatment. The patient shows great anxiety and intolerance when confronted with the idea of having a permanent erection. If the erection does not subside within days it can last months, even years, if left untreated. Also, the effect of an abnormal continuous high-flow state on the erectile capacity of the penis is not known, although there are a few anecdotal cases of maintained erectile function in patients with high-flow priapism lasting more than 20 years. It must be considered also, and this may be the most important consideration, that presently there are treatments available, like embolization of the lacerated artery, with excellent results with maintenance of erectile capacity [24–31]. Nevertheless, the experience with this treatment is in series of patients that have had priapism during days or weeks, but not years. It is possible that treatment outcome in patients with years of priapism will be different regarding the maintenance of the erectile capacity.

The lack of urgency in the treatment is important since supraselective pudendal artery angiography with embolization of the lacerated artery, may not be available in some medical centers, requiring the referral of the patient. The use of colour Doppler sonography allows an excellent visualization and localization of the arterio-lacunar fistula, which allows confirmation of the diagnosis [28] (Fig. 5). Angiography, an invasive technique, should not be used for the diagnosis of high flow priapism. When angiography is done it should be with the goal of resolving the priapism. In general the embolization should be done with reabsorbable material to produce temporary blockage of the artery that will eventually recanalize. In our experience, embolization with 3 ml of autologous clot is effective as definitive treatment in 4 out of 7 patients (Fig. 6). Two patients had recurrence of priapism, in hours or days, requiring a second embolization with an autologous clot. Finally, another patient with two recurrences, after two embolizations with autologous clots, was

Fig. 5. Colour Duplex sonography of the perineal area. Turbulent flow is observed which is created by an arterio-lacunar fistulae. This is a characteristic image in a patient with high flow priapism

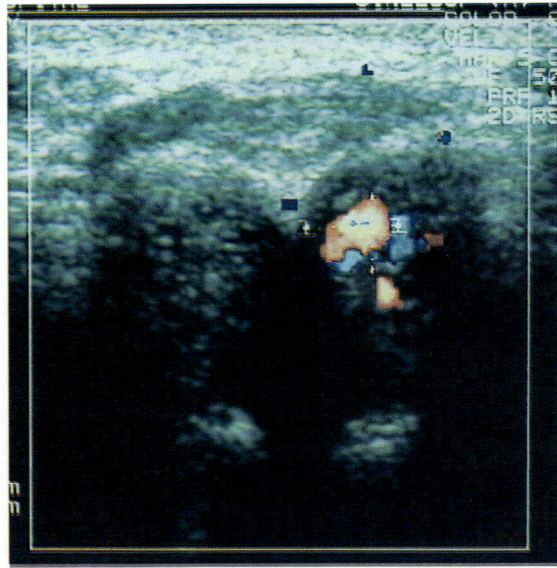

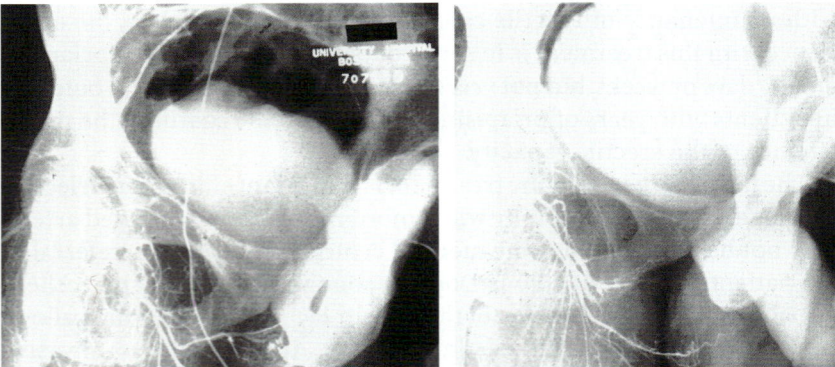

Fig. 6. Supraselective pudendal arteriography. *Left panel,* typical extravasation of contrast into the lacunar space; *right panel,* postautologous clot embolization of the lacerated artery. No further contrast extravasation is visualized

treated with a third embolization with gelatin foam without further recurrences. All patients regained the same erectile capacity as before. Nevertheless, a complete erectile capacity did not return, in some patients, until 3–4 months after treatment of priapism. Though the results of the treatment with embolization have been good, as a rule, complications may present. In our experience, infection of the clot in an adolescent patient, provoked a purulent cavernositis, with a complete erectile dysfunction subsequently.

Some cases of arterial priapism have been treated through surgical exploration of the corpora with direct ligature of the lacerated artery [32]. This form of treatment has the advantage that the lacerated artery is ligated distally, more selectively than with embolization. The ligation has, however, two important disadvantages: the possible damage of the cavernous tissue, and that the artery does not recanalize. The long term maintenance of the erectile capacity in patients treated through the arterial ligation is not known.

References

1. Lue TF, Wayne JG, Hellstrom WJG, McAninch JW, Tanagho EA (1992) Priapism: A refined approach to diagnosis and treatment. J Urol 136: 104
2. Winter CC, McDowell G (1988) Experience with 105 patients with priapism: update review of all aspects. J Urol 140: 980
3. Saenz de Tejada I, Kim N, Lagan I, Krane RJ, Goldstein I (1989) Regulation of Adrenergic Activity in Penile Corpus Cavernosum. J Urol 142: 1117
4. Bondil P (1990) Aspects physiopathologiques du priapisme. Maladie ou symptome? J d´Urologie 96: 115
5. Levine FJ, Saenz de Tejada I, Payton TR, Goldstein I (1991) Recurrent prolonged erections and priapism as a sequelae of priapism: pathophysiology and management. J Urol 145: 764
6. Tessier J, Saenz de Tejada I, Goldstein I (1991) Surgery of priapism. In: Marshall FF (ed) Operative Urology. Saunders, Philadelphia London Toronto Montreal Sydney Tokyo, pp 369–376
7. Porst H, van Ahlen H (1989) Pharmakon-induzierte Priapismen – ein Erfahrungsbericht über 101 Fälle. Urologe A 28: 84
8. Kim NN, Kim JJ, Hypolite J, García-Diaz JF, Broderick GA, Tornheim K, Daley J, Levin R, Saenz de Tejada I (1996) Altered contractility of rabbit penile corpus cavernosum smooth muscle by hypoxia. J Urol 155: 772–778
9. Kim N, Vardi Y, Padma-Nathan H, Daley JT, Goldstein I (1993) Oxygen tension regulates the nitric oxide pathway. Physiological role in penile erection. J Clin Invest 91: 437
10. Daley JT, Brown ML, Watkins MT, Traish AM, Huang YH, Moreland RB, Saenz de Tejada I (1996) Prostanoid production in rabbit corpus cavernosum: I. Regulation by oxygen tension. J Urol 155: 1482–1487
11. Spycher MA, Hauri D (1986) The ultrastructure of the erectile tissue in priapism. J Urol 135: 142

12. Daley JT, Watkins MT, Brown ML, Saenz de Tejada I (in press) Prostanoid production in rabbit corpus cavernosum: II. Inhibition by oxidative stress. J Urol

13. Padma-Nathan H, Goldstein I, Krane RJ (1986) Treatment of prolonged or priapistic erections following intracavernosal papaverine therapy. Sem Urol 4: 236

14. Saenz de Tejada I, Ware JC, Blanco R, Pittard JT, Nadig PW, Azadzoi KM, Krane RJ, Goldstein I (1991) Pathophysiology of prolonged penile erection associated with trazodone use. J Urol 145: 60

15. Kogeorgos J, de Alwis C (1986) Priapism and psychotropic medication. Brit J Psychiat 149: 241

16. Mitchell JE, Popkin MK (1982) Antipsychotic drug therapy and sexual dysfunction in men. Amer J Psychiat 139: 633

17. Siegel S, Streem SB, Steinmuller DR (1983) Prazosin-induced priapism: pathogenic and therapeutic implications. Brit J Psychiat 143: 332

18. Kaisary AV, Smith PJ (1986) Prazosin, priapism and management. Brit J Urol 58: 227

19. Fowler JE, Koshy M, Strub M, Chinn SK (1991) Priapism associated with sickle cell hemoglobinopathies: prevalence, natural history and sequelae. J Urol 145: 65–68

20. Hamre MR, Harmon EP, Kirpatrick DV, Stern MJ, Humbert JR (1991) Priapism as a complication of sickle cell disease. J Urol 145: 1

21. Macaluso JN, Sullivan JW (1985) Priapism: review of 34 cases. Urology 26: 233

22. Ekström B, Olsson AM (1987) Priapism in patients treated with total parenteral nutrition. Brit J Urol 59: 170

23. Fournier GR, Juenemann K-P, Lue TF, Tanagho EA (1987) Mechanisms of venous occlusion during canine penile erection: An anatomic demonstration. J Urol 137:163

24. Witt MA, Goldstein I, Saenz de Tejada I, Greenfield A, Krane RJ (1990) Traumatic laceration of intracorporal arteries: pathophysiology of nonischemic, high-flow priapism. J Urol 143: 129

25. Bastuba MD, Saenz de Tejada I, Dinlec CZ, Sarazen A, Krane RJ, Goldstein I (1994) Arterial priapism: Diagnosis, treatment, and long term followup. J Urol 151: 1231

26. Steers WD, Selby JB (1991) Use of methylene blue and selective embolization of the pudendal artery for high-flow priapism refractory to medical and surgical treatments. J Urol 146: 1361

27. Crummy AB, Ishizuka J, Madsen PO (1979) Posttraumatic priapism: Successful treatment with autologous clot embolization. AJR 133: 329

28 Gudinchet F, Fournier D, Jichlinski P, Meyrat B (1992) Traumatic priapism in a child: Evaluation with color flow doppler sonography. J Urol 148: 380

29. Dittrich A, Albrecht K, Bar-Moshe O, Vandendris M (1991) Treatment of pharmacological priapism with phenylephrine. J Urol 146: 323

30. Weiss JM, Ferguson D (1974) Priapism: the danger of treatment with compression. J Urol 112: 616

31. Wear JB, Crummy AB, Munson BO (1977) A new approach to the treatment of priapism. J Urol 117: 252

32. Ricciardi R, Bhatt GM, Cynamon J, Bakal CW, Melman A (1993) Delayed high-flow priapism: pathophysiology and management. J Urol 149: 119

Epidemiology and Diagnostics of Erectile Dysfunction

Wolf-Hartmut Weiske

Epidemiological data on the prevalence of erectile dysfunction are evidently based on estimates and therefore cannot be verified. The number of men in Germany suffering from erectile dysfunction is said to be 3–5 million. If an attempt is made to find out the source of those data, the trail usually disappears in the pseudoscientific jungle of an immense bulk of secondary literature.

Erectile dysfunction was defined in "NIH consense statement no. 10 of December 1, 1992, as follows: the inability to achieve and maintain an erection that is sufficient for satisfactory intercourse." This definition is limited to sexual ability, which, however, only partly accounts for sexual disorders. Psychologists [20] in particular point out the complexity of sexuality, which includes sexual interest and sexual activity in addition to sexual ability. Taking into account the complexity of sexuality is of utmost importance for reasonable diagnostic and therapeutic measures. In the past few years, the existing technical means for checking erectile function may quite often have led diagnosticians to concentrate too mechanistically on the functional aspects of erection, while paying little attention to the other aspects of sexuality mentioned above.

About 10 million American men have problems with their erectile function [5]. The point is to determine how many of these men have satisfactory sexual relationships despite their disorder and which of them wish to see a doctor to have their disorder diagnosed and treated. It has been reported that only 50% of men with erectile dysfunction were interested in an examination [13].

Greenstein's working group [3] investigated the question of which men would want their disorders of erectile function to be examined and which predictors there were. A questionnaire was submitted to 427 veterans (30–99 years old), and the answers were classified according to age, race, marital status, functional status, mood, health status, and prescribed medications. It was found that 136 men were interested in an examination of their erectile function and 291 men were not. The predictors were "inadequate erections" in addition to "loss of sexual interest or pleasure" with "retained orgasmic ability." The intact orgasmic ability was the strongest predictor of interest in evaluation of erectile dysfunction. It came as a surprise that age, partner availability, marital status, and functional status were unimportant as predictors.

The Frankfurt Study on the Virile Climacteric (Institute for Psychology of Frankfurt University) asked 240 working men between the ages of 35 and 64 about disorders that are usually attributed to the virile climacteric and for the causes of these disorders. The following answers were obtained among others:

Loss of libido	55%
Erection disorder	29%
Impairment of well-being	23%
Memory impairment	60%

The following causes of disorders were mentioned: stress during work (33%), personal problems (19%), and hormone deficit (4%).

Two results are noteworthy in this study regarding urologic and andrologic aspects. First, loss of libido is much more frequent than erectile dysfunction and, second, external stress is considered the principal cause by far. In an opinion poll by FOCUS (1995), stress during work was mentioned by 61%.

The probably most expressive normative data on the prevalence of erectile dysfunction were obtained in the Massachusetts Male Aging Study (MMAS), a multidisciplinary study involving 1709 men from the greater Boston area, aged between 40 and 70 years. Among numerous other questions concerning general medicine, 1290 men completely answered a sexual activity questionnaire that was evaluated by Feldmann et al. [1]. This revealed a combined prevalence of erectile dysfunction, classified as "minimal" (17%), "moderate" (25%), or "complete" (10%), in 52% of the men examined. This is equivalent to about 18 million men in the USA. The data show clearly that erectile dysfunction, while being strictly correlated with age, is not exclusively a symptom of old age. Complete impotence was demonstrated in 5% of the 40-year-old subjects and in 15% of those 70 years of age. Details are shown in Fig. 1. A correlation of erectile dysfunction with other conditions was found for heart disease, diabetes mellitus, hypertension, depression, and

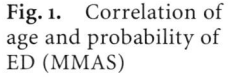 **Fig. 1.** Correlation of age and probability of ED (MMAS)

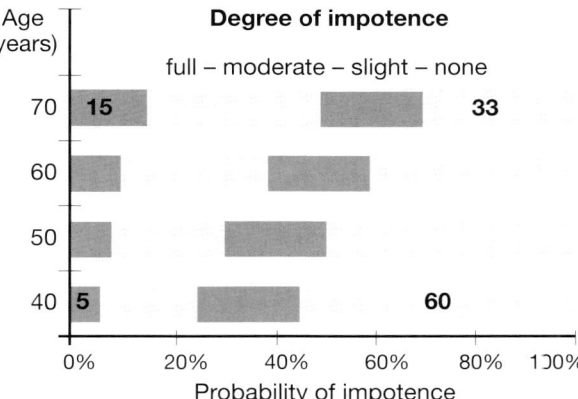

the administration of various drugs. For the diseases mentioned below, the probabilities in percent of suffering from erectile dysfunction in addition were as follows:

– Diabetes mellitus	up to 55%
– Heart disease	39%
– Heart disease and smoking	56%
– Hypertension	15%
– Depression	up to 90%
– Low HDL cholesterol	up to 25%

The incidence of erectile dysfunction following transurethral resection of the prostate because of benign prostatic hyperplasia (BHP) is – at 8.3% – relatively low, owing to advanced techniques [15]. An examination of 98 patients who had been classified as potent on the basis of the snap-gauge test prior to surgery showed 34 of them to be negative on the fourth postoperative day. After 3 months, however, only eight of the 98 patients were still affected (8.3%). On the whole, older age and greater weight of resected material were correlated with a higher risk of post-operative erectile dysfunction.

The multifactorial origin (Table 1) makes the diagnosis of erectile dysfunction very complex, and many of the methods are controversial. A general all-purpose tool for diagnosing erectile dysfunction that could serve as a kind of gold standard has not yet been found. A few generally accepted methods of diagnosis are available among a major number

Table 1. Pathogenesis of erectile dysfunction

Vascular:	arterial and/or venous (cavernous)
Drugs:	antihypertensives, H2-receptor antagonists, digoxin, neuroleptics, anti-depressants, clofibrate, narcotic drugs, chemotherapeutic drugs, etc.
Hormonal:	hypogonadism, diabetes mellitus, prolactinoma, sarcoidosis with affection of the pituitary-hypothalamic region
Neurologic:	cerebral insult, spinal cord injury, multiple sclerosis, peripheral or autonomic neuropathy, Parkinson´s disease
Psychologic:	sorrow, stress, anxiety, depression

Table 2. Diagnostic methods in erectile dysfunction (*CC* cavernous body, *PCM* dynamic pharmacocavernosometry, *VSS* visual sexual stimulation, *PCG* dynamic pharmacocavernosography, *NPT* nocturnal penile tumescence, *BCR* bulbocavernous reflex)

Generally accepted methods	Not generally accepted methods
• Pharmacological test	• Biopsy of cavernous body
	• Histomorphometry of CC
• Duplex sonography	• CT and NMR
	• CC-EMG
• PCM/PCG	• VSS
	• NPT
• Penile sonography	• Measurement of BCR latency time
	• Perfusion with radionuclides
• (Selective angiography)	• (Selective angiography)

of debated ones (Table 2). There is, however, no debate about the fact that enormous progress in diagnostics has been made during the past 10 years. This development has been sparked by the discovery and clinical use of vasoactive substances to induce erections [16].

State-of-the-art diagnosis of ED should be efficient and economical. This means that any diagnostic methods that will have no therapeutic consequence for the patient should not be carried out. Selective angiography of the penile arteries, for instance, is not indicated if surgical revascularization is contraindicated from the start or cannot be offered.

The examination scheme discussed below for erectile dysfunction has been used successfully for over 10 years in more than 2200 patients who were treated in a specialized medical office (Fig. 2). As required by a multidisciplinary diagnostic approach to erectile dysfunction, a psy-

Fig. 2. Diag-
nostic plan for
outpatient
evaluation of
erectile dysfunc-
tion. (*PGE*₁
Prostaglandin E₁,
SICI self-
intracavernosal
injection)

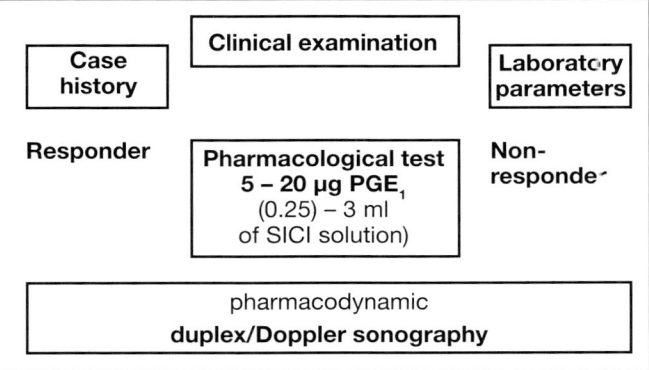

chologist familiar with the problem and a neurologist are available for
further diagnostics.

A comprehensive case history is of crucial importance. The first contact should enable the patient to establish a relationship with the clini-
cian that is characterized by personal confidence. Only if the patient
feels himself understood will he reveal to the treating physician the situations of conflict and the problems he finds difficult to bear. The sexual
case history is of particular importance and, as a part of it, the partner's
behavior – a factor that is neglected in most cases. Irrespective of the
extent of organic damage, there is always a causal or consequential psychological disorder of some degree. If obvious psychological problems
predominate the patient should be referred to a psychologist.

The physical examination should always include the vascular and
neurological status. Excluding the above-mentioned associated diseases
by means of adequate diagnostics is of particular importance. As to
hormonal disorders, which are seldom responsible for erectile dysfunction (< 5%), determination of the testosterone, prolactin, and, if necessary, of the thyroid hormone levels is sufficient.

In the clinical examination of the penis, attention must be paid to
indurations, plaques, and fibroses. Penile deviations associated with
erectile dysfunction are usually reported by the patient of his own
accord, so the recognition of Peyronie's disease does not generally pose
any difficulties. Sonography has proven particularly useful for the
diagnosis of local alterations in the penis, if linear transducers with 5
or, better, 7.5 MHz with a high image quality are used so that even minute

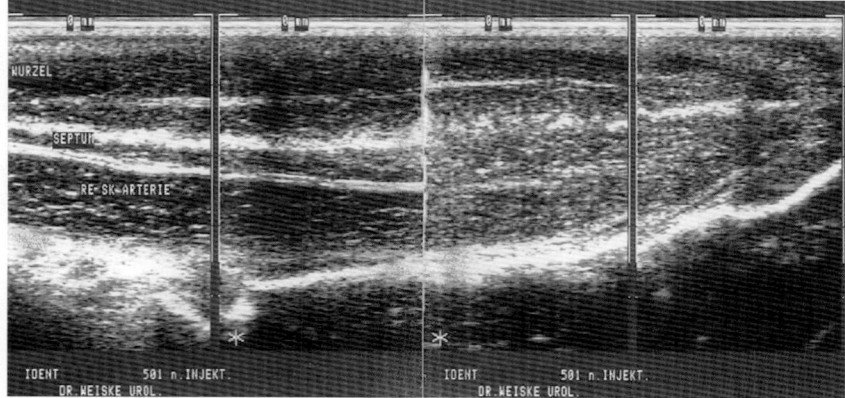

Fig. 3.   Sonographic imaging of the whole penis of a 40-year-old patient with erectile dysfunction. Transducer: 5 MHz. The two cavernous arteries and the septum are clearly circumscribed. The diffuse echoes in the distal portion correspond to the injected vasoactive substance (PGE_1) that has already spread diffusely in the two cavernous bodies

structures will be visualized (Fig. 3). The findings are sometimes disappointing in Peyronie´s disease, where sonographic imaging is reliable only in case of calcified plaques. A very good evaluation is possible for the cavernosal arteries. Plaques, stenoses, and particularly the pulsations can be visualized clearly. Most instruments are not sufficiently sophisticated to measure the very small vascular diameters (about 2 mm); this would require measurements accurate to 0.1 mm.

The spreading of vasoactive substances injected into the cavernous bodies can be observed very well. Admixed microscopic air bubbles cause the injected liquid to appear as an opaque (bright) area in the cavernous body. The diffuse spreading of the substance in the ipsilateral and particularly in the contralateral cavernous body depends on the condition of the cavernous tissue. In case of fibrosis, for instance, the opaque area remains unchanged for an extended time and will spread only very slowly, if at all. The principal rule is that a rapid diffusion of the injected liquid is prognostically good, whereas the opposite suggests an unfavorable outcome.

The clinical examination of erectile dysfunction is centered on the **pharmacological test** (Fig. 2, 4, 5). This test is used to investigate the response of the cavernous body to vasoactive substances. The drug of choice is prostaglandin E_1 (VIRILAN™, Schwarz Pharma Monheim) at

Fig. 4. Diagnostic scheme for responders to vasoactive substances. Pharmacodynamic duplex sonography of the cavernosal arteries is usually combined with the pharmacological test. More specific diagnostic measures should always be adapted to the available therapeutic possibilities. (*BCR* Bulbocavernous reflex)

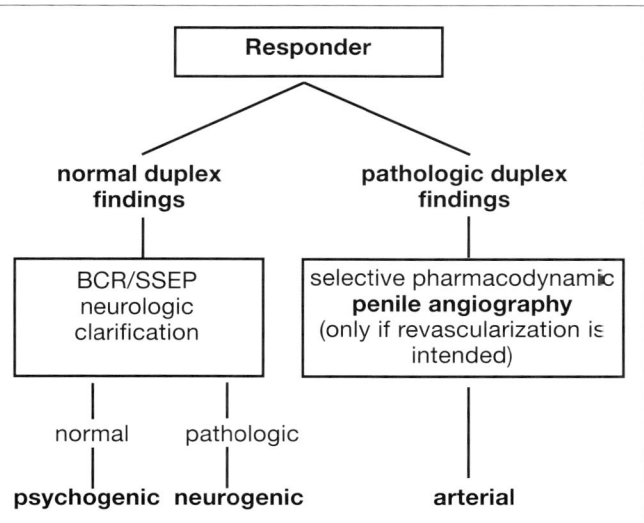

Fig. 5. Diagnostic scheme for nonresponders to the pharmacological test. For details see text

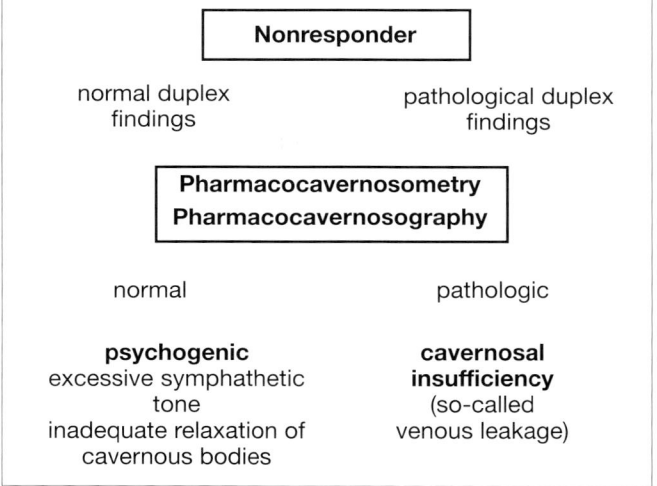

a dose of 5 or 10 µg. If there is strong suspicion of a neurologic or psychologic origin of the patient´s erectile dysfunction, a starting dose of 5 µg almost guarantees no prolonged erection (more than 4 h). If no erection of the cavernous bodies (response) follows the first injection, the test is repeated with a higher dose (up to 40 µg) during a second session. If even the highest dose fails to induce an erection, the addition of 1 ml of a papaverine/phentolamine solution (Androskat) as a triple drug is recommended to achieve adequate relaxation of the cavernous bodies (see chapter on vasoactive substances by Porst). The risk of priapism requiring treatment is extremely low if only PGE_1 is used (see chapters by Porst, Tejada). After more than 2000 first injections of PGE_1 into our own patients, we have had to treat prolonged erection with an antidote (Effortil™) only once. Spontaneous disappearance of a prolonged erection induced by PGE_1 can be expected after as long as 6 h. Damage of the cavernous tissue as a result of metabolic acidosis with a CO_2 surplus and an oxygen deficit must be feared at the earliest after 12 h (see chapter on prolonged erections by Tejeda).

If, for reasons of cost, the decision is made to use papaverine/phentolamine (Androskat™), the risk of prolonged erection is much higher (see Porst). The decisive disadvantage is that prolonged erections induced by this drug do not disappear spontaneously, but have to be treated. This can have quite unpleasant consequences for the daily work in the physician´s office and, in particular, for his night´s rest. The era of prolonged erections with all their possible complications (hypertensive crisis) ended when PGE_1 was introduced. Substances carrying a high risk of prolonged erections should therefore no longer be used for the pharmacological test.

Internationally, **pharmacodynamic duplex sonography** of the cavernosal arteries is the most widely accepted method for the diagnosis of erectile dysfunction (Fig. 6, 7). This may be due to the fact that all investigators obtain almost equal results, in particular, with respect to peak systolic velocity (PSV), although the instrument specifications differ greatly [11, 12]. The examination is performed during the tumescent stage following the intracavernosal injection of 10 µg PGE_1. There is no definable time for the execution of the examination. A full relaxation of the cavernosal smooth muscle has to be reached for the values to be reproducible. The measurements should therefore begin after about 2 min and be continued until the peak flow has been reached. This can be after 5, 10, or 20 min [2].

If relaxation is inadequate, either a second dose is given [9], or the measurement is performed with a higher dose of the vasoactive substance during a second examination on another day. Failure to note, an inadequate relaxation of the cavernosal muscles is among the most

Fig. 6. Pharmacodynamic duplex sonography in a 30-year-old patient with penile deviation but no erectile disorder. The intracavernosal injection of 10 µg PGE_1 induces full erection (E5). Extremely high systolic peak flow of 60 cm/measured after 20 min with a positive diastolic dip of 7 cm/s is a sign of high vascular elasticity

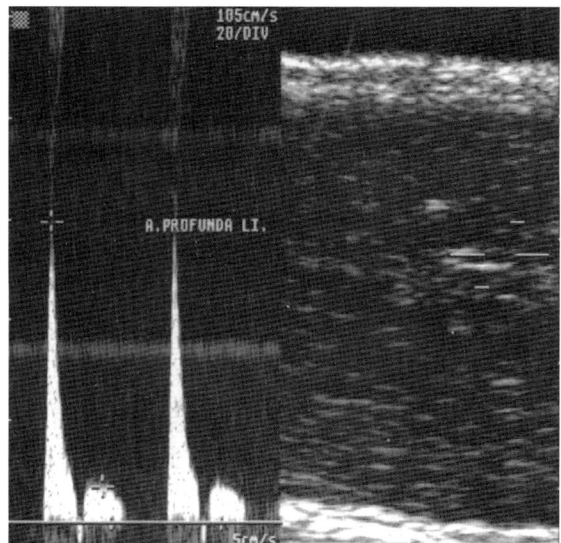

serious errors that can occur in pharmacodynamic duplex sonography. In case of uncertainty, the examination should be repeated.

The end-diastolic velocity (EDV) is determined at the same time. This parameter changes quite considerably in the course of the examination, since it depends upon the peripheral resistance (Fig. 7). In an intact cavernosal artery there will be at first a negative flow during the diastole (so-called diastolic dip), which will disappear completely as the examination is continued. A diastolic flow that remains high (> 5 cm/s) is indicative of low peripheral resistance in the cavernous body and is a reliable sign of a disorder in the occlusive mechanism, as occurs in cavernosal insufficiency in its extreme form. The cut-off values are defined as follows:

PSV > 25 cm/s, deep penile artery
PSV > 35 cm/s, dorsal penile artery

Meulemann et al. [8] observed values between 19 and 120 cm/s in healthy volunteers ($n = 44$), the time of examination being 5 min after the injection, however. This result shows that the PSV range is quite large, although the literature lacks reports on major populations of healthy

Fig. 7a

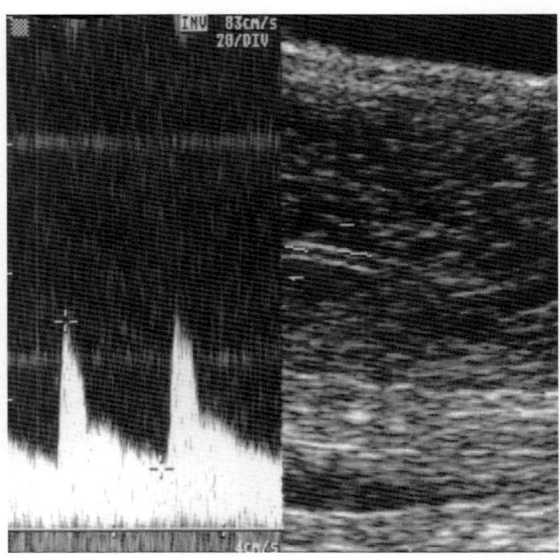

Fig. 7b

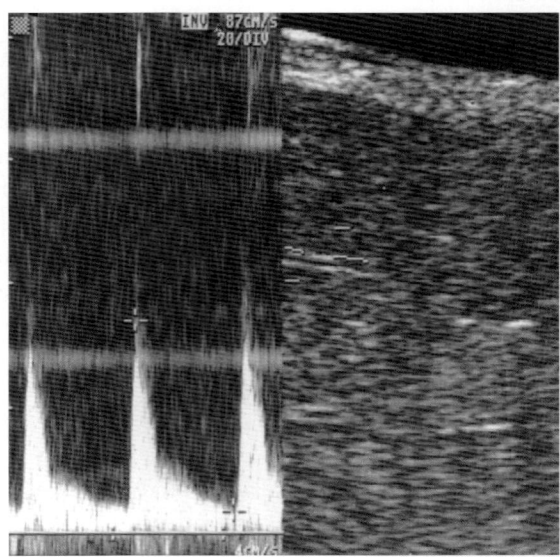

Fig. 7c

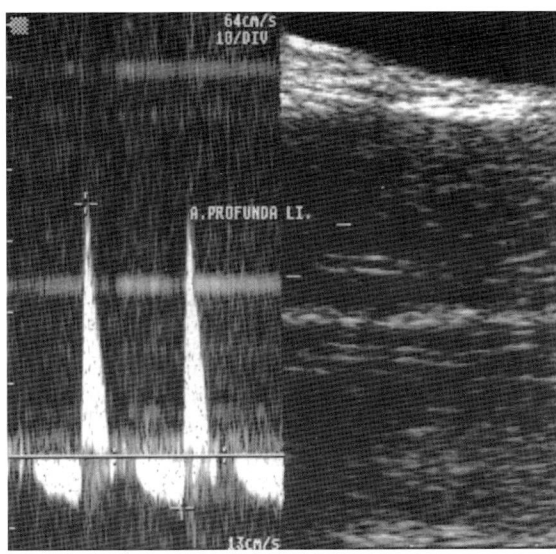

Fig. 7a–c. Duplex sonography of the cavernous arteries in a 58-year-old patient with psychogenic erectile dysfunction. The three recordings above the left cavernous artery, made over a period of half an hour following the intracavernosal injection of 10 µg PGE$_1$, show the whole spectrum of hemodynamics in the cavernous arteries during an erection. **a** In the tumescent stage (E2) the peak flow has already reached a normal level (PSV 33 cm/s), while the diastolic flow is still high (EDV 10 cm/s), because veno-occlusion of the cavernous bodies is still incomplete. **b** After several minutes, the end-diastolic flow decreases to 4 cm/s without a change in systolic peak flow (PSV), while the tumescence is developing into the beginning of erection (E3–E4). **c** There is now a full erection of medium rigidity (E4), and the PSV is high. The end-diastolic flow has become negative *(dip)* because of the arterial elasticity and the elevated peripheral resistance

subjects of different ages. Neither will such standard data be available in the future, since the diagnostic methods for erectile dysfunction are invasive. This is true not only for pharmacodynamic duplex sonography, but particularly for selective penile angiography and for dynamic pharmacocavernosometry (PCM) and pharmacocavernosography (PCG), which are discussed below.

Besides PSV and EDV, the peripheral resistance index and the systolic rise time (SRT) are used for eveluation of the penile vessels. The peripheral resistance index (RI) according to Pourcelot is calculated as follows [4, 3]:

$$RI = \frac{PSV - EDV}{PSV}$$

Contrasting PSV with SRT, Oates et al. [10] conclude that SRT allows a much more accurate distinction between pathologic and sound cavernosal arteries (standard error SRT, $p < 0.0001$; PSV, $p < 0.37$). The criterion used in this comparison was the selective angiography of the pudendal artery. What has to be evaluated critically is the PSV standard examination time of 5 min after the intracavernosal injection, a time that may not be sufficient to register the PSV. The present findings show only that after 5 min the SRT values (cut-off value 110 ms) correlate with the angiographic findings better than the PSVs. Whether the SRT will become an established new parameter for duplex sonography of the penile arteries cannot be foreseen today. The results would first have to be confirmed by other examinations, and the instruments would have to be improved such as to allow a safe SRT determination; this is probably not possible with most of the instruments on the market today.

Color-coded duplex sonography can demonstrate communications between the dorsal penile artery and the cavernous artery. Such communications are decisive for the surgical success of penile revascularization but are reported to be present in only about 14% of men suffering from arteriogenic impotence. This is, of course, a substantial limitation of the surgical indication for arterial revascularization, but it could be used to improve the postoperative results by patient selection. It is there-

Fig. 8a

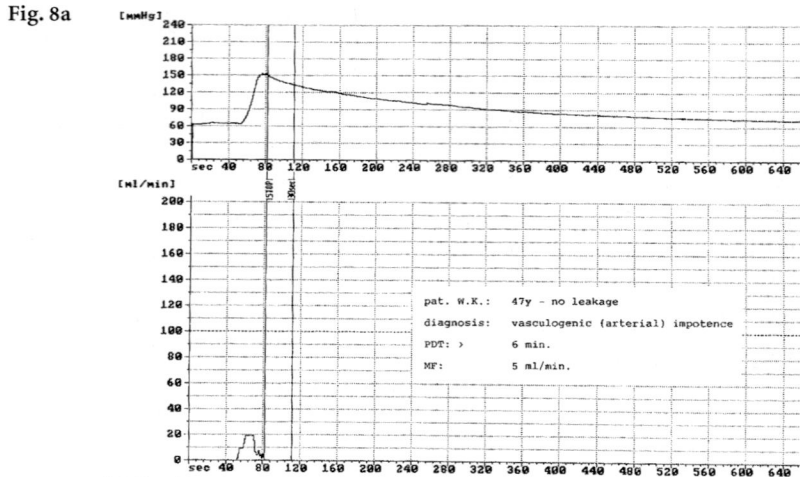

Fig. 8a, b. Findings of dynamic pharmacocavernosometry and pharmacocavernosography in a patient with intact veno-occlusion of the cavernous bodies. **a** Cavernosometry: maintenance-flow, 5 ml/min; time of pressure drop, 6 min. The intracavernosal pressure increases immediately to values above 150 mm Hg and begins to decrease very slowly after inflow through the cavernosal pump has stopped. **b** Cavernosography: visualization of the two completely intact cavernous bodies with communication in the middle third. No pathologic drainage is demonstrated

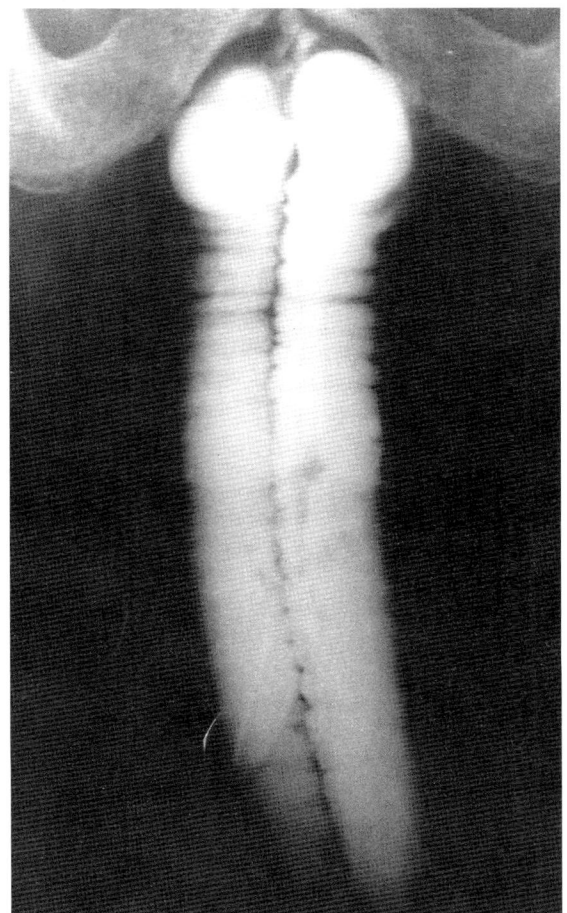

fore mandatory that revascularization surgery be performed only if such vascular communications can be demonstrated [18].

Due to Lue [6], the injection of vasoactive substances was introduced as a modification of the so-called artificial erection to visualize the cavernous bodies; the modified technique is generally used today in the form of dynamic **pharmacocavernosometry (PCM)** and **pharmacocavernosography (PCG)** (Fig. 9, 10). The injection of vasoactive substances leads to relaxation of the cavernosal smooth muscles and to a dilatation of the vessels, so the PCM can be executed in a more physiological way and using much lower volumes of infusion. PCM is indicated for nonresponders to the maximum dose of PGE$_1$ (40 µg), or to 3 ml of the papaverine/phentolamine mixture (papaverine hydrochloride 15 mg/phentolamine mesylate 0.5 mg/ml aqueous solution), or to a mixture of the three substances (triple drug) and for the purpose of imaging the cavernous bodies in case of pathologic alterations such as Peyronie´s disease, deviations, penile fracture, fibroses of the cavernous bodies, plaque formation. PCM is used to examine venous drainage, i.e., the occlusive function of the cavernous bodies, while PCG is used to localize the site of venous drainage, apart from visualizing the cavernous bodies. Only rarely is an ectopic vein demonstrated as the possible cause of erectile dysfunction (below 5%).

PCM and PCG techniques: Following the intracavernosal injection of PGE$_1$ 20 µg, butterfly needles are inserted into both cavernous bodies during the tumescent stage. One needle is used to administer Ringer´s solution at body temperature and radiopaque medium, while the other needle is connected with a transducer. The two variables of inflow and intracavernosal pressure can thus be measured and recorded continuously.

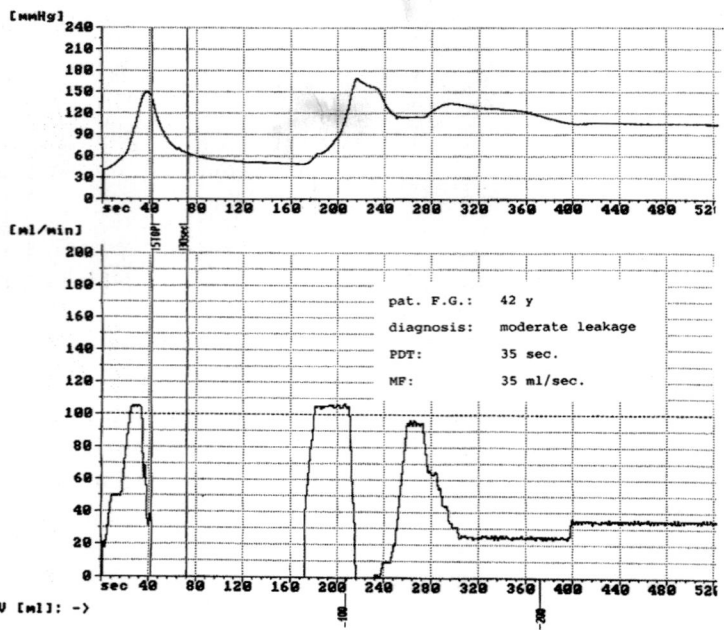

Fig. 9a

Fig. 9a,b. Findings of dynamic pharmaco-cavernosometry and pharmacocavernoso-graphy in a patient with moderate venous leakage. **a** Cavernosometry: maintenance-flow, 35 ml/min; time of pressure drop, 35 s. **b** Cavernosography: visualization of the left external pudendal vein

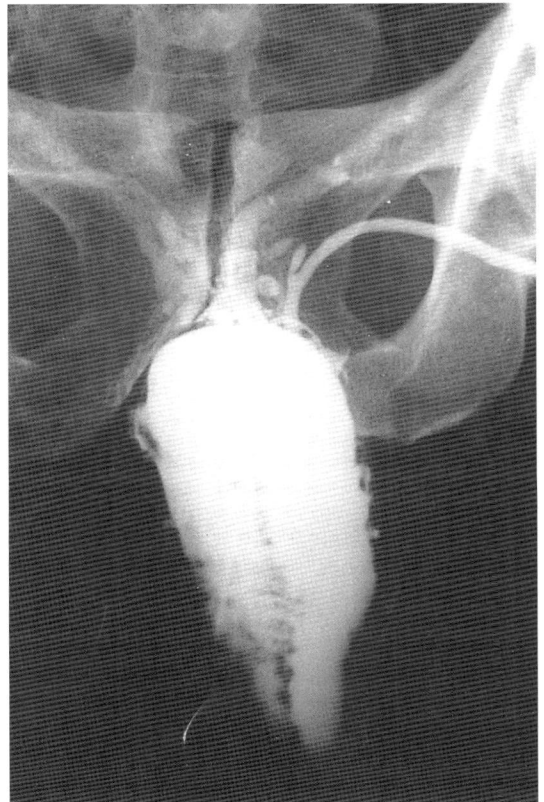

The maintenance flow in milliliters per second is the most expressive parameter of PCG, if the flow is measured at an intracavernosal pressure of 80–90 mm Hg under the condition of an adequate relaxation of the cavernosal muscles and the best possible exclusion of foreign influences liable to cause anxiety. In case of inadequate relaxation, a second dose of the vasoactive substance should be given, especially if the reaction of the cavernous body is lower than in the pharmacological test. Patients´ ability to cope with the stress occasioned by the technical circumstances and the insertion of the needles into the penis varies. In particular, younger men with excessive sympathetic tone can show false-negative results due to stress; this may lead to the diagnosis of cavernosal insufficiency, which would, however, not be compatible with spontaneous erections in the morning and full erections after the intracavernosal injection of vasoactive substances at home. These are the weak points of the method as such, and the investigator´s experience is required when such false-negative results are obtained.

Another parameter is the time of pressure drop. The time necessary for the intracavernosal pressure to fall from 150 to 50 mm Hg is measured. While the pressure drop takes several minutes in case of a normal occlusive mechanism, cavernosal insufficiency is associated with a fall in pressure of only several seconds (Fig. 6). The standard values that have proven suitable after more than 1000 examinations of our own patients during the past 10 years [19]:

Maintenance flow	< 15 ml/s	normal
	15–30 ml/s	suspicion of venous leakage
	> 30 ml	definite cavernosal insufficiency
Time of pressure drop (150 to 50 mm Hg)	> 1 min	normal
	30–60 s	moderate leakage
	< 10 s	serious cavernosal insufficiency

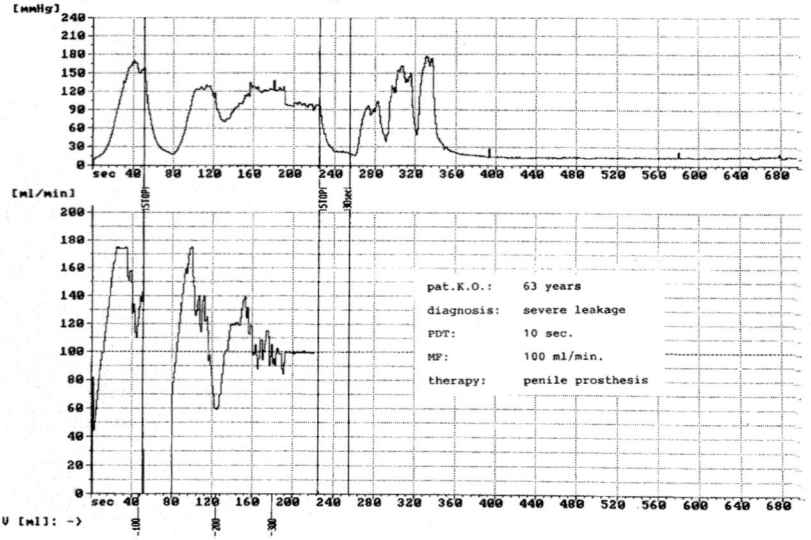

Fig. 10a

Fig. 10a, b. Findings of dynamic pharmacocavernosometry and pharmacocavernosography in a patient with cavernosal insufficiency. **a** Cavernosometry: maintenance flow 100 ml/min; time of pressure drop, 10 s. The intracavernosal pressure falls rapidly immediately after inflow through the cavernosal pump has stopped. **b** Cavernosography: visualization of all possible physiologic paths of venous drainage including a caverno-balanic shunt. Most conspicuous is the massive outflow through the prostaticovesical plexus. The only therapeutic option is the implantation of a penile prosthesis

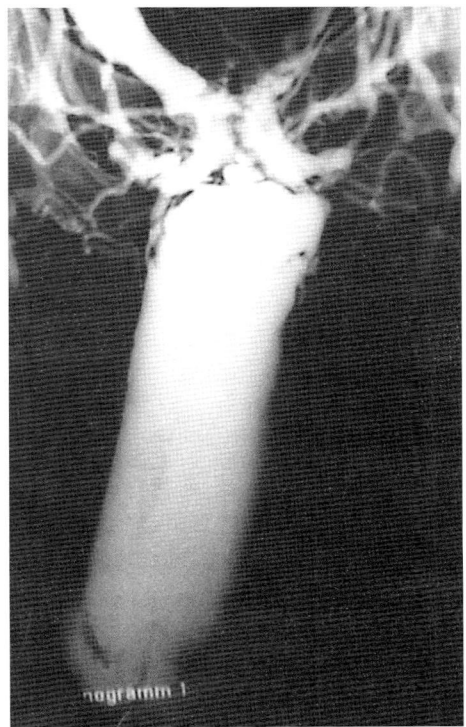

After PCM, the PCG examination is performed: If the maintenance flow is high and the time of pressure drop short, the venous drainage system will usually be visualized, as can well be expected in disorders of cavernosal veno-occlusion. An ectopic vein will be found only very rarely in cases of moderately elevated maintenance flow. The PCG examination is further used to image cavernosal fibroses (Fig. 11); knowledge of the extent of fibrosis can be useful if the implantation of a penile prosthesis is intended. PCG is also a safe means of documenting deviations.

PCM and PCG are investigative methods that are associated with few complications, if performed by a trained physician, and do not require hospitalization. Major hematomas and penile edemas occur only during the training stage and can be prevented. Insignificant small hematomas, not requiring therapy, as a result of the puncture are seen in about 10% of cases. Pulmonary edema was never seen in over 1000 PCM/

Fig. 11. Cavernosography of a
53-year-old (diabetic) patient with
marked cavernosal fibrosis following
self-intracavernosal-injection
therapy with papaverine/phen-
tolamine

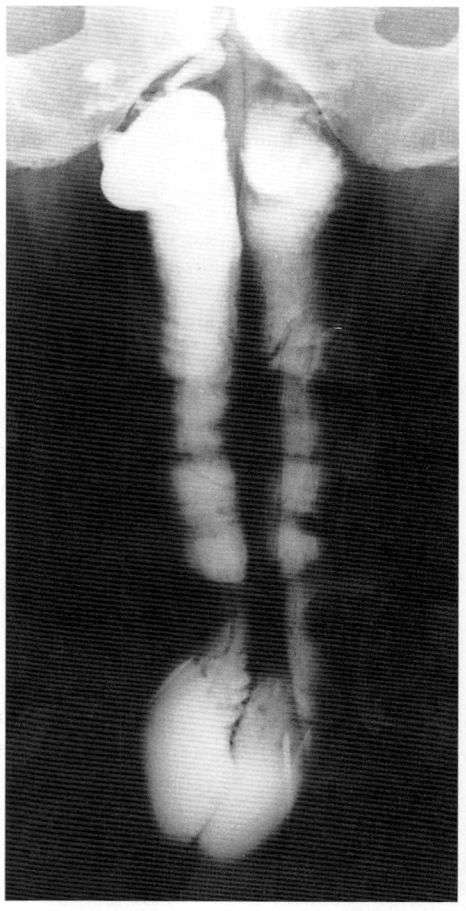

PCG examinations with infusion volumes of up to 500 ml (average 200–300 ml), nor were threatening reactions to contrast media observed after infusions of 90–180 ml of a nonionic contrast medium. Mild nausea occurred in 1.6% of patients [19].

The diagnosis of **neurogenic erectile dysfunction** is problematic, as there is no test to examine the autonomic nervous system. The measurement of **bulbocavernous reflex (BCRL) latency** is probably the most widely used neurophysiologic test. It can, however, reveal only lesions of the somatic penile innervation (pudendal nerve), but not of the autonomic innervation (parasympathetic and sympathetic nerves).

Wagner and Gerstenberg [17] reported on the measurement of electric potentials in the cavernous body. Such a method should theoretically be suitable for detecting autonomic neuropathy of the cavernous body and smooth muscle dysfunction as a result of degeneration. If the recorded potentials could be attributed to certain causes of erectile dysfunction, this would be an ideal method for diagnosing it, as the measurement would be made in the actually affected organ. Unfortunately, however, the so-called **Corpus cavernosum EMG (CC-EMG)** cannot meet this demand to date despite improvement of the instruments and a certain standardization. In particular, there are artifacts that have so far prevented reliable and reproducible diagnostic statements. There is hope that intelligent software will be capable in the future of identifying and eliminating these artifacts. Currently, however, the CC-EMG is not a routine method in the diagnosis of erectile dysfunction.

In conclusion, there is presently no generally accepted gold standard for the diagnosis of erectile dysfunction. Pharmacological testing and pharmacodynamic duplex sonography of the penile vessels are the most reliable methods of examination and probably the least controversial internationally. Standard values obtained in potent men of various age-groups are not available, for reasons mentioned above.

The examinations and, above all, the interpretation of their results depend partly upon the investigator's personal experience and his technical equipment. The methods described above have revolutionized the diagnostics of erectile dysfunction in the past 10 years and, combined with basic research in this area, they have brought enormous improvement in the understanding of the underlying disorders. While the diagnostics were formerly limited to determination of the testosterone level and long psychological examinations, medical science has gained a much better understanding of the vascular and cavernosal causes of erectile dysfunction, although a great deal of uncertainty remains. The fact that aspects of sexual medicine are now considered in addition to so-called organic causes is certainly a change of great benefit to the patient.

We, the physicians in charge, should always bear in mind that erectile dysfunction, i.e., impotentia erigendi et coeundi, means always substantial impairment of the quality of life, a consequence that becomes particularly important against the background of an aging population. In the past 10 years alone, the expectation of life has increased by 2.6 years and has reached 75.9 years for men in Germany (Switzerland: 77.5; Sweden: 77.7 years). This will necessarily lead to an increase in the number of men with potency problems who consult a doctor for help. This is not only a challenge for the physicians who have to tackle these problems; it will also bring with it immense economic problems for the health system.

References

1. Feldman HA, Goldstein I, Hatzichristou DG, Krane RJ, McKinlay JB (1994) Impotence and its medical and psychosocial correlates: Results of the Massachusetts Male Aging Study. J Urol 151: 54–61
2. Govier FE, Asase D, Hefty TR, McClure RD, Pritchett TR, Weissman RM (1995) Timing of penile color flow duplex ultrasonography using a triple drug mixture. J Urol 153: 1472–1475
3. Greenstein A, Chen J, Perez ED, Mulligan T (1994) Characteristics of men interested in evaluation of erectile dysfunction. Int J Impotence Res 6: 199–204
4. Jünemann KP, Siegismund M, Löbelenz M, Alken P (1990) Doppler-Sonographie der Penisarterien. Urologe A 29: 113–119
5. Krane RJ, Goldstein I, Saenz de Tejada I (1989) Impotence. N Engl J Med 321: 1648–1659
6. Lue TF, Hricak H, Marich KW, Tanagho EA (1985) Vasculogenic impotence evaluated by high-resolution ultrasonography and pulsed Doppler spectrum analysis. Radiology 155: 777
7. Meuleman EJH, Bemelmans BLH, van Asten WNJC, Doesburg WH, Skotnicko SH, Debruyne FMJ (1990) The value of combined papaverine testing and duplex scanning in men with erectile dysfunction. Int J Impotence Res 2: 87–98
8. Meulemann EJH, Bemelmans BLH, van Asten WNJC, Doesburg WH, Skotnicko SH, Debruyne FMJ (1993) Assessment of penile blood flow by duplex ultrasonography in 44 men with normal erectile potency in different phases of erection. J Urol 149: 51–56
9. Nehra A, Hakim LS, Abobakr RA, Krane RJ, Goldstein I (1995) A new method of performing duplex Doppler ultrasonography: the effect of re-dosing of vasoactive agents on hemodynamic parameters. J Urol 153 Nr.4: 332A (abstract 415)
10. Oates CP, Pickard RS, Powell PH, Murthy LN, Whittingham TAW (1995) The use of duplex ultrasound in the assessment of arterial supply to the penis in vasculogenic impotence. J Urol 153: 354–357
11. Porst H, Jünemann KP (1991) Duplex- und Farbduplexsonographie der penilen Gefäße. In: Jünemann KP, Weiske W-H (eds) Dopplersonographie in der Urologie. VHC Verlagsgesellschaft, edition medizin, Weinheim, pp 41–72
12. Porst H (1993) Die Duplexsonographie des Penis. Urologe (A) 32: 242–249
13. Slag MF, Morley JE, Elson MK, Trence DL, Nelson CJ, Nelson AE, Kinlaw WB, Beyer HSM, Nutall FQ, Shafer RB (1983) Impotence in medical clinic outpatients. JAMA 249: 1736–1740
14. Stief CG, Jünemann KP, Kellner B, Gerstenberg T, Merckx L, Wagner G (1994) Consensus and progress in corpus cavernosum-EMG (CC-EMG). Int J Impotence Res 6: 177–182

15. Tscholl R, Largo M, Poppinghaus E, Recker F, Subotic B (1995) Incidence of erectile impotence secondary to transurethral resection of benign prostatic hyperplasia, assessed by preoperative and postoperative snap-gauge test. J Urol 153: 1491–1493
16. Virag R (1982) Intracavernous injection of papaverine for erectile failure. Lancet 2: 938
17. Wagner G, Gerstenberg T (1988) Human in vivo studies of electrical activity of corpus cavernosum. J Urol 139: 327A
18. Wegner HEH, Andresen R, Knispel HH, Banzer D, Miller K (1995) Evaluation of penile arteries with color-coded duplex sonography: prevalence and possible therapeutic implications of connections between dorsal and cavernous arteries in impotent men. J Urol 153: 1469–1471. Comment in: J Urol 153: 1482
19. Weiske W-H (1990) Pharmakokavernosometrie und Pharmakokavernosographie bei erektiler Dysfunktion. Urologe (A) 29: 126–134
20. Zilbergeld B (1994) Die neue Sexualität der Männer. Dgvt-Verlag, Tübingen

Pharmacology of Penile Smooth Muscle

Iñigo Saenz de Tejada and Ignacio Moncada

The contractile activity of the penile muscle (arterial and trabecular) is regulated by several factors: adequate levels of agonists (neurotransmitters, hormones, and endothelium-derived substances), adequate expression of receptors, integrity of the transduction mechanisms, calcium homeostasis, interaction between contractile proteins, and effective intercellular communication among smooth muscle cells (gap junctions) [1]. Ultrastructural examination of the muscle cell reveals filamentous structures that may be thin, thick, or intermediate. The thin filaments are composed mainly of actin, whereas the thick ones are composed of myosin. The intermediate filaments contain either desmin or vimentin. After the phosphorylation of myosin by ATP, bridges form between the globular heads of the light chain of myosin and actin. These attachments ("cross-bridges") confer the contractile tone to the smooth muscle [2, 3]. Tone can be maintained at a low energy expense; this is due to an interaction among contractile proteins that is known as "latch-state," during which the bridges between actin and myosin are largely maintained, despite being in a dephosphorylated state [3]. To maintain this state, a high concentration of free intracellular calcium seems to be required [1].

Penile Smooth Muscle Contraction

The contraction of smooth muscle depends on the rise, relatively rapid, of the intracellular concentration of free calcium. This concentration must be kept above baseline level for the maintenance of the contractile tone. Several mechanisms are activated favoring entry of calcium from the extracellular compartment and/or the release of calcium accumulated in intracellular organelles, mainly the sarcoplasmic reticulum [4].

Alpha-Adrenergic Mechanisms

Locally, the detumescence of the erect penis is mediated by adrenergic nerve terminals whose neurotransmitter, norepinephrine, activates adrenergic receptors. It has been proposed that the contraction of the human cavernous artery that follows stimulation of the adrenergic nerves is mediated, mainly by α_2 receptors, while in trabecular muscle neurogenic contraction is mediated largely by α_1 adrenergic receptors [4, 5]. The $\alpha_1 d$ and $\alpha_1 a$ subtypes are the ones expressed with higher density in the trabecular muscle [6]. The α-adrenergic receptors can also be stimulated by circulating catecholamines (norepinephrine as well as epinephrine) (Fig. 1). Contraction mediated by α_2-receptors depends on the entry of calcium from the extracellular compartment, while the ac-

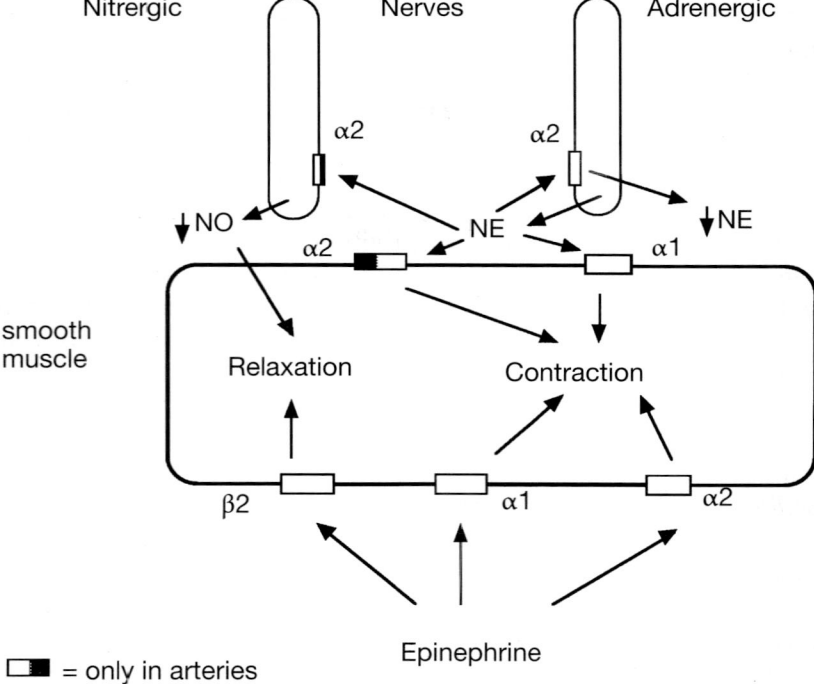

Fig. 1. Adrenergic mechanisms of penile smooth muscle (arterial and trabecular). Pre- and postjunctional mechanisms regulated by adrenergic receptors are schematically represented. (*NE* norepinephrine)

tivation of α_1-receptors provokes the release of intracellular calcium initially, with subsequent extracellular calcium entry for the mainte- nance of the contractile tone.

Adrenergic stimulation causes vasoconstriction of the penile arter- ies and contraction of the trabecular muscle, resulting, respectively, in reduction of the arterial inflow and in collapse of the lacunar spaces. The contraction of the trabecular muscle causes decompression of the drain- age venules from the cavernous bodies, allowing the venous drainage of the lacunar spaces [7–9]. Even though the role of the adrenergic neuroeffector system as mediator of detumescence of the erect penis has been demonstrated, its role in the maintenance of penile flaccidity is not clearly defined. An important argument against an α-adrenergic mecha- nism in maintaining flaccidity of the penis is the observation that the intracavernosal injection of an α-adrenergic receptor blocker, in the absence of other stimuli, does not cause an erection. However, α-adren- ergic blockers are effective in prolonging the duration of an already established erection.

The peptide endothelin and some eicosanoids (PGF$_2\alpha$, thromboxane A$_2$) are candidates to participate in the maintenance of penile flaccid- ity. Endothelin-1 is a member of a family of three peptides, discovered in 1988 [10]. This peptide is a potent constrictor synthesized by the lacunar endothelium and, possibly, by the trabecular muscle itself [11, 12]. Its presence and constrictor activity in human cavernous tissue suggests the participation of this peptide in the regulation of trabecu- lar smooth muscle contractility. It has been also demonstrated that endothelin potentiates the constrictor effects of catecholamines on trabecular smooth muscle [13]. Two receptors for endothelin, ET$_A$ and ET$_B$, mediate the biological effects of endothelin in vascular tissue. ET$_A$ is the principal mediator of the contraction in response to endothelin, while ET$_B$ prevails in endothelium, mediating an endothelium-depend- ent vasodilator response. The mechanism of intracellular transduction for both receptors is the activation of the metabolism of inositol-phos- phate, with release of intracellular calcium and activation of protein kinase C (PKC). Several constrictor prostanoids, including PGH$_2$, PGF$_2\alpha$, and thromboxane A$_2$ (TXA$_2$), are synthesized by the human cavernous tissue. In vitro studies have demonstrated that prostanoids are respon- sible for the tone and the spontaneous activity of isolated trabecular muscle [14]. Also, it has been observed in vitro that constrictor prosta- glandins, simultaneously released with nitric oxide, attenuate the dilator effect of this substance [15]. The correlation of these in vitro findings with the physiological regulation in vivo is not yet established.

Penile Smooth Muscle Relaxation

Dilation of the penile arteries (cavernous artery and helicine arteries), is the first event in the development of erection. Its consequence is an increase of blood flow and pressure into the lacunar spaces. Following arterial dilation, the trabecular muscle relaxes, increasing the compliance of the lacunar spaces to its expansion and facilitating the accumulation of blood. The relaxation of the muscle depends on endocrine (circulating substances) and paracrine mechanisms (neurogenic and endothelial), and possibly on autocrine mechanisms (release of vasodilator substances generated in the muscle).

Role of Nitric Oxide and the cGMP Pathway

Nitric oxide (NO) is a free radical (the molecule has an electron in excess); therefore, it is a highly reactive and chemically unstable molecule. It is known now that this molecule is synthesized in different types of cells in mammals and that is a modulator of several biological activities including endothelium-dependent dilation of blood vessels, inhibition of platelet aggregation, and macrophage cytotoxic activity, and it also plays role as a neurotransmitter in the peripheral and central nervous system [16].

The constitutive forms of nitric oxide synthase (NOS), located in nerves (nNOS) and endothelium (eNOS), use the amino acid arginine and molecular oxygen to produce nitric oxide and the amino acid citrulline [17, 18]. This reaction requires a series of co-factors, among them NADPH, tetrahydrobiopterin, and calcium-activated calmodulin. The inducible form of this enzyme, whose expression in cells occurs after stimulation with cytokines, does not require calcium-activated calmodulin as a co-factor [17, 18]. While the constitutive isoforms of NOS have been identified in the cavernous body, the presence or the possible physiological role of the inducible form in this tissue is yet to be determined.

Unlike many other regulatory substances, such as the classic neurotransmitters (acetylcholine, noradrenaline) or growth factors, NC does
not have a specific receptor on the cellular membrane. NO crosses the
plasma membrane of the cells targeting the enzyme guanylate cyclase,
producing a conformational change in the molecule that increases its
activity. Activated guanylate cyclase catalyzes the conversion of guano-
sine-5"-triphosphate (GTP) to $3',5'$ cyclic guanosine monophosphate
(cGMP). The accumulation of cGMP sets in motion a cascade of events
at the intracellular level which induce a loss of contractile tone. These
include: hyperpolarization, closure of voltage-activated calcium channels, sequestration of calcium by intracellular organelles, decrease in
intracellular calcium, and, probably, changes in the affinity of the contractile apparatus for calcium (Fig. 2). There are many experiments that

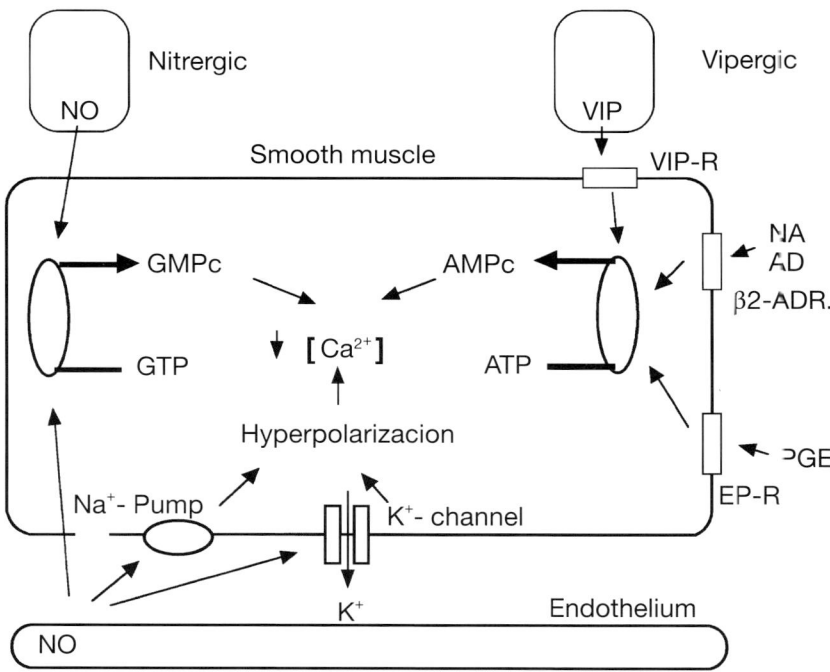

Fig. 2.   The three pathways that regulate penile smooth muscle relaxation: cGMP, cAMP,
and hyperpolarization. (*NA* noradrenaline, *AD* adrenaline, β_2-*ADR* = β_2-adrenergic receptor, *EP-R* prostaglandin E receptor, *VIP-R* vasoactive intestinal peptide receptor. *Na$^+$-
pump* Na$^+$-K$^+$-ATPase, *NO* nitric oxide)

demonstrate, in vivo and in vitro, an essential role for NO in the erection of the penis.

In Vitro Experiments

Exposure of cavernous tissue to acetylcholine (an endothelium-dependent vasodilator) or electrical stimulation of nonadrenergic noncholinergic dilator nerves causes accumulation of cGMP and the formation of nitrites, a product of the oxidation of NO [19, 20]. Neurogenic relaxation and endothelium-dependent relaxation are inhibited in the presence of NOS inhibitors (e.g., N^G-ethyl-methyl-L-arginine, N^G-nitro-L-arginine), inhibitors of the soluble isoform of the guanylate cyclase/superoxide-generating substances (methylene blue), and substances that, because of their high affinity for NO, are its scavengers (e.g., oxyhemoglobin) [19–21]. It has also been demonstrated that NO and NO donors are potent dilators of penile arteries and trabecular smooth muscle [19–22].

Immunohistochemical studies with anti-nNOS and anti-eNOS antibodies have demonstrated positive immunoreactivity in autonomic nerves and in the endothelium of arteries and trabecular tissue [23]. At the same time, autonomic nerves and the endothelium demonstrate positive NADPH-diaphorase activity, an enzymatic activity characteristic of NOS [23, 24]. Finally, considerable NOS enzymatic activity can be demonstrated, with the citrulline assay, in homogenates of corpus cavernosum tissue [21, 25].

In Vivo Studies

Studies with experimental animals have demonstrated that erection induced by electrical stimulation of the pelvic nerve/pelvic plexus or the sacral roots is blocked by the intravenous or intracavernosal administration of NOS inhibitors [26, 27]. It has been demonstrated as well that the intracavernosal administration of NO donors induces erection [28–30].

Despite this experimental evidence, a key role for NO in erection has recently been questioned, as transgenic mice lacking nNOS or the eNOS genes maintained their reproductive capacity [31, 32]. Nevertheless, reproduction being an essential biological function, it is possible that compensatory mechanisms are developed to correct for specific deficiencies. In support of this concept, it has been demonstrated that mice lacking nNOS overexpress the endothelial isoform of this enzyme (eNOS) in corpus cavernosum tissue. Also, in the penis, another transduction pathway exists for the relaxation of the smooth muscle, the one dependent on cAMP, that could compensate in part deficiencies in the NO/cGMP pathway.

The cAMPc Pathway

Vasoactive intestinal peptide (VIP) in the autonomic nerves, prostaglandin E (PGE_1 and PGE_2) synthesized by the smooth muscle, and neural or circulating catecholamines (norepinephrine and epinephrine), stimulate specific receptors coupled to Gs proteins with stimulation of the adenylate cyclase that catalyzes the formation of cAMP (Fig. 2). This is an efficient route for the relaxation of the smooth muscle of the penis, as demonstrated by the erectogenic effect of intracavernosal PGE_1 administered for the treatment of impotence. It is probable that the coordinated activation of both pathways, cGMP and cAMP, participates in the physiology of erection.

During the 1980s, great attention was given to VIP as the possible mediator of erection. This proposal was based on the observation of nerve fibers that contained VIP in cavernous tissue and the finding that exogenous VIP was a potent relaxant of the smooth muscle of the penis [33–35]. Furthermore, the intracavernosal administration of VIP caused tumescence and rigid erection in some individuals [36].

The discovery of the role of NO diverted the interest from VIP to the new molecule. Recently, the co-localization of VIP and nNOS in nerves within the corpus cavernosum was reported [37]. This has revived once more the concept of co-transmission in this tissue and the interest in VIP. The two molecules, VIP and NO, would induce relaxation in the muscle by two different and potentially synergistic pathways. Selective release of neurotransmitters depending on the stimulation frequency has been demonstrated. Thus, for example, NO would be released at low frequencies, while the largest release of VIP would occur with high frequencies. The precise physiological role of this modulation in the release of neurotransmitters in erection is not known. VIP receptors in the cavernous body are coupled to Gs proteins that stimulate the catalytic activity of adenylate cyclase with formation of cAMP.

Prostaglandis E_1 and E_2 are the most abundant prostanoids synthesized by the smooth muscle of the penis. It is not known if the endogenous prostanoids participate in the regulation of penile smooth muscle contractility, although preliminary evidence from our laboratory supports such a role for PGE. The receptor(s) that mediates relaxation to PGE is designated the EP receptor. The specific subtype, of the four that exist in the EP family, has not been determined. The EP_2 and EP_4 subtypes are the most likely candidates, since they are coupled to Gs proteins which stimulate adenylate cyclase.

Finally, the stimulation of β-adrenergic receptors by catecholamines causes relaxation of arterial and trabecular smooth muscle. The $β_2$ subtype is probably the most important receptor mediating these effects [38–40]. Adrenaline has a high affinity for this receptor, whose stimulation counteracts in part the constrictor effects of this catecholamine, which are mediated by α-adrenergic receptors. There is evidence in the vascular system that the expression of $β_2$-adrenergic receptors decreases with age; therefore, in the erectile tissue the constrictor mechanisms α-adrenergic) would progressively prevail.

Relaxation Through Hyperpolarization of the Muscular Cell

One of the mechanisms by which the cyclic nucleotides induce relaxation of the smooth muscle is through the opening of potassium channels, hyperpolarizing the cell. This effect on K^+ channels can be provoked by the cAMP-dependent protein kinase (PKA), by the cGMP-dependent protein kinase (PKG), or by GMPc itself. The activation of potassium channels (of the "maxi-K^+" type) by the action of the PGE_1, an effect mediated by AMPc, has been demonstrated [41]. It has also been demonstrated that relaxation of penile arteries is inhibited, in part, upon blocking of calcium-dependent K^+ channels [22]. Hyperpolarization causes the closure of voltage-dependent calcium channels, therefore reducing the calcium entry from the extracellular compartment, with a decrease in the concentration of intracellular free calcium and subsequent relaxation of the muscle.

Independently of this mechanism, provoked by the action of the cyclic nucleotides, it has been proposed that in arteries, NO can stimulate directly the opening of potassium channels as well as the sodium-potassium ATPase (the sodium pump). This last mechanism has been demonstrated in the trabecular muscle [42] (Fig. 2). The sodium-potassium ATPase pump is electrogenic due to the fact that it extracts three positive charges from the cell while introducing only two. Therefore, the cell hyperpolarizes, initiating the same mechanisms of closure of calcium channels described after the activation of K^+ channels. This process therefore represents a mechanism for relaxation that does not depend on cyclic nucleotides.

Regulation of the Balance Between the Dilator and Constrictor Mechanisms

Cholinergic Nerves

Erection is initiated by a sacral parasympathetic nerve input, the preganglionic neurotransmitter of which is acetylcholine. Because of this fact, it was initially assumed that postganglionic cholinergic nerves were the direct mediators of penile smooth muscle relaxation. As already explained above, it is now known that the relaxation of the smooth muscle is mediated by one or more nonadrenergic, noncholinergic (NANC) neurotransmitters. Nevertheless, cholinergic nerves are present in the cavernous body and seem to have a modulator role on the other neuroeffector systems. Adrenergic nerves receive inhibitory interneuronal cholinergic modulation. The interaction of acetylcholine with muscarinic receptors in the adrenergic nerves reduces their release of noradrenaline [5, 43]. This prejunctional regulation, therefore, would favor erection through the decrease of constrictor adrenergic tone. Cholinergic nerves also seem to modulate NANC nerves, but in this case they facilitate or potentiate the vasodilator response mediated by these nerves [43]. The specific underlying mechanism of this facilitation remains unidentified. In summary, cholinergic activity in the cavernous body would have a modulatory role facilitating erection, on the one hand reducing constrictor tone (adrenergic) and on the other facilitating NANC-mediated relaxation.

Regulation of the Adrenergic Activity by Prostanoids

The precise physiological role of the endogenous prostanoids has not been clearly established. Prostacyclin, the most abundant prostanoid in the cavernous tissue, is produced by the endothelium and participates, probably together with the nitric oxide, in the regulation of homeostasis between the trabecular wall and the blood. E prostaglandins (E_1 and E_2) are the most abundant prostanoids synthesized by the cavernous muscle. In addition to their role as relaxants of trabecular muscle, previously mentioned, and as regulators of collagen synthesis [44], the PGEs modulate adrenergic nerves through a prejunctional mechanism. It has been demonstrated in human cavernous tissue that PGE_1 inhibits the release of noradrenaline by adrenergic nerves [45]. E prostaglandins, therefore promote erection by their direct relaxing effect in the muscle and indirectly by reduction of adrenergic tone. Certain prostanoids such as PGD_2 have the opposite effect, since they facilitate the release of noradrenaline by adrenergic nerves [45].

Adrenergic Regulation of NANC Nerves

In intracavernosal arteries from experimental animals, prejunctional regulation of NANC nerves by α_2-adrenergic receptors has been demonstrated. The activation of these adrenergic receptors inhibits vasodilation induced by NANC nerves [46]. This regulation suggests that termination of the erection by the increased adrenergic activity would have two components: one direct, constrictor, on the smooth muscle, mediated by α_1 and α_2 receptors and other one indirect, in which the vasodilator effect of NANC nerves is inhibited by a prejunctional, α_2-adrenergic-mediated mechanism.

Molecular Oxygen as a Modulator of Penile Erection

The partial oxygen pressure (pO_2) in the blood of the cavernous body during the flaccid state is similar to that of venous blood (≈ 35 mm Hg). However, during an erection, due to the increase in arterial blood entering the lacunar spaces, the pO_2 increases to approximately 100 mm

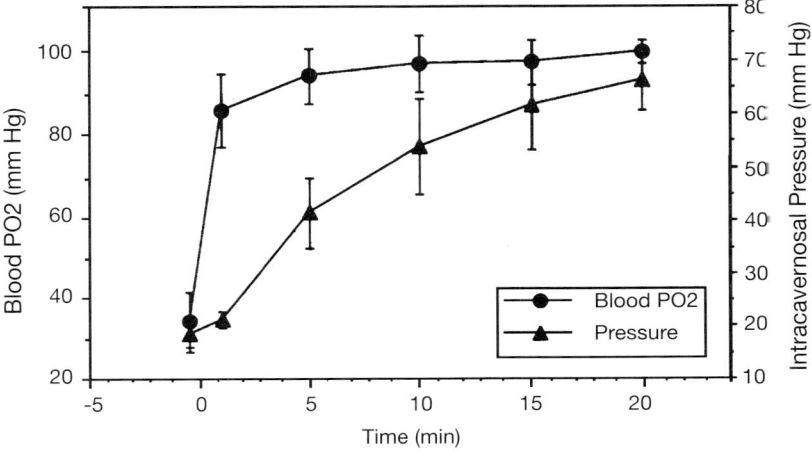

Fig. 3. Simultaneous determination of oxygen tension *(filled circles)* and intracavernosal pressure in flaccidity *(time 0)* and during erection, over time *(filled triangles)*. Graph represents the mean response in a group of ten patients who underwent intracavernosal injection of papaverine-phentolamine. In flaccidity pO$_2$ is similar to that of venous blood; after intracavernosal injection pO$_2$ increases to arterial levels that are maintained for the duration of erection

Hg (i.e., the corpora cavernosa are arterialized) [25] (Fig. 3). Molecular oxygen is a substrate, together with L-arginine, for the synthesis of NO mediated by NOS. In corpus cavernosum tissue, it has been demonstrated that the synthesis of NO is directly regulated by the oxygen concentration [25]. At the low oxygen concentrations that are measured in the cavernous body of the flaccid penis, the synthesis of NO is profoundly inhibited, therefore, blocking, endothelium and neurogenic relaxation of the trabecular muscle. This would help in the maintenance of penile flaccidity since it facilitates constrictor tone by suppressing relaxation.

After arterial vasodilatation, the oxygen concentration in the cavernous bodies rises providing sufficient substrate (O$_2$) for the synthesis of NO. It has been estimated, following in vitro studies, that the minimal concentration of oxygen in the cavernous bodies necessary to reach full activity of the NO synthase is between 50 and 60 O mm Hg. Inferior concentrations would induce a partial synthesis of NO with subsequent partial relaxation of the trabecular muscle. Similar, to the NO synthase,

Fig. 4. Effect of various oxygen tensions on the production of prostacyclin (*6-keto-PGF$_{1\alpha}$ is the stable metabolite of PGI$_2$ in rabbit corpus cavernosum tissue). Prostacyclin synthesis is almost completely inhibited when the corpus cavernosum is exposed to venous-like oxygen tensions

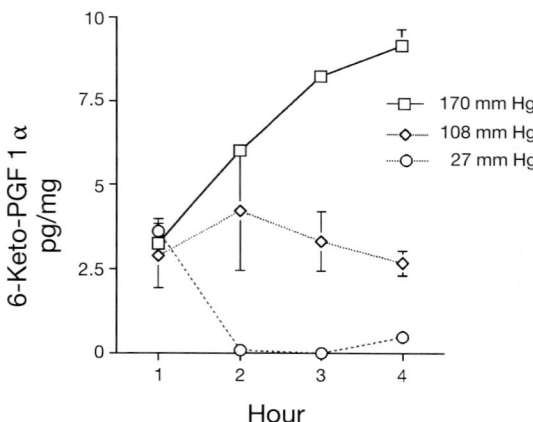

the prostaglandin H synthase (cyclo-oxygenase) is also an oxygenase and uses oxygen as substrate for the synthesis of prostanoids. It has been demonstrated that the oxygen concentration to which the cavernous bodies are exposed regulates the synthesis of prostanoids [47] (Fig. 4). In the case of PGE, the relaxing prostaglandin of the trabecular muscle, physiological variations in the oxygen concentration will condition its endogenous production: it is inhibited in flaccidity and stimulated in erection.

The synthesis of the vasoconstrictor endothelin is also subject to modulation by the oxygen concentration. In this case low oxygen concentrations promote its synthesis and high levels (arterial) inhibit it. This capacity of the molecular oxygen for regulating the synthesis of endogenous vasoactive substances make it an important modulator of the erectile activity of the penis.

Pharmacology of Commonly used Intracavernosal Drug

Papaverine

Activity and Kinetics. Papaverine is derived from *Papaver somniferum*, the opium plant, and is a nonselective inhibitor of phosphodiesterases [48, 49]. Three isoenzymes have been identified in human corpus cavernosum: types III, IV, and V of the seven that constitute the family of phosphodiesterases [50]. Therefore, papaverine is able to potentiate the accumulation of cGMP and cAMP after the activation of guanylate cyclase and adenylate cyclase, respectively.

It has been demonstrated in the tracheal smooth muscle that papaverine inhibits (closes) L-type voltage-dependent calcium channels [51]. It is possible that this mechanism also contributes to the relaxation of the penile smooth muscle. In vitro, papaverine relaxes trabecular and arterial muscle of cavernosal and helicine arteries. Since the main activity of papaverine is to amplify a signal facilitating relaxation, its activity may be limited if the signal is small. Therefore, if there is a deficiency in the synthesis or availability of nitric oxide, or in the mechanisms that activate adenylate cyclase (VIP, β-adrenergic receptors, or the EP receptors for the PGE), papaverine may not be effective in inducing erection. Papaverine has a short half-life in plasma, from 1 to 2 h, and is metabolized in the liver. Papaverine is not metabolized in the cavernous body and reaches a maximum concentration in plasma 30 min after intracavernosal administration [52].

Toxicity. Papaverine can cause arterial hypotension and hepatic toxicity. The elevation of hepatic enzymes in patients treated with papaverine is frequent, especially when it is used in high doses as a single drug; therefore, it is advisable to perform periodic biochemical controls. Nevertheless, the incidence of papaverine-induced hepatitis is less than 1/1000, and the described increase in liver enzymes is usually resolved upon stopping treatment with papaverine [53].

Local complications include a high incidence of priapism and fibrosis. The lack of local metabolism is thought to contribute to the high incidence of priapism, and the acidity of the solution ($\approx$ pH 3.0) probably contributes to the tissue damage that leads to fibrosis [53]. Nevertheless, the damage attributed to acidity is not, in the opinion of other authors, the cause of the fibrosis associated with the papaverine, but is attributed to the intrinsic characteristics of this molecule.

Formulation. Papaverine solutions have great stability, decaying less than 10% within 4 years at ambient temperature. It has been observed that solutions using saline (0.9% NaCl) tend to show a precipitate with time; this does not occur when a 5% glucose solution is used [54].

Phentolamine

Activity and Kinetics. Belonging to the group of imidazolines, phentolamine is a competitive antagonist of α-adrenergic receptors, with a similar affinity for the α_1 and α_2 subtypes(Fig. 2). Some additional effects of phentolamine have been described, including blockade of serotonin receptors and blockade of potassium channels [52]. Nevertheless, these effects have not been studied in the penile smooth muscle. An additional indirect effect of phentolamine is that, as it blocks all α-adrenergic receptors, circulating catecholamines or those released by the adrenergic nerves have available only β-adrenergic receptors (β_2 for the most part), which facilitate relaxation of the smooth muscle of the penis. This would explain, in part, the synergy between phentolamine and papaverine, since the stimulation of the β-adrenergic receptors activates adenylate cyclase, with the production of cAMP. Papaverine would potentiate this effect by inhibiting the degradation of this cyclic nucleotide.

Phentolamine has a half-life of 30 min, considerably shorter than phenoxybenzamine [52]. Following its intracavernosal injection, a maximum serum concentration is reached at 30 min, diminishing quickly to undetectable levels [52].

Toxicity. Although the intracavernosal injection of phentolamine may be accompanied by arterial hypotension and tachycardia, it is a well-tolerated drug. Normally, it is not used as a single drug but in combination with papaverine, with PGE_1, or with both. For this reason, little is known about its specific contribution to the local toxicity. Nevertheless, the improvement by phentolamine of the erectile response induced by papaverine or PGE_1 makes it possible to reduce the concentration of these substances and potentially their toxicity.

Formulation. Solutions of phentolamine hydrochloride or mesylate are stable at room temperature. It has been demonstrated that solutions with papaverine or PGE_1 or both, protected from the light and at cool temperature (when there is PGE_1), are stable for months [54]. The usual concentration of phentolamine in the mixtures is 0.5–1 mg/ml.

Alprostadil

Activity and Kinetics. Alprostadil is the synthetic form of prostaglandin E_1, a natural prostanoid synthesized from dihomo-g-lynoleic acid, a membrane phospholipid [55]. The prostanoids of the E series (E_1 and E_2) are the ones most abundantly synthesized by trabecular muscle and the only prostanoids that cause its relaxation. Considering that prostacyclin (PGI_2) does not cause relaxation of the trabecular muscle, although it does cause relaxation of the arterial muscle, it is most probable that the relaxation induced by PGE_1 is mediated by a specific receptor for prostaglandin E (the EP receptors). As discussed above, the EP_2 and the EP_4 receptors are the most likely candidates for mediating relaxation to PGE_1.

The intracellular mediator for relaxing response to the PGE_1 is cAMP. Through the activation of multiple regulatory mechanisms for the homeostasis of intracellular Ca^{2+}, either directly by cAMP or by the cAMP-dependent protein kinase, a decrease in the concentration of this ion is produced, which favors relaxation. Also, it is probable that interactions between calcium-calmodulin-contractile proteins are modified, facilitating the loss of contractile tone.

In addition to these direct actions on the muscle, as discussed above, PGE_1 reduces the adrenergic constrictor tone by inhibiting the release of noradrenaline through prejunctional receptors in adrenergic nerve endings [45]. The combination of these effects would explain the high efficacy of this molecule in the treatment of impotence when it is used as a single drug.

The half-life of PGE_1 in plasma is very short, less than 1 min, due to the action of 15-hydroxy-PGE_1 dehydrogenase [55, 56]. At a systemic level, metabolism occurs principally in the lung, 60–80% during the first pass by the pulmonary circulation. In 1991, an alternative metabolic route was discovered in which 15-oxo-PG-reductase intervened, with formation of PGE_0 (13, 14, dehydro-PGE_1) [57]. This route is important, since PGE_0 has biological activity and is considerably more stable than PGE_1. Therefore, it is possible that PGE_0 is partly responsible for the therapeutic effects attributed to PGE_1.

Human cavernous body tissue contains 15-hydroxy-dehydrogenase activity, suggesting the possibility of local metabolism (intracavernosal) of PGE_1. One study on the kinetics of PGE_1 administered by the intracavernosal route demonstrates local intracavernosal metabolism of this molecule [58]. This perhaps explains the low incidence of priapism with PGE_1.

Formulation. Alprostadil is supplied as a sterile lyophilized powder, that is reconstituted with saline. The lyophilized substance contains lactose and sodium citrate (which require refrigeration) or alpha cyclodextrin (which can be stored at room temperature).

References

1. Christ GJ (1995) The penis as a vascular organ. The importance of corporal smooth muscle tone in the control of erection. Urol Clin North Am 22 (4): 727
2. Steers WD (1994) Smooth muscle physiology. AUA Update Series Less 30
3. Hai CM, Murphy RA (1988) Crossbridge phosphorylation and regulation of the latch state in smooth muscle. Am J Physiol 255: C86
4. Hedlund H, Andersson K-E (1985) Comparison of responses to drugs acting on adrenoceptors and muscarinic receptors in human isolated corpus cavernosum and cavernous artery. J Auton Pharmacol 5: 81
5. Saenz de Tejada I, Kim N, Lagan I, Krane RJ, Goldstein I (1989) Modulation of adrenergic activity in penile corpus cavernosum. J Urol 142: 1117
6. Traish AM, Netsuwan N, Daley JT, Padma-Nathan H, Goldstein I, Saenz de Tejada I (1995) A heterogeneous population of alpha 1 adrenergic receptors mediates contraction of human corpus cavernosum smooth muscle to norepinephrine. J Urol 153: 222
7. Saenz de Tejada I, Moroukian P, Tessier J, Kim JJ, Goldstein I, Frohrib D (1991) The trabecular smooth muscle modulates the capacitor function of the penis. Studies on a rabbit model. Am J Physiol 260 (Heart and Cir Physiol 29): H1590
8. Hatzichristou DG, Saenz de Tejada I, Kupferman S, Namburi S, Pescatori ES, Udelson D, Goldstein I (1995) In vivo assessment of trabecular smooth muscle tone, its application in pharmaco-cavernosometry and analysis of intracavernous pressure determinants. J Urol 153: 1126
9. Fournier GR, Jünemann K-P, Lue TF, Tanagho EA (1987) Mechanisms of veno-occlusion during canine penile erection: An anatomic demonstration. J Urol 137: 163
10. Inoue K, Yanagisawa M, Kimura S, Kasuya Y, Miyauchi T, Goto K, Masaki T (1989) The human endothelin family: three structurally and pharmacologically distinct isopeptides predicted by three separate genes. Proc Natl Acad Sci USA 86: 2863
11. Saenz de Tejada I, Carson MP, de las Morenas A, Goldstein I, Traish AM (1991) Endothelin: Localization, synthesis, activity and receptor types in the human penile corpus cavernosum. Am J Physiol 261 (Heart Circ Physiol 30): H1078
12. Holmquist F, Andersson K-E, Hedlund H (1990) Actions of endothelin on isolated corpus cavernosum from rabbit and man. Acta Physiol Scand 39: 113
13. Christ GJ, Lerner SE, Kim DC, Melman A (1995) Endothelin-1 as a putative modulator of erectile dysfunction: I. Characteristics of contraction of isolated corporal tissue strips. J Urol 153: 1998
14. Christ GJ, Maayani S, Valcic M, Melman A (1990) Pharmacological studies of human erectile tissue: Characteristic of spontaneous contractions and alteration in

α-adrenoceptor responsiveness with age and disease in isolated tissues. Br J Pharmacol 101: 375

15. Azadzoi KM, Kim N, Brown ML, Goldstein I, Cohen RA, Saenz de Tejada I (1992) Modulation of penile corpus cavernosum smooth muscle tone by endothelium-derived nitric oxide and cyclooxygenase products. J Urol 47: 220

16. Moncada S, Palmer RMJ, Higgs EA (1991) Nitric oxide: physiology, pathophysiology and pharmacology. Pharmacol Rev 43: 109

17. Moncada S (1992) The L-arginine-nitric oxide pathway. The 1991 Ulf von Euler Lecture. Acta Physiol Scand 145: 201

18. Moncada S, Palmer RMJ, Higgs EA (1989) Biosynthesis of nitric oxide from L-arginine. Biochem Pharmacol 38: 1709

19. Ignarro LJ, Bush PA, Buga GM, Wood KS, Fukoto JM, Rajfer J (1990) Nitric oxide and cyclic GMP formation upon electrical stimulation cause relaxation of corpus cavernosum smooth muscle. Biochem Biophys Res Commun 170: 843

20. Kim N, Azadzoi KM, Goldstein I, Saenz de Tejada I (1991) A nitric oxide-like factor mediates nonadrenergic noncholinergic neurogenic relaxation of penile smooth muscle. J Clin Invest 88: 112

21. Holmquist F, Andersson K-E, Hedlund H (1992) Characterization of inhibitory neurotransmission in the isolated corpus cavernosum from the rabbit and man. J Physiol Lond 449: 295

22. Simonsen U, Prieto D, Saenz de Tejada I, Garcia-Sacristan A (1995) Involvement of nitric oxide in non-adrenergic non-cholinergic neurotransmission of horse deep penile arteries: Role of charybdotoxin-sensitive K+-channels. Br J Pharmacol 116, 2582

23. Burnett AL, Tillman SL, Chang TSK, Epstein JI, Lowenstein CJ, Bredt DS, Snyder SH, Walsh PC (1993) Immunohistochemical localization of nitric oxide synthase in the autonomic innervation of the human penis. J Urol 150: 73

24. Keast JR (1992) A possible neural source of nitric oxide in the rat penis. Neurosci Lett 143: 69

25. Kim N, Vardi Y, Padma-Nathan H, Daley J, Goldstein I, Saenz de Tejada I (1993) Oxygen tension regulates the nitric oxide pathway: Physiological role in penile erection. J Clin Invest 91: 437

26. Holmquist F, Stief CG, Jonas U, Andersson K-E (1991) Effects of the nitric oxide synthase inhibitor NG-nitro-L-arginine on the erectile response to cavernous nerve stimulation in the rabbit. Acta Physiol Scand 143: 299

27. Burnett AL, Lowenstein CJ, Bredt DS, Chang TSK, Snyder SH (1992) Nitric oxide: a physiologic mediator of penile erection. Science 257: 401

28. Porst H (1993) Prostaglandin E1 and the nitric oxide donor linsidomine for erectile failure: a diagnostic comparative study of 40 patients. J Urol 149: 1280

29. Wang R, Domer FR, Sikka SC, Kadowitz PJ, Hellstrom WJG (1994) Nitric oxide mediates penile erection in cats. J Urol 151: 234

30. Hellstrom WJG, Monga M, Wang R, Domer FR, Kadowitz PJ, Roberts JA (1994) Penile erection in the primate: induction with nitric oxide donors. J Urol 151: 1723

31. Huang PL, Huang Z, Mashimo H, Bloch KD, Moskowitz MA, Bevan JA, Fishman MC (1995) Hypertension in mice lacking the gene for endothelial nitric oxide synthase. Nature 377: 239

32. Huang PL, Dawson TM, Bredt D, Snyder SH, Fishman MC (1993) Target discription of the neuronal nitric oxide synthese gene. Cell (United States), Dec. 31 1993, 75(7) p 1273–1286

33. Larsen JJ, Ottesen B, Fahrenkrug J, Fahrenkrug L (1981) Vasoactive intestinal polypeptide (VIP) in the male genito-urinary tract, concentration and motor effect. Invest Urol 19: 211

34. Larsson LI, Fahrenkrug J, Schaffalitzky de Muckadell OB (1977) Occurrence of nerves containing vasoactive intestinal polypeptide immunoreactivity in the male genital tract. Life Sci 21: 503

35. Hedlund H, Andersson K-E (1985) Effects of some peptides on isolated human penile erectile tissue and cavernous artery. Acta Physiol Scand 124: 413

36. Ottesen B, Wagner G, Virag R, Fahrenkrug J (1984) Penile erection: Possible role for vasoactive intestinal polypeptide as a neurotransmitter. Br Med J 288: 9

37. Ehmke H, Jünemann K-P, Mayer B, Kummer W (1995) Nitric oxide synthase and vasoactive intestinal polypeptide colocalization in neurons innervating the human penile circulation. Int J Impotence Res 7: 147

38. Dhabuwala CB, Ramakrishna VR, Anderson GF (1985) Beta-adrenergic receptors in human cavernous tissue. J Urol 133: 721

39. Carati CJ, Goldie RG, Warton A, Henry PJ, Keogh EJ (1985) Pharmacology of the erectile tissue of the canine penis. Pharmacol Res Commun 17: 951

40. Hedlund H, Andersson K-E (1985) Comparison of the responses to drugs acting on adrenoceptors and muscarinic receptors in human isolated corpus cavernosum and cavernous artery. J Autonomic Pharmacol 5: 81

41. Christ GJ, Brink PR, Brook S, Ney P (1996) PGE1-induced alterations in maxi-K^+-channel activity in cultured human corporal smooth muscle cells. J Urol 155: 678A (abstract# 1468)

42. Gupta S, Moreland RB, Munarriz R, Daley J, Goldstein I, Saenz de Tejada I (1995) Possible role of Na^+-K^+ ATPase in the regulation of human corpus cavernosum smooth muscle contractility by nitric oxide. Br J Pharmacol 116: 2201

43. Saenz de Tejada I, Blanco R, Goldstein I, Azadzoi K, de las Morenas A, Krane RJ, Cohen RA (1988) Cholinergic neurotransmission in human corpus cavernosum. I. Responses of isolated tissue. Am J Physiol (Heart Circ Physiol 23): H459

44. Moreland RB, Traish A, McMillin, Smith B, Goldstein I, Saenz de Tejada I (1995) PGE$_1$ suppresses the induction of collagen synthesis by transforming growth factor-β1 in human corpus cavernosum smooth muscle. J Urol 153: 826

45. Molderings GJ, Gothert M, Van Ahlen H, Porst H (1992) Modulation of noradrenaline release in human corpus cavernosum by presynaptic prostaglandin receptors. Int J Impotence Res 4: 19

46. Simonsem Ulf. Personal communication

47. Daley JT, Brown ML, Watkins MT, Traish AM, Huang Yue-Hua, Moreland RB, Saenz de Tejada I (1996) Prostanoid production in rabbit corpus cavernosum: I. Regulation by oxygen tension. J Urol 155: 1482

48. Ferrari, M (1974) Effects of papaverine on smooth muscle and their mechanisms. Pharmacol Res Commun 6: 97

49. Poch G, Kukovetz WR (1971) Papaverine-induced inhibition of phosphodiesterase activity in various mammalian tissues. Life Sci 10: 133

50. Taher A, Meyer M, Schulz-Knappe P, Forssmann W, Stief CG, Jonas U (1993) Phosphodiesterase activity in human cavernous tissue and the effect of various selective inhibitors. J Urol 149: 285A (abstract # 285)

51. Iguchi M, Naakajima T, Hisada T, Sugimoto T, Kurachi Y (1992) On the mechanism of papaverine inhibition of the voltage-dependent Ca++ current in isolated smooth muscle cells from the guinea pig trachea. J Pharmacol Exp Ther 263: 194

52. Hakenberg O, Wetterauer U, Koppermann U, Luhmann R (1990) Systemic pharmacokinetics of papaverine and phentolamine: Comparison of intravenous and intracavernous application. Int J Impotence Res 2: 247

53. Hedlund H (1993) Pharmacology of PGE$_1$ and other agents. In: Goldstein I, Lue T (eds) Role of alprostadil in the diagnosis and treatment of erectile dysfunction. Excerpta Medica, Inc. Princeton, NJ, p 17

54. Torrado-Valeiras JJ, Montaner J, Torrado-Duran JJ (1991) Preparación, análisis y estabilidad físico-química de una mezcla de fentolamina con papaverina para la administración parenteral. An R Acad Farm 57: 547

55. Porst H (1996) The rationale for prostaglandin E1 in erectile failure: a survey of worldwide experience. J Urol 155: 802

56. Roy AC, Adaikan PG, Sen DK, Ratnam SS (1989) Prostaglandin 15-hydroxydehydrogenase activity in human penile corpora cavernosa and its significance in prostaglandin-mediated penile erection. Br J Urol 64: 180

57. Peskar BA, Hesse WH, Rogatti W, Diehm C, Rudofsky G, Schweer H, Seyberth HW (1991) Formation of 13, 14-dihydroprostaglandin E$_1$ during intravenous infusions of prostaglandin E$_1$ in patients with peripheral arterial occlusive disease. Prostaglandins 41: 225

58. van Ahlen H, Peskar BA, Sticht G, Hertfelder H-J (1994) Pharmacokinetics of vasoactive substances administered into the human corpus cavernosum. J Urol 151: 1227

Current Status of Noninvasive Pharmacological Therapy for Erectile Dysfunction

A. Morales and J. P. W. Heaton

The enormous success achieved by vasoactive intracavernosal therapy for erectile failure has precluded, in many ways, more emphasis and development in the search for non-invasive approaches. Only recently we have began to see some clear paths for clinical application for the oral and transcutaneous routes. It is very likely that oral medication will never be effective beyond those cases in which the physiological mechanisms of erection in the penis are either intact or only mildly affected by disease. It is reasonable to assume that severe penile abnormalities may respond to intracavernosal injections or vacuum devices while the worst cases will remain candidates for prosthetic implants and a few will be candidates for vascular surgery.

Erectolytic Agents

During history taking, it is essential to know the drugs that the patient may be taking since many are known to interfere with erectile function. After all, impotence coexists, not uncommonly, with other conditions requiring medication. Recreational erectolytic agents include tobacco, alcohol, cannabis, LSD and cocaine. Iatrogenic erectolytic agents include the following:

- Hormonal, e.g., estrogens, antiandrogens, luteinizing hormone-releasing hormone (LHRH) analogues, 5-α reductase inhibitors
- Antihypertensives, e.g., diuretics, β-blockers, methyldopa, CA^{2+} antagonists
- Psychotropics, e.g., major tranquilizers, monoamine oxidase (MAO) inhibitors, tricyclic antidepressants
- Others, e.g., histamine receptor antagonists, antihyperlipidemics)

Many additional drugs have been implicated, but consistent evidence is lacking.

Erectogenic Drugs

The ideal pharmacological agent for the treatment of impotence should exhibit the following characteristics:

1. Effective
2. Useful "on demand"
3. Free of side effects
4. Easy to administer (oral or topical)
5. Affordable

Such miracle drug has not been invented, although for some cases of hypogonadism and for patients with hyperprolactinemia, noninvasive, effective treatment is available. The next few pages will summarize the current state of knowledge on recognized medications and on those with initial promising results and which may become available for clinical use. A few, not readily available, will be mentioned for the sake of completeness.

Hormones

Testosterone

Hypogonadism is not a common cause of erectile dysfunction; it is, however, the easiest one to document and treat if the physician is familiar with the biochemical parameters and the handling and consequences of the various testosterone preparations available. Supplemental androgens should be supplied exclusively to men with biochemical documentation of hypogonadism or those with the sequelae of advanced age in whom hypotestosteronemia may be the cause. There is no evidence that supplemental testosterone (T) is of any benefit to eugonadal men. On the contrary, the evidence suggest that impotent men with normal or only marginally low levels of serum T are poor responders to exogenous

Table 1. Commercially available testosterone preparations

Preparation	Advantages	Disadvantages
Injectable esters (cypionate, enanthate, propionate)	Well tolerated, effective, universally recommended, approximately monthly administration	I.M. injection, "roller-coaster" effect, tachyphylaxis
Methyl testosterone	Oral administration	Limited effectiveness, serious liver toxicity
Testosterone undecanoate	Equivalent to I.M. esters, no "roller-coaster effect," oral administration	Administration T.I.D. costly
Transdermal T	Easy to use, circadian curve	Daily application, scrotal shaving (for some preparations)

androgenic steroids. Profound hypogonadism offers the best opportunity for success. The practical pros and cons of commonly used preparations are summarized in Table 1.

The use of supplemental androgens is aimed at achieving physiological levels of T in plasma. Nevertheless, a number of concerns exist about the safety of administering supplemental T to a population of men usually over 50 years of age. They include changes in body composition, bone metabolism, lipid profile, and hematological and biochemical parameters. Early studies have shown that testosterone supplementation in aging males results in an increase in erythropoiesis and lean body mass. More recent studies by Tenover [1] have confirmed these findings, but have further shown that patients receiving exogenous T exhibit a significant decline in total cholesterol and low density lipoprotein cholesterol. Her observations have been further supported by Friedl et al. [2], Marin et al. [3], and Barret-Connor [4]. In addition, the recent study by Phillips et al. [5] investigated parameters of sex hormones and their influence in the occurrence of myocardial infarction (MI) showed that "the correlations found in this study between testosterone and the degree of coronary artery disease and between testosterone and other risk factors for MI raise the possibility that in men hypotestosteronemia may be a risk factor for coronary arteriosclerosis." Therefore, the currently available evidence does not support concerns about negative effects on lipid profile for patients receiving exogenous T supplementation.

Perhaps the most frequent concerns about supplemental androgen therapy relates to its effects on the prostate gland. There is a serious body of information on which to base an opinion in this regard. Experimental evidence has been presented showing that canine prostatic epithelial cells cultured in vitro in the presence or absence of several sex steroids exhibit the same growth pattern regardless whether steroids are present or not. The same studies demonstrated that the proliferative response was dependent on the time and concentration of serum. Therefore, these investigators [6] concluded that humoral factors, other than steroids may be of importance in the activation of epithelial cells leading to the development of prostatic hyperplasia. Franchi and Kicovic [7] in an 11-month study found no increase in prostatic size or deterioration of voiding symptoms, but their evaluation was primarily subjective. More recent studies also employing testosterone undecanoate (TU) help to clarify the picture. Holmang et al. [8] again found no significant increase in serum prostate specific antigen (PSA) during 8 months of treatment, while Gooren [9] documented a mild reduction in urine flow but no increase in prostate size and no evidence of cancer development. A recently published investigation by Behre et al. [10] has shed a great deal of light in our perception of the role of exogenous T on the prostate gland. In this large and well designed study hypogonadal men not previously treated with T were compared with age matched hypogonadic and normal men. The authors concluded that "effective testosterone treatment of hypogonadic men results in prostate volume and prostatic specific antigen levels comparable to age matched normal men. Therefore, testosterone-induced prostate growth should not preclude hypogonadal men from testosterone substitution therapy." Short-term clinical studies in aging men treated with injectable testosterone enanthate (100 mg every 3 weeks for 3 months) did not induce a significant increase in prostate size or the amount of post-void residual but there was a significant increase in PSA, which, however, remained within normal limits [1]. The oral undecanoate form of T has been evaluated in long-term clinical trials. In a controlled study it was found to result in a modest (12%), but statistically significant increase in the gland volume but no changes in the values of serum PSA between the pre-, peri-, and post-treatment readings [3]. The discrepancies in findings between these two studies go beyond the differences between the forms of T used.

Marin et al. [3] treated the patients for a longer period of time, had the PSA samples positioned next to each other in the assay run and performed the volumetric evaluation of the gland by transrectal ultrasonography. Tenover [1], on the other hand, determined the PSA values as they were obtained and the volumetric measures were performed by suprapubic transvesical sonography. These and other studies are reassuring but not conclusive as to the safety of supplemental T on the biological behavior of the gland. Controlled studies with larger cohorts and long periods of treatment and follow-up are mandatory to elucidate these important issues [11].

The serious attention given to hepatic toxicity (cholestatic hepatitis and hepatic carcinoma) is based on the well-documented cases in whom steroids with a 17α-methyl substituent were employed [12, 13]. Multiple studies have shown that the risk is minimal with the chronic use of the injectable esters or the oral undecanoate preparation [14, 15].

For physicians treating men with erectile dysfunction, it is important to be familiar with the individual merits and drawbacks of the currently available T preparations when treating hypogonadic patients. The most acceptable to the patients are the oral compounds. Of these, methyl-T requires repeated daily administration, results in supraphysiological levels of circulating total T (tT) with dissociated values of free T (fT) [14]. Its major drawbacks include erratic absorption [15] and the previously mentioned hepatic toxicity. TU also requires daily doses at 8-h intervals, results in more physiological levels of both serum tT and fT. Its lymphatic absorption requires it to be ingested with meals; this circumvents the first hepatic passage thus preventing liver toxicity and rapid aromatization. In our experience, it produces better subjective responses than its methyl counterpart. Both oral forms offer the advantage of a stable levels of serum T, thus preventing the ups and downs frequently observed with the injectable esters. Testosterone patches are relatively new and represent an appealing concept. In an investigation of four patients, McClure et al. [16] reported that their use achieved normal levels of both T and dihydrotestosterone (DHT), resulted in no hepatic toxicity and there were no appreciable changes in the lipid profile although the high density lipoproteins decreased slightly; this was a short study of 12 weeks. Longer studies using the transdermal administration confirm the safety of these preparations [17]. The application of a patch results in a physiological curve of serum T that imitates the circadian serum levels of the hormone. Drawbacks of the transdermal testosterone use include the need for daily application, for some formulations to the scrotal skin where the absorption of the drug is particularly effective and the need to shave the area frequently in order to facilitate its transdermal delivery. More recent preparations do not require scrotal application.

T injectable esters were recommended as the only acceptable form by the panel of the Consensus Conference on Impotence [18]. This view, of course, was based on concerns about the toxicity of some oral preparations and disregard for new forms of delivery. The injectable drugs (cypionate, enanthate or propionate) are generally well tolerated and remain the gold standard for effectiveness. Drawbacks of this preparations include the need for periodic intramuscular administration (every 2–3 weeks), the high activity observed in the first 10 days after administration which is followed by a noticeable decrease towards the end of the cycle [19]. Patients find this "roller-coaster" effect disturbing and unpleasant.

If, after a 3-month course of supplemental T, there is no response, other causes for the erectile difficulties should be ruled out diligently.

Hyperprolactinemia

Hyperprolactinemia is a rare cause of impotence and frequently it is associated with hypogonadism. After documentation of persistent high levels of serum prolactin (with or without evidence of a prolactinoma by magnetic resonance imaging, MRI), the initial treatment involves the oral administration of prolactin inhibitors.

Obviously, extrapituitary causes should be sought diligently and treated accordingly. The preferred management of prolactinomas remain controversial and, in large part depends on the expertise available at the treating institution.

Surgical Treatment.   Transsphenoidal microsurgery is an effective approach for the treatment of microprolactinomas resulting in long term remissions although recurrences of the tumor are likely [20]. Limited success is reported with this procedure in the treatment of large (> 1.5 cm) tumors. Transfrontal craniotomy is rarely employed and reserved for patients with major extrasellar extension of the tumor resulting in dangerous compression of adjacent structures (optic chiasma, internal carotid artery) (Fig. 1).

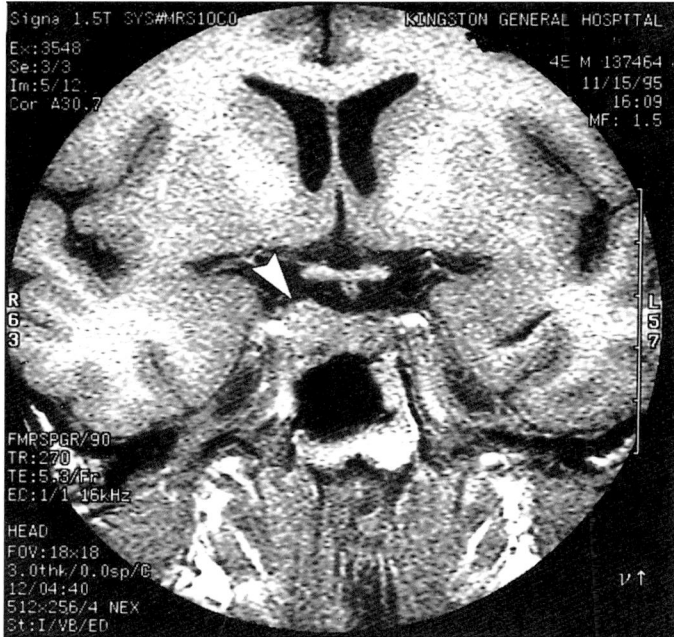

Fig. 1.   Magnetic resonance imaging (MRI) of the pituitary gland showing a tumor *(arrow head);* the stalk of the pituitary is deviated to the left. This man had a 2-year history of decreased libido. Biochemical investigations documented abnormally high levels of serum prolactin in association with hypogonadism

Medical Treatment.   Medical management continues to gain in popularity because of its effectiveness and relatively low risk. It should be mentioned, however, that successful pharmacological management is limited to a reduction to a normal range of serum prolactin levels and resolution of the symptoms. Elimination of the tumor does not occur, since virtually all patients exhibit biochemical and clinical evidence of recurrence following interruption of therapy even in those cases (> 60%) in which a reduction in tumor size is documented. With the exception of large tumors presenting immediate danger to vital structures, medical therapy is often the preferred initial choice; it is also indicated after incomplete removal of an adenoma.

A number of compounds fall into the category of **dopamine agonists,** including bromocriptine, pergolide, metergolin and lisurid. Bromocriptine is a full agonist at D_2 receptors and a mixed agonist at D_1 receptors, while pergolide, also a full agonist at D_2 receptors, is ten times more potent than bromocriptine. It is worth mentioning here the effect of **apomorphine,** another dopamine agonist, on men with a primarily psychogenic erectile dysfunction. Recent studies at our institution have demonstrated it to be an effective erectogenic agent [21]; however, none of these patients have evidence of hyperprolactinemia, which suggests that dopamine agonists may have a dual effect on erectile function.

Bromocriptine (Parlodel, Pravidel) is administered orally. Because of undesirable side effects, it is best to start at reduced doses such as 1.25 mg once a day until reaching 2.5–10 mg/day in three divided doses. Side effects common to all dopamine agonists (bromocriptine, pergolide, and apomorphine) include nausea, vomiting, dizziness, and postural hypotension. Side effects usually resolved with continuation of treatment.

Pergolide mesylate (Permax) is used less frequently than bromocriptine in the treatment of hyperprolactinemia. Administration of the drug should be initiated with a single daily dose of 0.5 mg, which is increased progressively to a dose of 1–1.5 mg/day in three divided doses. Since pergolide is significant more active than bromocriptine the progressive increase in dosage should be slower. Further dopamine agonists and prolactin inhibitors, available in Germany and other European countries, are lisurid (Dopergin) or metergolin (Liserdol).

Radiotherapy.   This modality is restricted as an adjuvant to surgery when there is insufficient resolution of the manifestations of the adenoma.

Follow-up.   Following institution of therapy, it is important to establish a firm schedule of follow-up since these tumors are rarely, if ever, completely eliminated. Periodic measures of serum prolactin as well as MRI of the sella turcica are indicated. In the presence of a satisfactory biochemical response but persistence of the erectile problem or lack of improvement in libido, it is important to ascertain that a concomitant hypogonadism is not present. Patients who failed to show an improvement when one or both endocrinopathies have been treated, deserve a more complete evaluation to rule out the presence of comorbidity.

Neuropharmacological Agents

It is believed that most agents in this group have a beneficial effect by influencing the central mechanisms of erections. Most of the experience, but not all, has evolved around the treatment of patients in whom organic causes are not documented or if present, are of moderate severity. For purposes of clarity, they will be presented as class compounds with their relative merits and drawbacks.

Adrenergic Receptor Antagonists

Phentolamine.   Although it is most commonly used in combination for intracavernosal injections, there was early but limited evidence that its *buccal* administration exhibits erectogenic activity [22]. These results have been confirmed more recently in a multicenter controlled study [23]. The dose employed was 20–40 mg in a strip of filter paper 15 min prior to intercourse. There was a 30%–40% response to buccal phentolamine compared to the placebo of only 15–20%. Side effects were limited to burning feeling in the oral mucosa.

Yohimbine.   A large experience exists with the use of this drug [24]. As anticipated, its effectiveness is limited in cases of organic impotence but, as compared to placebo, a significant difference has been documented in those men with a primarily psychogenic etiology [25]. These early results have been supported by the report of a recent controlled trial of yohimbine versus placebo (H. J. Vogt 1996). The drug is recommended as first line of treatment for a limited period (i.e., 1 month). Currently we used the dose of 10 mg orally. There appears to be a synergistic effect when used in combination with trazodone (see below). Side effects include palpitation, gastric intolerance, and Headache. Larger doses (20–30 mg) used "on demand" are said to be effective. However, the safety and effectiveness of this approach have not been studied.

Delaquamine.   This is a new compound developed by Syntex. The compound was found initially to have erectogenic properties but when it reached the dose-response stages of evaluation, the pharmaceutical company that develop it was acquired by a different company which felt that further research on the drug was not warranted.

Dopamine Receptor Agonists

Various drugs in the category of dopamine receptor agonists are available, but not frequently used in the treatment of erectile dysfunction.

Some were cited in the treatment of hyperprolactinemia. Apomorphine is a promising one. It has been shown to induce bouts of yawning and penile erections in animals and humans when administered by subcutaneous injection. Our group [21] has developed a proprietary formulation in a buccal tablet which has been recently shown, in a pilot study, to be effective in the majority of patients treated on "p.r.n. basis". The dose has not been firmly established, but ranges between 4 and 8 mg. The product is not yet available for general use. Toxicity includes hypotension, nausea, and vomiting at larger doses.

Serotoninergic Receptors

Trazodone.   Commonly used as an antidepressant, trazodone was fortuitously found to induce priapism. A number of recent publications have documented significant erectogenic activity for this compound [26] in impotent patients. The commonly used dose varies between 100 and 200 mg once daily. Adverse effects include drowsiness, orthostatic hypotension, hypertension, nausea, vomiting, and urinary retention. It may have a synergistic effect when combined with yohimbine (see above).

Oxytonergic Receptors

Oxytocin is included here for the sake of completeness. There is clear evidence that the drug exhibits erectogenic properties in rodents. It may have clinical applications in the future.

Peripheral Agents

Besides the drugs mentioned above, other oral and transcutaneous agents have profound effects on penile function. There is indisputable evidence that **nitric oxide** (NO) is the fundamental, but not the exclusive, mediator of relaxation of cavernosal smooth muscle as well as other vascular beds. Nitrovasodilator-induced relaxation is the result of signal transduction involving cyclic adenosine monophosphate *(cAMP)* and cyclic guanosine monophosphate *(cGMP)*. Both cAMP and cGMP activate Ca^{2+} and K^+ channels at the cellular level, resulting in hyperpolarization of the cell and eventual relaxation. This oversimplification of a rather complex process must be kept in mind to understand the mechanisms of the next compounds.

Nitroglycerine Paste.   The drug (considered an NO donor) is capable of inducing marked dilatation of the cavernosal arteries when applied directly to the penis or to the perineum (to avoid partner contamination). It results in modest increases in tumescence, but not in usable rigidity [27]. This information was gathered under laboratory conditions which, as anticipated, are not the most conducive for penile performance. No credible data exists on domestic use of nitroglycerine. It may be effective in improving marginal arterial insufficiency. Usual dose is 2 cm of 2% paste applied to the shaft of the penis or perineum. Side effects include hypotension and severe headache. Partner contamination may result in the development of a headache of industrial proportions, with disastrous consequences for sexual performance! The main disadvantage is its limited activity. It is not approved for use in impotence.

Minoxidil.   Widely known for its capacity to reverse alopecia androgenetica, this vasodilator was reported to be more effective than nitroglycerine in inducing erections. Further studies have failed to confirm its activity. The jury is still out, but the available evidence does not support a significant benefit from its use. The recommended dose is 1 ml topical solution applied to the penis. Adverse effects are mostly dermatological reactions (pruritus, burning sensation). Systemic effects may occasionally occur. It is said that in combination with capsaicin it works better. Information in this regard is still very sparse [28].

Phosphodiesterase Inhibitors.   As mentioned above, cAMP and cGMP are fundamental in the production of cavernosal smooth muscle relaxation. They are inactivated by phosphodiesterases (PDE). It follows, then, that if these diesterases are inhibited, the activity of cAMP and cGMP would be enhanced. Oral administration of the **PDE V inhibitor** (also designated Sildenafil) has been found to exhibit erectogenic properties in a limited clinical trial. The dose remains undetermined. Toxicity is also undetermined. A concern, of course, is that a systemic drug would result in a generalized alteration of a variety of regulatory mechanisms, particularly in the vascular system. A recent report has shown that the **PDE III inhibitor milrinone** is effective and, in the short term, carries minimal side effects [29].

L-Arginine.   This aminoacid is a precursor of NO and for this reason was tried orally in the treatment of impotence. The only study available is very small. Out of 15 men treated, six reported improvement. The drug is very well tolerated [30].

Prostaglandin E₁.   This drug has found a prominent niche in the intracavernosal treatment of impotence. It is currently the most widely used because of its superior pharmacological profile (excluding pain). It is included here because there is initial evidence that its transmucosal (intraurethral) administration is effective at large doses [31]. This delivery for the prostaglandin E_1 (PGE$_1$) system results in marked smooth muscle relaxation. The quality of the induced erections requires further evaluation. The dose employed is large: 500–1000 µg (as opposed to the 10–20 µg used for intracavernosal injection). Cost may be a problem. Side effects include pain (a prominent feature of the drug) and hypotension. Among the negative factors are the need for a device to introduce the urethral pellet and the use of protection to avoid partner contamination.

Conclusion

The current status of noninvasive pharmacotherapy of erectile failure is at the bronze age of its development and presents a confusing picture. There are many compounds with variable effectiveness and many claims with little scientific support. It is encouraging, however, to see that serious interest exists in the study of these class compounds and that some progress is being made in finding clinical applications for old and new drugs. However, we are not close to finding universally effective noninvasive drug for therapy of impotence. The reasons for the difficulties are multiple, the most important being the complexity of neurohormonal interactions at higher centers and the structural abnormalities in the target organ (penis). Continuing research in these areas will translate into the resolution of some causes of erectile dysfunction as long as we do not remain complacent with the imperfect noninvasive therapies available at present.

References

1. Tenover JS (1992) Effects of testosterone supplementation in the aging male. J Clin Endocr Metab 75: 1092–1098
2. Friedl KE, Hannan CJ, Jones RE, Playmate SR (1990) High-density lipoprotein cholesterol is not decreased if an aromatizable androgen is administered. Metabolism 39: 69–74
3. Marin P, Holmang S, Jonsson L, Sjostrom L, Kvist H, Holm G, Goran L, Bjontorp, P (1992) The effects of testosterone treatment on body composition and metabolism in middle-aged obese men. Int J Obesity 16: 991–997
4. Barret-Connor E (1992) Lower endogenous androgen levels and dyslipidemia in men with non-insulin-dependent diabetes mellitus. Ann Intern Med 117: 807–811
5. Phillips GB, Pinkernell, BH Jing T (1994) The association of hypotestosteronemia with coronary artery disease in men. Arterioscler Thromb 14: 701–705
6. Chevalier S, Bleau G, Roberfts KD, Chapdelaine A (1984) Non-steroidal serum factors involved in the regulation of the proliferation of canine prostatic epithelial cells in culture. Prostate 5: 503–508
7. Franchi F, Luisi M, Kicovic PM (1978) Long-term study of testosterone undecanoate in hypogonadal males. Int J Androl 1: 270–276
8. Holmang S, Marin P, Lindstedt G, Hadelin H (1993) Effect of long-term oral testosterone undecanoate treatment on prostate volume and serum prostate-specific antigen concentration in eugonadal middle-aged men. Prostate 23: 99–104
9. Gooren LJG (1994) A ten-year safety study of the oral androgen testosterone undecanoate. J Androl 15: 212–215
10. Behre HM, Bohmeyer J, Nieschlag E (1994) Prostate volume in testosterone-treated and untreated hypogonadal men in comparison to age-matched controls. Clin Endocr 40: 341–346
11. Vermeulen A (1991) Androgens in the aging male. J Clin Endocr Metab 73: 221–224
12. Henderson JT, Richmond J, Summerling MD (1973) Androgenic-anabolic steroid therapy and hepatocellular carcinoma. Lancet I: 934
13. Westaby D, Ogle JD, Paradinas FJ, Randell JB, Murray-Lyon LM (1977) Liver damage from long term methyltestosterone. Lancet 2: 261–263
14. Morales A, Johnston B, Heaton JPW, Clark A (1994) Oral androgens in the treatment of hypogonadal impotent men. J Urol 152: 115–118
15. Wilson JD, Griffth JD (1980) The use and misuse of androgens. Metabolism 29: 1278–1295
16. McClure RD, Oses R, Ernest ML (1991) Hypogonadal impotence treated by transdermal testosterone. Urology 37: 224–227
17. Orwoll E, Oviatt S, Biddle J et al (1992) Transdermal testosterone supplementation in normal older men. Abstracts of the 74th Annual Meeting of the Endocrine Society, p 319
18. NIH Consensus Conference on Impotence (1993) NIH Consensus Development Panel on Impotence. JAMA 270: 83–87
19. Snyder PJ, Lawrence DA (1980) Treatment of male hypogonadism with testosterone enanthate. J Clin Endocr Metab 51: 1335–1341
20. Cunnah D, Besser M (1991) Management of prolactinomas. Clin Endocr 34: 231–235
21. Heaton JPW, Morales A, Adams MA, Johnston B, El-Rashidy R (1995) Recovery of erectile function by the oral administration of apomorphine. Urology 45: 200–204

22. Gwinup G (1988) Oral phentolamine in non-specific erectile insufficiency. Ann Intern Med 109: 162–164
23. Wagner G, Lacy S, Lewis R, Zorgniotti A (1994) Buccal phentolamine: a pilot trial for male erectile dysfunction at three separate clinics. Int J Impot Res Suppl 1: D78
24. Morales A, Surridge DA, Marshall PG, Fenemore J (1982) Non-hormonal pharmacological treatment of organic impotence. J Urol 128: 45–48
25. Reid K, Surridge DH, Morales A, Fenemore J (1987) Double blind trial of yohimbine in the treatment of psychogenic impotence. Lancet 2: 421–422
26. Kurt U, Ozkardes H, Ugur A, Germiyanoglu C, Gurdal M, Erol D (1994) The efficacy of antiserotoninergic agents in the treatment of erectile dysfunction. J Urol 152: 407–411
27. Heaton JPW, Morales A, Owen JA, Fenemore J (1990) Topical glyceriltrinitrate causes measurable penile arterial dilatation in impotent men. J Urol 143: 729–733
28. Cavallini G (1994) Minoxidil and capsaicin: an association of transcutaneous active drugs for erection facilitation. Int J Impotence Res Suppl 1: D70
29. Stief CG, Uckert S, Truss, MC, Becker AJ, Jonas U (1995) Cyclic nucleotide PDE isoenzymes in human cavernous smooth muscle. Int J Impotence Res 7 [Suppl 1]: 6
30. Zorgniotti AW, Lizza EF (1994) Effect of large doses on nitric oxide precursor, L-arginine, on erectile failure. Int J Impotence Res 6: 33–35
31. Padma-Nathan H, Keller T, Proppiti R, Lue T, Tam P, Place V (1994) Hemodynamic effect of intra-urethral alprostadil: the medicated urethral system for erection (MUSE). Int J Impotence Res Suppl 1: D42

Transurethral Drug Therapy for Erectile Dysfunction

Harin Padma-Nathan

The transurethral system for erection was developed to deliver vasoactive compounds to the urethral mucosa to treat men with erectile dysfunction. The urethral epithelium just beyond the fossa navicularis shifts from stratified squamous to complex columnar tissue where vasoactive compounds may be absorbed. Following absorption into the corpus spongiosum surrounding the urethra, medications may be subsequently transferred to the corpora cavernosa via collateral vessels.

The transurethral system for erection is a polypropylene applicator prefilled with one dose of medication (Fig. 1). Following urination, the

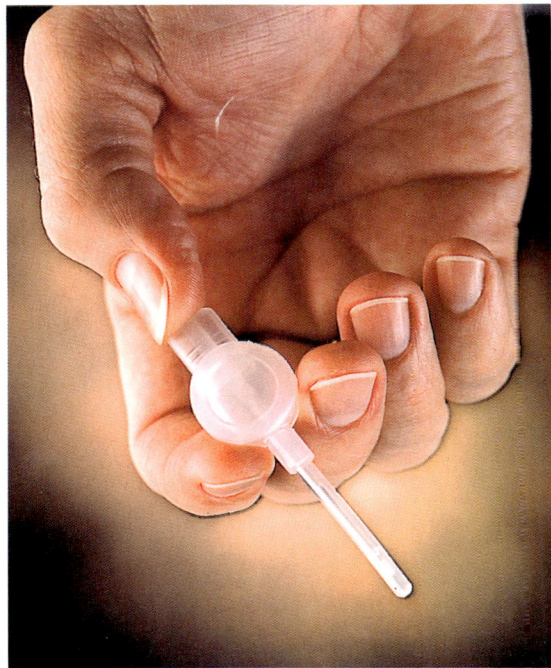

Fig. 1. Transurethral system for erection; polypropylene applicator with a hollow stem containing a semisolid pellet of medication

Fig. 2a.   After urination, the
MUSE is gently inserted into
the urethra.

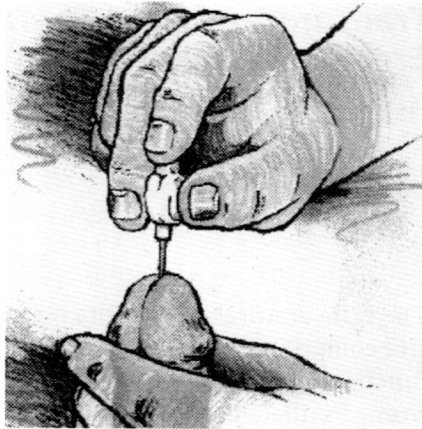

Fig. 2b.   A button is pressed
to release medication into the
urethra.

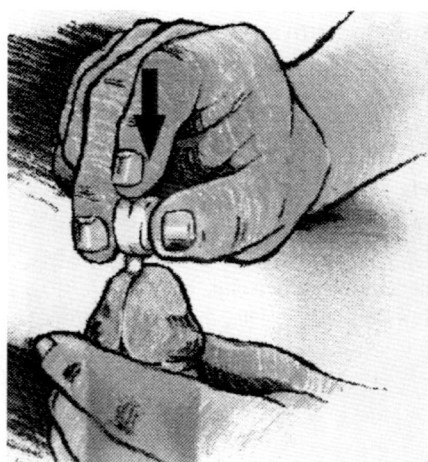

Fig. 2c.   The patient then
rolls the penis between the
hands for 10 s to distribute
the medication along the
urethra

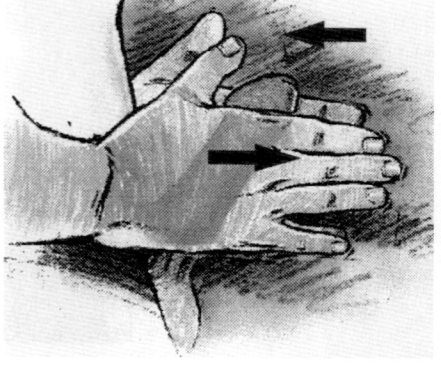

stem of the applicator is gently inserted 3 cm into the urethra (Fig. 2a). Residual urine may provide a lubricant for the applicator and a solvent for the medication. A button on the end of the applicator is pressed to release a semisolid pellet of medication onto the urethral mucosa (Fig. 2b). The applicator is removed and the patient massages the penis to help disperse the pellet (Fig. 2c).

A color duplex ultrasonography study of 21 patients with erectile dysfunction demonstrated significant hemodynamic changes in the penis following transurethral administration of alprostadil (synthetic prostaglandin E_1). The peak flow and end diastolic velocities were measured with an ATL Ultramark9 HD 80 (7.5–10 MHz wand) following intraurethral administration of 500 µg, alprostadil. Measurements were made at baseline and 5 and 15 min after drug administration. The mean peak flow and mean end diastolic velocities changed significantly from baseline after 5 and 15 min ($p < 0.001$) [1]. These hemodynamic changes can be seen in the color flow image and Doppler spectrum (Fig. 3), which are representative of arterial inflow 15 min following transurethral alprostadil. These results were generally comparable to data collected from the same patients following intracavernosal injection of 10 µg alprostadil.

During a randomized, double-blind, placebo-controlled, multicenter, in-clinic study, 234 patients received intraurethral administrations of alprostadil (125–1000 µg) and prazosin (250–2000 µg), alone and in combination; patients also received placebo. Full erections were achieved by 76.5% of patients on active medication and 2.7% of patients on placebo

Fig. 3. Color flow image and Doppler spectrum of hemodynamic changes in the penile cavernosal arteries following transurethral alprostadil

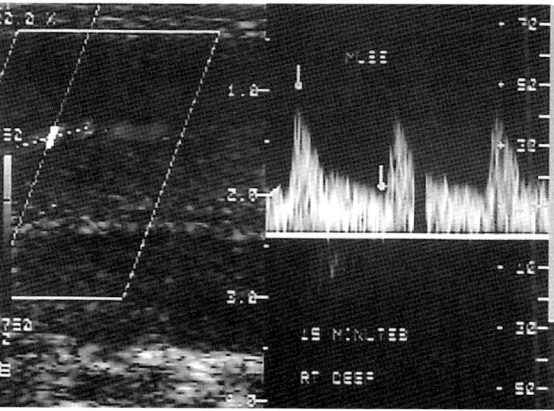

[2]. The first 68 patients to complete the study self-administered eight blinded doses of alprostadil or alprostadil/prazosin combinations at home. The response was similar, with 81.8% of patients reporting full enlargement of the penis and 71.2% reporting intercourse on active medication compared to 15.4% reporting full enlargement and 12.3% reporting intercourse on placebo ($p < 0.001$ for each comparison) [3]. Side effects included penile pain, minor urethral abrasion, and hypotension in a small percentage of patients.

The color duplex ultrasonography study has demonstrated that 500 µg alprostadil administered intraurethrally resulted in significant hemodynamic changes in peak flow velocity and end diastolic velocity without the risk of developing prolonged erections. The in-clinic and home studies showed that transurethral therapy can restore penile erections resulting in sexual intercourse. Transurethral alprostadil or MUSE (VIVUS, Inc., Menlo Park, CA) may provide a less invasive alternative in the diagnosis and treatment of patients with erectile dysfunction.

References

1. Padma-Nathan H, Keller T, Poppiti R, Lue TF, Tam P, Place V (1994) Hemodynamic effects of intraurethral alprostadil: the medicated urethral system for erection (MUSE). J Urol 151: 469A
2. Padma-Nathan H, Bennett A, Gesundheit N, Hellstrom W, Henry D, Lue TF, Morley J, Peterson C, Prendergast JJ, Tam P, Teresi A, Place V, VIVUS-MUSE Study Group (1995) Treatment of erectile dysfunction by the medicated urethral system for erection (MUSE). J Urol 153: 473A
3. Hellstrom W, Bennett A, Gesundheit N, Kaiser F, Lue TF, Padma-Nathan H, Peterson C, Tam P, Todd L, Vasady J, Place V, VIVUS-MUSE Study Group (in press) A double-blind, placebo-controlled evaluation of the erectile response to transurethral alprostadil. Urology

Twenty Years of Vacuum Therapy for Erectile Dysfunction in the United States

R. Lewis

The history of the use of vacuum therapy for erectile dysfunction is summarized in Table 1. Although this is a simple noninvasive treatment, it did not gain popularity until recently and this was primarily through the work of the two American pioneer urologists. Initially, they were often greeted with a great deal of skepticism in their early advocacy for this therapy for the patient with erectile dysfunction.

Table 1. History of vacuum devices

Reference	Year	Event
John King [1]	1874	Small "exhausting pump" (vacuum) to excite new activity in penile blood vessels
Otto Lederer [2]	1917	US patent for a device to produce erection by vacuum
Geddings D. Osbon [3]	1960	Developed vacuum device for his own personal use
	1974	Formed a company to market the device
	1982	Given permission by US Food and Drug Administration to distribute and market a noninvasive treatment for impotence
Perry Nadig [4]	1986	First article published by physician regarding his own practice of patients using vacuum therapy for impotence
Roy Witherington [5]	1989	Published paper with results of satisfaction questionnaire from patients using vacuum therapy

Patient Selection

Almost all patients suffering from erectile dysfunction are suitable candidates for the use of vacuum therapy to treat their erectile dysfunction.

This selection of therapy can be made after the first office encounter where the discussion with the patient and preferably the partner is made and the various options of therapy are explained to them. Patients who have severe penile scarring of the corpora cavernosa may not get an acceptable penile engorgement with the vacuum device. An example of this type of patient are those who may have had priapism secondary to sickle cell trait or severe intracavernosal fibrosis after infection associated with removal of penile prosthesis. Patients with severe curvature from Peyronie´s disease may not be able to obtain a rigid penis because of the confines of the cylinder. In patients with severe phimosis, a circumcision may be necessary before using the vacuum device. The contraindications to the use of vacuum therapy are few and relative. Patients with a history of unexplained priapism or diseases prone to priapism or patients with bleeding disorders or those on anticoagulation therapy, particularly in those who have enhanced capillary fragility should be cautioned regarding the use of the vacuum device.

Patients who have had implants that were removed may obtain satisfactory erections with subsequent use of the vacuum device [6,7]. The vacuum therapy has also been reported to enhance sexual activity in patients with an indwelling penile implant [7]. The vacuum device can be used successfully in patients with veno-occlusive disorder [8]. There has been one report in the literature that presented low satisfaction with vacuum therapy in patients with psychogenic impotence and also those who had previously used injection therapy with subsequent use of the vacuum device [9]. Others have suggested using vacuum devices to enhance injection therapy [10, 11].

Function and Use of Vacuum Devices

There are many types of vacuum systems available (see Table 2 for a list of different vacuum therapy products available in the United States). There has been one published paper comparing different devices [12]. Components of the vacuum system are essentially three: the cylinder, the pump and the tension or occlusion bands or rings (see Fig. 1 for examples of some of the varying products that are available). Cylinders vary in construction but essentially are made of clear plastic so the penis can be observed during the application of the vacuum. The vacuum pump is hand

Table 2. External vacuum devices

Device	Manufacturer
Catalyst vacuum system	Dacomed Corporation, Minneapolis, MN
E/P System	NuMedTec, Inc., Vernon Hills, IL
ErecAid system	Osbon Medical Systems, Ltd. Augusta, GA
Pos-T-Vac vacuum therapy	Post-T-Vac, Dodge City, KS
Response Touch vacuum constriction	Mentor, Goleta, CA
VED vacuum erection device	Mission Pharm, San Antonio, TX
VET vacuum erection technologies	Vetco, Birmingham, AL
VTU system	Encore, Louisville, KY
Innovital system	Innocept GmbH, Germany

or battery operated for those patients who might have difficulty in using a hand pump. The vacuum pump is connected to the cylinder by plastic tubing and held in the hand separately or attached to the distal of the

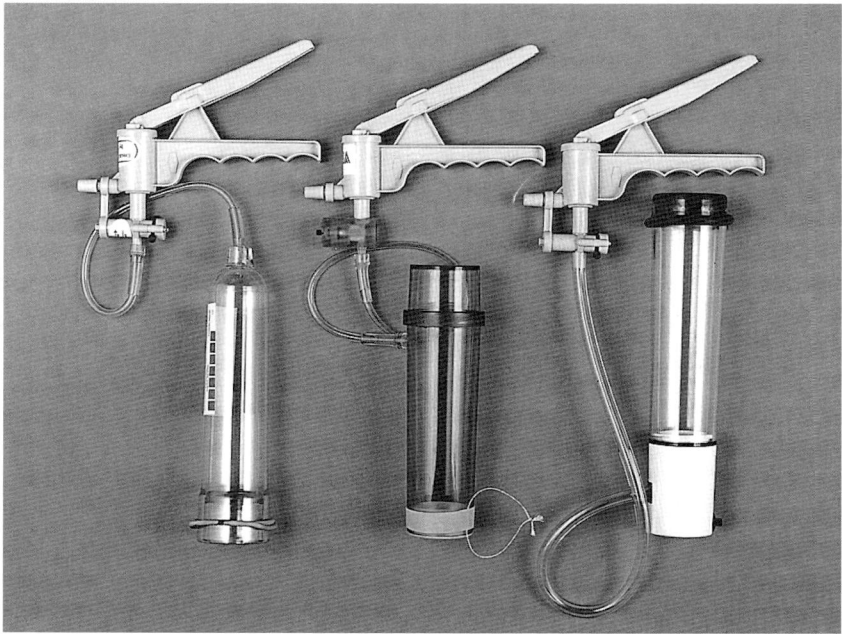

Fig. 1a.   Examples of devices that are connected to the cylinder with tubing. Left, the old model of the Osbon Erec Aid; middle, the Mission Pharmaceuticals VED; right, the Mentor Piston device. (Photograph supplied by Dr. Wayne J. G. Hellstrom, Tulane University, New Orleans, LA).

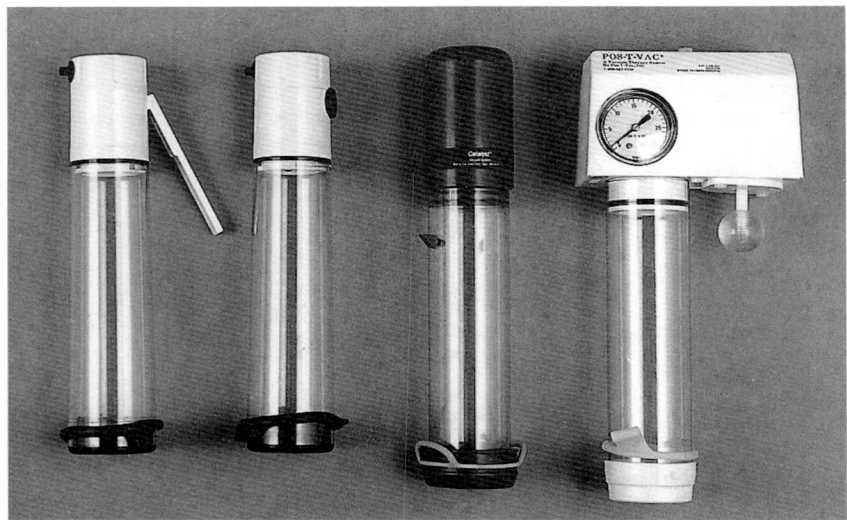

Fig. 1b. Examples of devices with the pump connected to the end of the cylinder. From left to right: Mentor Response system, Mentor Touch system (a battery-powered pump), a Dacomed Catalyst system, and Pos-T-Vac system. (Photograph supplied by Dr. Wayne J. G. Hellstrom, Tulane University, New Orleans, LA).

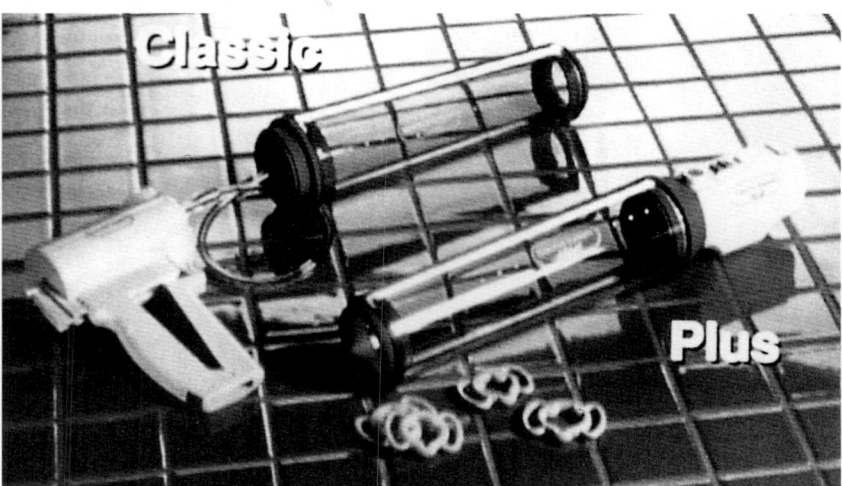

Fig. 1c. An example of the revised model of the classic Osbon Erec Aid and the Erec Aid Plus (a battery powered device) along with an example of notched tension rings.

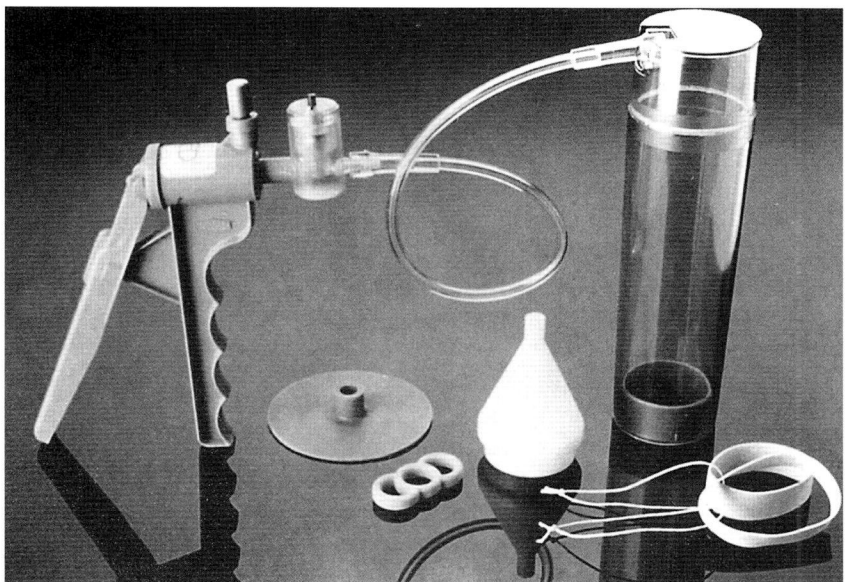

Fig. 1d.   A Mission Pharmaceutical VED showing three types of tension devices.

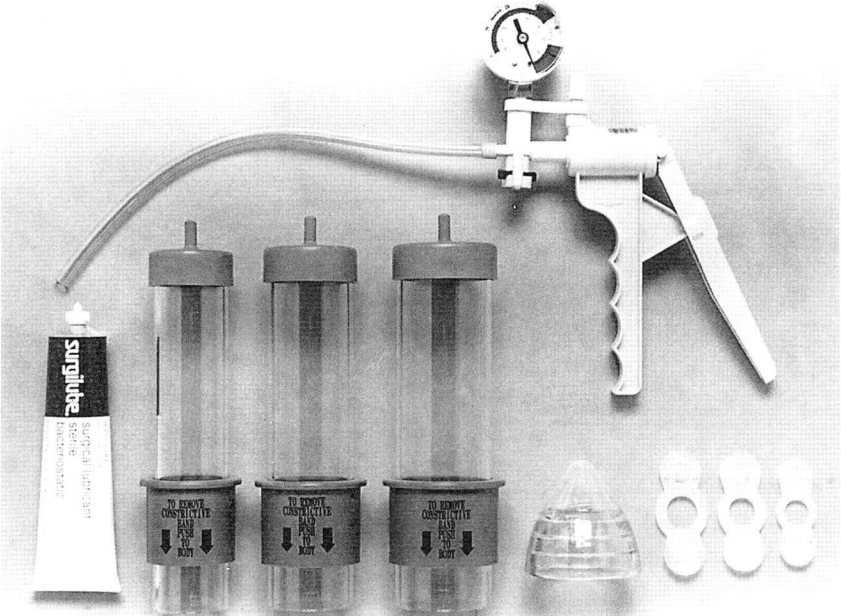

Fig. 1e.   A NuMedTec E/P system

cylinder end with a pump handle attached to it. Most devices have a release valve which acts after a certain negative pressure is reached (200–300 mm Hg). To produce an adequate rigidity of the penis, the vacuum pressure must exceed 90 mm Hg. All devices have release mechanisms built into the pump for release of negative pressure when adequate penile engorgement has been obtained and tension bands have been placed around the base of the penis. The tension devices vary somewhat. The costs of the different devices vary from area to area and the physician must find out this information for his particular region. Some of the larger companies cite the availability of a 24-h telephone line for consultation by a trained professional staff for patient questions and support as a value feature for their device. Most of the devices come with a video tape that explains the use of that particular device.

The patient first assembles the components of the device according to the instructions of the company. The base of the cylinder is loaded with the appropriate tension band. The proximal end of the cylinder is usually lubricated very generously with a water-soluble lubricant to obtain a better seal to the skin surrounding the base of the penis. If there is difficulty in obtaining a tight seal due to excessive pubic hair, it may have to be partially cut away. The cylinder is placed around the penis and held against the skin surrounding the base of the penis and the patient begins to pump (see Fig. 2). The number of pumps neces-

Fig. 2. An example of a patient using the vacuum device to create an erection

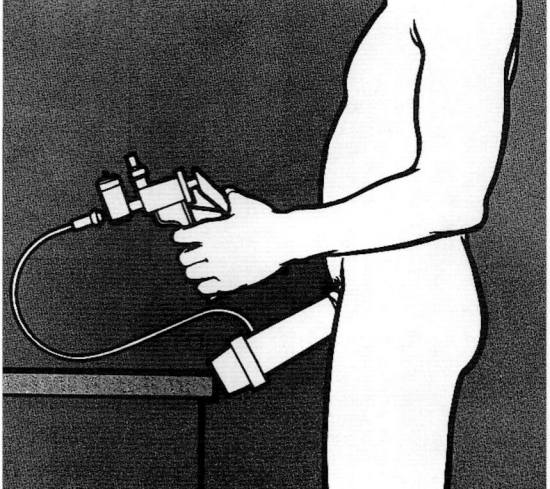

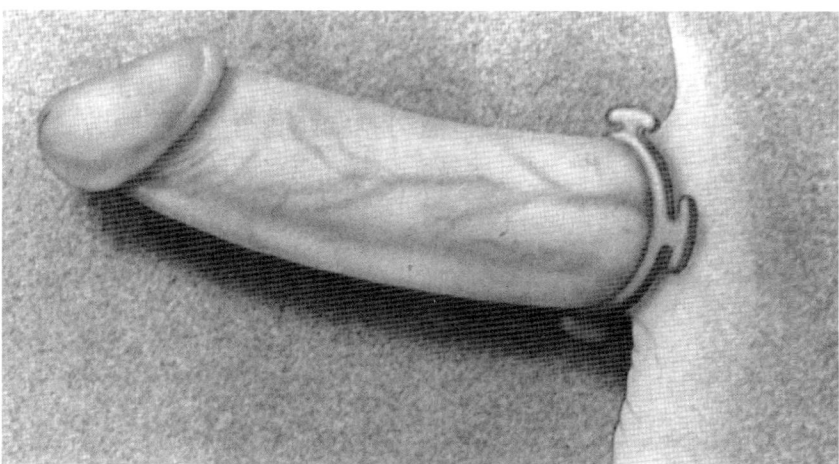

Fig. 3.   An erect penis with the tension ring in place

sary with manual pumping devices and the time to produce an adequate erection vary. Adequate rigidity may be obtained in as quick as 30 s or may take as long as seven minutes. Some manufacturers advise pumping for 1–2 min, releasing the pressure, and then resuming pumping for 3–4 min. Once adequate penile engorgement and rigidity is obtained, the preloaded bands are slipped off the proximal end of the cylinder onto the base of the penis, the vacuum released, and the cylinder removed. The patient is then ready for intercourse. The patient is cautioned not to leave the tension bands in place for more than 30 min (see Fig. 3). The rigidity obtained with the vacuum device is engorgement of all the tissues of the penis with trapped blood. There is usually some hinging of the penis since the more proximal corpora beneath the tension band do not become engorged with blood. The penis may be slightly cool and obtain a slightly cyanotic color. Occasionally, there is some numbness. Pain of such an intensity to discontinue the use of the device is extremely rare. Sometimes there is mild pain on obtaining rigidity of the penis. With ejaculation and orgasm, fluid may be expulsed from the end of the penis, but also may not because of the tension band. It is recommended by most of the companies selling these devices that the patients and partner practice with the device before sexual intercourse.

Results of Vacuum Therapy

Dr. Perry Nadig, one of the early pioneers of the device, reported on his personal series of patients using vacuum therapy in the *Journal of Urology* in 1993 [13]. The device was used regularly in approximately 70% of the patients with greater than 80% patient and partner satisfaction. The quality of the erection obtained with the device, when questioned regarding hardness, length of penis, and circumference of penis, was graded as quite adequate in 90% of the patients for each of these parameters. In that article, the readers are referred to the side effects patients complained of. Other authors have reported success rate from the use of the device from 70%–85% [14, 15]. Both of these studies reported a 20% drop out rate of patients followed over time. There have been two reports of less success with the vacuum device [9, 16]. Dr. Roy Witherington published the first results of the retrospective survey of the Osbon vacuum devices in 1989 [5].

Recently, the Impotence Resource Center of the Geddings Osbon Foundation conducted a questionnaire survey of 34 777 registered owners of the Osbon vacuum products. The survey was a stratified, disproportionate sample of owners (see Table 3). Seven thousand seventy-five (20.3%) returned the questionnaire. Of these, 5847 were considered valid for interpretation of the results of the use of vacuum device (see Table 4).

Table 3. Stratified survey

Year acquired	Surveyed (%)
1974–1988	100
1989	50
1990	35
1991	30
1992	25

Table 4. Results of questionnaire

	Questionnaires	
	(*n*)	(%)
Mailed	34 777	100.0
Required	3 478	10.0
Returned	7 075	20.3
Scannable	6 902	19.8
Not used	959	2.8
Valid	5 847	16.8

The respondent's ages are seen in Table 5. Table 6 shows the number of partners who participated in selecting therapy, and Table 7 shows who provided training if training or support was utilized. The continuous users are shown in Table 8. Table 9 shows the reasons for ceasing use of

Table 5. Age of respondents

Age-group	Respondents	
	(n)	*(%)*
< 40	42	0.7
41–50	192	3.3
51–60	688	11.8
61–70	2254	38.5
71–80	2191	37.5
> 80	351	6.0

Table 6. Partner participation in selecting therapy among 5847 respondents

	Patients	
	(n)	*(%)*
Accompanied man to see physician	1297	22.2
Influenced decision to procure vacuum device	2028	34.7

Table 7. Training and/or support in 5847 respondents

	Patients	
	(n)	*(%)*
Prescribing physician	1456	24.9
Certified technician	1158	19.8
Telephone hotline	1554	26.6
Total	4168	71.3

Table 8. Continuous users (5847 respondents)

Year acquired	Users	
	(n)	*(%)*
1974–1988	941	16.1
1989	606	10.4
1990	763	13.0
1991	951	16.3
1992	1229	21.0

Table 9. Reason for ceased vacuum device use not related to device (1357 patients)

Reason	Patients (n)	(%)
No partner	231	17.0
Natural erections returned	146	10.8
Health problems	126	9.3
No desire for sex	79	5.8

Table 10. Reason for ceased vacuum device use – 1357 related to device (1357 patients)

Reason	Patients (n)	(%)
Inability to achieve adequate erection	580	42.7
Pain or discomfort	555	40.9
Too much trouble	487	35.9
Partner nonacceptance	280	20.6
Switched to another treatment	214	15.8
Fear of injury	157	11.6

Table 11. Satisfaction parameters (4490 continuous users)

	Users (n)	(%)
Sex as often as desired	3749	83.5
Improved self-image	2936	65.4
Improved relationship with partner	3125	69.6

the vacuum device that were not related to the device in 1357 patients. Table 10 shows reason for discontinuing of device that could be attributed to the device itself. There is obviously more than one reason for each patient´s discontinued use. Table 11 shows the satisfaction parameters that were obtained in the 4490 continuous users.

There have been a couple of papers in the literature comparing vacuum therapy to other types of therapy in the patient with erectile dysfunction [17, 18].

Complications are rare and of a minor nature. Some patients develop minimal bruising or petechiae of the superficial skin of the shaft of the penis. Some patients complain that the scrotum may be drawn into the cylinder when the vacuum is applied. Damage to the penis due to ischemia may occur if the occluding band is left in place too long. This is why this is a very high caution to users of the device. There has been a report of skin necrosis in one patient [19] and development of Peyronie's disease in another patient [20].

References

1. King J (1874) American Family Physician/Domestic Guide to Health. Streight/ Douglass, Indianapolis, p 384
2. Nadig PW (1994) External devices for erectile dysfunction. In: Whitehead ED, Nagler HM (eds) Management of Impotence and Infertility. Lippincott, Philadelphia, p 99
3. Lewis RW (1996) Vacuum devices. In: Mulcahy JJ (ed) The Diagnosis and Management of Male Sexual Dysfunction. Igaku-Shoin Medical Publishers, New York
4. Nadig PW, Ware JC, Blumoff R (1986) Noninvasive device to produce and maintain an erection-like state. Urology 27: 126–131
5. Witherington R (1989) Vacuum constriction device for the management of erectile dysfunction. J Urol 141: 320–322
6. Moul MW, McLeod DG (1989) Negative pressure devices in the explanted penile prosthesis population. J Urol 142: 729–731
7. Korenman SG, Viosca SSP (1992) Use of a vacuum tumescence device in the management of impotence in men with a history of penile implant or severe pelvic disease. JAGS 40: 61–64
8. Blackard CE, Borkon WD, Lima JJ et al (1993) Use of vacuum tumescence device for impotence secondary to venous leakage. Urology 41: 225–230
9. Meinhardt W, Lycklama a Nijeholt AAB, Kropman RF et al (1993) The negative pressure device for erectile disorders: when does it fail? J Urol 149: 1285–1287
10. Marmar JL, DeBenedictis TJ, Praiss DE (1988) The use of a vacuum constrictor device to augment a partial erection following an intracavernous injection. J Urol 140:975–979
11. Chen J, Godschalk MF, Katz PG et al (1995) Combining intracavernous injection and external vacuum as treatment for erectile dysfunction. J Urol 153: 1482
12. Salvatore FT, Sharman GM, Helstrom WJ (1991) vacuum constriction devices and the clinical urologist: an informed selection. Urology 38: 323–327
13. Cookson MS, Nadig PW (1993) Long-term results with vacuum constriction device. J Urol 149: 290–294
14. Sidi AA, Becher EF, Zhang G et al (1990) Patient acceptance of and satisfaction with an external negative pressure device for impotence. J Urol 144: 1154–1156
15. Turner LA, Althof SE, Levine SB et al (1991) External vacuum devices in the treatment of erectile dysfunction: a one-year study of sexual and psychosocial impact. Jour Sex Mar Therapy 17: 81–93
16. Gilbert HW, Gingell JC (1992) Vacuum constriction devices: second-line conservative treatment for impotence. Br J Urol 70: 81–83
17. Gould JE, Switterd DM, Broderick GA et al (1992) External vacuum devices: a clinical comparison with pharmacologic erections. World J Urol 10: 68–70

18. Turner LA, Althof SE, Levine SB et al (1992) Twelve-month comparison of two treat-
    ments for erectile dysfunction: self-injection versus external vacuum devices. Urol-
    ogy 39: 138–144
19. Meinhardt W, Kropman RF, Lycklama a Nijeholt AA et al (1990) Skin necrosis caused
    by use of negative pressure device for erectile impotence. J Urol 144: 983
20. Kim JH, Carson CC (1993) Development of Peyronie´s disease with the use of a
    vacuum constriction device. J Urol 149: 1314–1315

Vasoactive Substances in Erectile Dysfunction – A Survey of 10 Years´ Global Experience

Hartmut Porst

Historical Development

Papaverine, a raw opium alkaloid, was first mentioned in the literature by Merck in 1884, but it was not until 37 years later, in 1921, that Pal described the vasodilator properties of the substance [references in 11] (Table 1). The combination of papaverine and yohimbine was successfully used in erectile dysfunction 2 years later (references in [11]). After another almost 60 years, in 1982, Virag [38] was the first to report on intracavernosal injections of papaverine for patients suffering from erectile dysfunction. This report was the basis for the development of a completely new therapy of erectile dysfunction, i.e., intracavernosal injection therapy. When Zorgniotti and Lefleur [42] reported the successful treatment of a large number of patients with a combination solution of papaverine and phentolamine, intracavernosal injection therapy became known throughout the world and began to weaken, in particular, the position of prosthetics, which had been an established therapy till then. Two years previously, Brindley [6] had already pointed out the successful induction of erections by intracavernosal injections of phenoxybenzamine, which he had attempted partly using himself as a subject.

The publications by Porst [24] and Stackl [31] propagated alprostadil (PGE$_1$) as an alternative to the mixture of papaverine and phentolamine, the solution commonly used so far; 2 years earlier, at the Second World Meeting on Impotence held in Prague in 1986, both Adaikan and Ishii had reported on the use of PGE$_1$ in erectile dysfunction. Several other substances such as moxisylyte, VIP, CGRP (calcitonin gene-related peptide), linsidomine, and VIP/phentolamine or CGRP/PGE$_1$ combinations had been examined for their therapeutic benefit in erectile dysfunction since 1988, but except for moxisylyte (Icavex), none of these was developed to the stage of official approval, owing in part to their insufficient efficacy.

Table 1. Historical survey of vasoactive substances used to treat erectile dysfunction

Year	Author	Source	Substance
1884	Merck	Lieb. Ann Phys	Papaverine
1921	Pal	Berlin K. Wochenschr.	Papaverine
1923	Fleischer	Münch. Med. Wochenschr.	Papaverine/yohimbine
1982	Virag	Lancet	Papaverine
1983	Brindley	Br. J. Psychiatry	Phenoxybenzamine
1985	Zorgniotti	J. Urol.	Papaverine/phentolamine
1986	Ishii	2nd World Meeting on	PGE_1
	Adaikan	Impotence, Prague	PGE_1
1987	Wagner	World J. Urol.	VIP
1988	Porst	Urologe A	PGE_1
1988	Stackl	J. Urol.	PGE_1
1989	Buvat	J. Urol.	Moxisylyte
1990	Goldstein	J. Urol.	Pap./phentol./PGE_1 (triple drug)
1991	Stief	J. Urol.	CGRP
1992	Gerstenberg	J. Urol.	VIP/phentolamine
1992	Stief	J. Urol.	SIN-1 (linsidomine)
1993	Porst	J. Urol.	SIN-1

Because of the high efficacy and the low cost of manufacture, the so-called triple-drug solution of papaverine/phentolamine and PGE_1 was able to maintain its position in the USA against PGE_1 monotherapy, which is not true for Europe.

Results of Basic Research

Papaverine

Papaverine is a nonselective phosphodiesterase inhibitor of cyclic nucleotide phosphodiesterase and therefore leads to the elevation of the intracellular concentrations of $3´,5´$-cAMP and $3´,5´$-cGMP. Activating voltage-dependent calcium channels, these nucleotides increase the calcium efflux out of the cell and, at the same time, the calcium influx from the cytoplasm into the calcium stores of the endoplasmic reticulum (references in [28]). Both mechanisms result in a calcium depletion of the cytoplasm, and therefore in a relaxation of the muscle cell. This means that papaverine has relaxant effects on all smooth muscle cells, and it was therefore given for instance, in cases of ureteral and biliary colic and of vascular spasm, before being used for erectile dysfunction.

Prostaglandin E$_1$ and Prostanoids

Prostaglandin E$_1$ is an endogenous substance produced in many regions of the organism, among them the prostate gland, from which the name of the substance is derived. Various animal and human experiments with cavernous tissue have shown that prostanoid (PGE$_1$) receptors with a high binding affinity can be demonstrated in particular in man, whereas they are either absent or present only in very low concentrations in the cavernous tissue of monkeys or rabbits [28]. This explains the fact that PGE$_1$ results, at best, in tumescence following intracavernosal injection into animals, while leading to full erections in about 70% of cases in man.

Via the activation of adenylate cyclase, PGE$_1$ leads to an increase in the intracellular concentration of $3',5'$-cAMP, which triggers the mechanisms already described for papaverine that effect a reduction of the intracellular concentration of calcium and thus the relaxation of smooth muscle cells. PGE$_1$ further activates presynaptic PGE$_1$ receptors of adrenergic nerve fibers and subsequently inhibits the release of norepinephrine from the vesicles in synaptic nerve terminals at the α_1 receptors [28]. Besides effecting the direct relaxation of smooth muscle cells, PGE$_1$ therefore also has antiadrenergic properties that contribute to the markedly higher efficacy of that substance as compared with papaverine.

In the vascular system, PGE$_1$ leads, among other effects, to a relaxation of the arterial resistance vessels, which means a substantial increase in blood flow. In the venous vasculature, however, PGE$_1$ leads to contraction. There is no final proof whether this is also true for the penile veins.

PGE$_1$ further inhibits platelet aggregation and platelet function and LDL receptor activity. Either mechanism imparts to the substance marked antithrombotic properties [28].

Hedlund and Andersson [15] carried out in vitro trials with human cavernous tissue to examine the efficacy of various prostanoids. PGE$_1$ had the greatest relaxant effect on the smooth cavernosal musculature and on the penile arteries. PGE$_2$, on the other hand, had only weak relaxant effects on the cavernosal muscles. PGE$_{2\alpha}$, PGI$_2$, and Thromboxane A$_2$ agonists led to dose-dependent muscle contraction.

Oxidative biochemical reactions that degrade PGE_1 form several metabolites; of these PGE_0 shows biologically similar, but lower activities than PGE_1. Part of the PGE_1 injected into the cavernous body is metabolized in the cavernous body itself [29]; part of it reaches the systemic circulation and is subject to the known metabolic processes there [20].

Alpha-Blocking Agents

Phenoxybenzamine

Phenoxybenzamine was first proposed for the indication of erectile dysfunction in Brindley´s publication [6], and he performed a heroic test on himself during the 1983 AUA annual meeting. Phenoxybenzamine is a nonselective α_1- and α_2-receptor blocker that cannot be antagonized by α-adrenergic agonists. This explains the disadvantages of the substance, which has a plasma half-life of more than 24 h and therefore a markedly higher potential for inducing priapism. In animal experiments, the substance further led to considerable inflammatory tissue reactions [32], so no further research into its use for erectile dysfunction was done.

Phentolamine

Phentolamine also effects a blockade of the α_1 and α_2 receptors and is further reported to possess inhibitory properties where the 5-HT and the serotonin receptors are concerned [3]. Like papaverine, phentolamine led to relaxation of the peripheral resistance vessels and, as a result, to an increase in blood flow in animal experiments [18], but, contrary to papaverine, no additional blockade of venous drainage due to the relaxation of the smooth cavernosal muscles was observed [41]. Since the injection of phentolamine alone into the cavernous body led only to slight tumescence [5], it was very soon combined with papaverine; this combination solution held a leading position throughout the world in the 1980s, but PGE_1 has begun to supersede papaverine/phentolamine more and more in the past few years.

The combination of phentolamine and VIP at a dosage of 0.5–2 mg phentolamine and up to 30 µg VIP also produced promising results in erectile dysfunction [13], but it was not developed further by the pharmaceutical industry.

Multicenter studies are underway to examine the efficacy and safety of phentolamine in the form of oral on-demand tablets in a large number of erectile dysfunction patients, since recent results have shown oral phentolamine at a dose of 20 mg to be markedly superior to placebo, the responder rates being 30–40% for phentolamine vs. 15–20% for placebo [40].

Moxisylyte (Synonym Thymoxamine)

Moxisylyte has selective α_1-receptor-blocking properties that persist for 3–4 h. Although in vitro trials with this substance showed it to lead to a lesser degree of relaxation of the smooth cavernosal muscles than phentolamine [17], it was developed for use in self-intracavernosal-injection therapy by Buvat et al. [8] and has meanwhile been approved officially in France under the name of Icavex at a dosage of 10–20 mg. The advantages of the substance are the low incidences of priapism (< 1%) and of local fibrotic alterations (< 1%). A considerable disadvantage, however, is its low efficacy, which limits the use of moxisylyte to, among other conditions, psychogenic disorders and neurogenic and slight arterial lesions.

Vasoactive Intestinal Polypeptide

Vasoactive intestinal polypeptide (VIP) is a neurotransmitter of the nonadrenergic, noncholinergic nerve fibers and was demonstrated in human cavernous tissue in coexistence with nitric oxide synthetase (NOS) by Juenemann et al. [19]. When injected into the cavernous body alone, VIP was not capable of inducing a sufficient erection [39]. Combined with phentolamine, VIP was used somewhat successfully in Denmark under the name of Vasopotin [13], but for unknown reasons, it was not developed into a marketable product.

Calcitonin Gene-Related Peptide

Using immunohistochemic methods, Stief et al. [33], demonstrated the neurotransmitter calcitonin gene-related peptide (CGRP) in very close proximity to the cavernosal arteries and the smooth cavernosal muscle cells. Injected into the cavernous body at a dose of 500 ng, CGRP leads to an increase of arterial blood flow and to some relaxation of the cavernosal muscles, and thus to a reduction in venous drainage, which induces tumescence, but not a rigid erection [33]. Only when combined with PGE_1 (20 µg) did CGRP (5 µg) induce rigid erections; this combination solution led to sufficient erections even in 30% of the so-called nonresponders to PGE_1 40 µg or to 60 mg papaverine plus 2 mg phentolamine so it was suggested as a last-resort therapy [30]. Currently, however, the clinical data are insufficient to confirm the reported results.

Nitric Oxide (NO) Donors

After Aronson et al. [4] had proven that NO is the endothelial mediator of smooth muscle relaxation in cavernous tissue as well, interest was aroused in NO donors in cases of erectile dysfunction.

Linsidomine (SIN-1)

Although Stief et al. [35] had reported quite promising preliminary data on the intracavernosal injection of SIN-1 at a dosage of 1–2 mg, this substance, as compared with PGE_1, showed a markedly lower responder rate of 10–20% both in our own trials [26] and in trials performed by other authors [2, 21]. Due to a lack of efficacy, SIN-1 is therefore not suitable for the majority of patients suffering from erectile dysfunction, but it may be useful in particular groups of patients (i.e., those with psychogenic or neurogenic erectile dysfunction). This is also the reason why no data on long-term results from fairly large numbers of patients are available.

Sodium Nitroprusside

Martinez-Pineiro et al. [23] compared the efficacy of 300–400 mg sodium nitroprusside, a NO donor, with that of 20 µg PGE_1 and found a better reaction to PGE_1 in 21 patients and a better reaction to sodium nitroprusside in 12; the duration of erection was markedly longer with PGE_1 (88 min) than with sodium nitroprusside (53 min). These promising reports conflict with observations by Brock et al. [7], who discontinued a therapeutic attempt with sodium nitroprusside in three patients after no rigid erection could be induced in any of them. All three patients, however, showed a marked decrease in blood pressure, with "absence of pressure" in one case. Developing the substance for routine use in erectile dysfunction therefore does not seem to be reasonable.

Vasoactive Substances in Long-term Follow-up Studies

Research shows that only a few vasoactive substances have been introduced into routine use by hospitals and practitioners. Most important among them are papaverine, the papaverine/phentolamine combination solution, PGE_1, and – in the USA – the so-called triple drug (synonym: trimix solution) of papaverine, phentolamine, and prostaglandin E_1. Parallel with these, moxisylyte has gained a certain importance in France, but it has not prevailed – at least thus far – in other European countries.

Personal Experience

The author has used various vasoactive substances for the diagnosis and therapy of erectile disorders since 1985. Besides papaverine and the papaverine/phentolamine combination solution that were used among other substances until late 1987, my interest focused on prostaglandin E_1, which became the substance of choice from late 1987 onwards. This was due, on the one hand, to the frequent induction of priapism after papaverine and papaverine/phentolamine [25] and, on the other hand, to the higher efficacy of prostaglandin E1. Minor numbers of patients were also treated with NO donor linsidomine and the α-receptor blocker moxisylyte to test these substances (Table 2).

Diagnostic Use

Up to May 1995, vasoactive substances were used in a total of 5800 patients for diagnostic reasons; the responder rates are shown in Table 2.

Table 2. Diagnostic use of vasoactive substances in erectile dysfunction

Substance	No of patients (our own series)	Responders (%)
Papaverine (50 mg)	950	39
Papaverine/phentolamine (50 mg + 2 mg)	249	61
Prostaglandin E$_1$ (20 µg)	4577	70
SIN-1 (1 mg)	65	15
Moxisylyte (20 mg)	10	10

Side Effects

Priapism (> 6 h) was not observed after moxisylyte and linsidomine but did occur in 0.26% of cases (12/4577) after PGE$_1$, in 5.3% (51/950) after papaverine, and in 5.2% (13/249) after papaverine/phentolamine.

The induction of painful erections after PGE$_1$ was seen in 9.2% of cases (422/4577). Immediately after the intracavernosal injection of papaverine, about 80% of the patients felt a temporary, fairly intense burning pain in their glans penis; however, this ceased after several minutes and did not influence the subjective sensation of the pharmacologically induced erection any further. This temporary burning pain in the glans or at the site of injection occurred much more rarely after papaverine/phentolamine. Of the patients receiving moxisylyte, more than half complained of brief burning pain after the injection, but this had no negative effects on the further development of the erection. While none of the patients treated with SIN-1 reported relevant sensations of pain in the penis, 9% (6/65) complained of transitory headache. No other complications were observed during the diagnostic use of the aforesaid substances.

Hemodynamic Parameters

Doppler sonography and, from 1987 on, duplex sonography of the penile arteries were performed in all patients 5–15 min after intracavernosal administration of the vasoactive substance. This examination produced comparable results regarding the increase in flow amplitude, peak flow velocity,, and resistance index for papaverine, papaverine/phentolamine, and PGE_1. Linsidomine, however, proved significantly worse in a comparative study with PGE_1; i.e., the majority of the patients who had normal hemodynamic parameters after PGE_1 showed pathologic values after linsidomine, a fact that would have led to the wrong diagnosis of arterial blood flow disorders in such patients [26]. Because of these results, the continued diagnostic use of SIN-1 proved no longer reasonable.

Intracavernosal Injection Therapy

Since papaverine and papaverine/phentolamine were used by the author only from 1985 and were replaced by PGE_1 in 1987, the long-term experience with intracavernosal injection therapy refers only to PGE_1.

Cavernosal Interval Therapy

A number of patients received a total of 6–10 PGE_1 injections at 8- to 14-day intervals as cavernosal stimulation therapy ("bodybuilding of the cavernosal muscles"). Irrespective of the etiology of erectily dysfunction – the therapy was used in patients with psychogenic, arteriogenic, or neurogenic disorders – more than 62% of the patients were satisfied or very satisfied with this therapy (Table 3).

Table 3. Results obtained after prostaglandin E_1 interval therapy in 124 patients	Patients	
	(n)	(%)
Very satisfied	61	49.2
Satisfied	16	12.9
Moderately satisfied	18	14.5
Not satisfied	29	23.4

Whereas almost 60% of the patients reported complete inability to perform sexual intercourse before beginning therapy, only 17% had the same problems after the therapy was discontinued (Table 4). The results reported by the patients were impressively corroborated by the duplex sonographic measurements, the average peak flow velocity in the cavernous arteries having risen by 27% after therapy (Table 5).

Table 4.   Results of the prostaglandin E_1 interval therapy in 124 patients

	Before	After
	therapy (%)	
Completely incapable of sexual intercourse > 6 months	59.7	16.9
Intercourse < 1 x/month	21.8	3.3
Intercourse 1–2 x/month	11.3	8.7
Intercourse 1–2 x/week	7.2	71.1

Table 5. Results of duplex ultrasonography during PGE_1 interval therapy in 124 patients

	Dorsal artery		Deep artery	
	Left	Right	Left	Right
	(cm/s)		(cm/s)	
Beginning	50.6	47.7	31.7	33.6
End	63.0	61.1	40.4	42.6
Difference (%)	24.5	28.1	27.4	26.8

Self-intracavernosal Injection Therapy

Another group of patients wanted the self-intracavernosal-injection (SICI) therapy to start immediately and were therefore instructed in this method comprehensively. A retrospective study from August 1987 to December 1992 evaluated 178 patients who were performing SICI therapy with PGE_1 at home (Table 6). Based on an average follow-up period of 25 months (6–64 months) and a mean number of 64 injections per patient, the dropout rate was 38% (68/178) and the rate of local complications 10%.

Table 6.   Results of PGE_1 injection therapy: retrospective study, August 1987– December 1992

Number of enrolled patients	178
Average follow-up period (months)	25
Average number of injections	64
Dropout rate (%)	38
Complications (%):	10
Nodules, indurations	5
Deviations	3
Penile pain	2

Prospective Controlled Long-term Studies

Both Schwarz Pharma and Pharmacia/Upjohn have for some years been performing prospective long-term studies with alprostadil according to GCP regulations in the USA and Europe. These studies are now going to be or have been terminated, but the final results have not yet been published. Interim results, however, have already been presented and discussed at various meetings [22, 27]. The results were comparable with respect to both dropout rates and, among other parameters, the incidence of local complications and depended upon the duration of therapy and the frequency of injections (Tables 7 and 8). It was conspicuous in this connection that half of the local fibrotic alterations occurred only after an injection average of > 50/patient [27].

A shortcoming of the SICI therapy, also reported by other authors, is the high dropout rate often amounting to more than 40% after 1 1/2–2 years. In our own three studies it was 12.8% after 6 months, 28.4% after

Table 7. Comparison of prospective European multicenter studies with alprostadil (PGE$_1$) in respect of fibrotic complications

Author	Number of patients	Follow-up period (months)	Fibrotic complica-tions (%)	Remission of fibrotic complica-tions (%)	Persistence of fibrotic complica-tions (%)
Linet et al.	1777	18	4.7 (84/1777)	29 (24/84)	3.4 (60/1777)
Porst et al.	162	36	11.1 (18/162)	50 (9/18)	5.6 (9/162)

Table 8. Categories of local fibrotic complications in prospective European multicenter studies with alprostadil (PGE$_1$)

Author	Total complica-tions (%)	Nodules (%)	Peyronie´s disease, plaques (%)	Penile deviations, with or without plaques (%)
Linet et al.	4.7 (18 months)	0.6	2.4	1.7
Porst et al.	11.1 (36 months)	4.9	2.5	3.7

Table 9. Reasons for dropout from self-intracavernosal-injection therapy with alprostadil (results from three different studies)

	Multicenter GER, prospective	Monocenter GER, retrospective	Multicenter Europe, prospective, GCP
Mean follow-up period (months)	6	25	12
Dropout rate (%)	12.8	38	28.4
Reappearance of spontaneous erections (%)	21	29	4
Serious concomitant diseases	12	25	22
Therapy ineffective dissatisfaction	17	22	–
Partner problems (%)	17	9	11
Other reasons for discontinuation (%)	21	11	20
Noncompliance (%)	12	4	37

12 months, and 38% after 25 months; the most frequent reasons for dropout are summarized in Table 9.

Results of Intracavernosal Injection Therapy Reported in the Literature

Since Virag [38] published his report on intracavernosal injections of papaverine in 1982, hundreds of publications dealing with the intracavernosal injection of vasoactive substances in erectile dysfunction have appeared. The results of an extensive literature research that was occasioned by the composition of a review article [28] are shown in Tables 10–12. It can be seen from table 10 that, based on the international literature, PGE_1 is markedly superior to both papaverine and the papaverine/phentolamine combination solution, with respect to efficacy and rate of priapism as well as to the development of local fibrotic complications. The average priapism rate with PGE_1, for instance, was only 0.25%, while papaverine and the papaverine/phentolamine combination solution showed rates of 6.8% and 6%, respectively (Table 10). The dropout rates, on the other hand, were almost comparable for all three sub-

Table 10. Efficacy and complications of vasoactive substances used in the diagnosis of erectile dysfunction: survey of published results[a]

Substance	Total no. of patients	Dosage	Response (full erection)	Priapism (> 6 h)	Pain
Papaverine (19 authors)	2 161	30–110 mg	61.0% (987/1616)	6.8% (144/2108)	No data
Our own series	950	12.5–50 mg	39% (370/950)	5.3% (50/950)	No data
Papaverine/ phentolamine (12 authors)	3 016	15 mg + 1.25 mg 60 mg + 2 mg	68.5% (2065/3016)	6.0% (73/1210)	No data
Our own series	249	15 mg + 1 mg 50 mg + 2 mg	60.6% (151/249)	5.2% (13/249)	No data
PGE$_1$ (27 authors)	10 353	5–40 µg	72.6% (7519/10 353)	0.25% (26/10 353)	11.5% (881/7637)
Our own series	4 577	5–20 µg	70.0% (3206/4577)	0.26% (12/4577)	9.2% (422/4577)

[a]From [28]

stances, ranging between 37% for PGE$_1$ and 46.6% for papaverine Table 11).

A more detailed analysis of the results given in the literature, intended to make them comparable with communicated data available from the prospective PGE$_1$ long-term studies and with our own results, reveals conspicuous serious insufficiencies of the various publications. The complication of priapism is not detailed in 31% of all the publications dealing with papaverine/phentolamine, while this is the case for only 3% of the publications on PGE$_1$. Local fibrotic complications are disregarded in 31% of the publications concerning papaverine and in 19% of the publications on papaverine/phentolamine. Averages of injections > 50/ patient were found in only 13% of the publications on PGE$_1$ and in 26% of the publications concerning papaverine/phentolamine, so the vast majority of the cases reported lack any indication of long-term complications. Most of the cited publications carry no information on the average number of injections per patient altogether. This fact must be borne in mind for interpretation of Tables 10–13.

Table 11. Complications of self-intracavernosal-injection therapy with vasoactive substances in erectile dysfunction: survey of published results[a]

Substance	Total no. of patients	Priapism (> 6 h)	Nodules, indurations, fibroses	Infection	Pain	Hematoma	Increase in liver enzymes
Papaverine (15 authors)	1527	7.1% (92/1300)	5.7% (60/1056)	0% –	4.0% (18/452)	11.4% (98/858)	1.6% (5/314)
Papaverine/ phentolamine (22 authors)	2263	7.8% (122/1561)	12.4% (228/1843)	1.0% (10/1014)	11.6% (141/1215)	25.6% (250/976)	5.4% (43/799)
PGE$_1$ (10 authors)	2745	0.36% (10/2745)	0.8% (18/2180)	0% –	7.2% (40/558)	6.6% (86/1309)	0% –
Our own series	162	0%	1.3% (2/155)	0%	1.3% (2/155)	not evaluated	0% –

[a]From [28]

Table 12. Dropout rates of the self-intracavernosal-injection therapy with vasoactive substances: survey of published results[a]

Substance	Total no. of patients	Percentage (number) of dropouts
Papaverine (9 authors)	895	46% (417/895)
Papaverine/phentolamine (19 authors)	2005	45% (903/2005)
PGE$_1$ (10 authors)	2778	37.0% (608/1641)
Our own series	162	41.3% (67/162)

[a]From [28]

Table 13. Obvious insufficiencies of the published studies with vasoactive substances used to treat erectile dysfunction

Priapism	not considered	PGE$_1$ 3% Papaverine/phentolamine 31%
Fibrotic complications	not considered	Papaverine/phentolamine 19% Papaverine 31%
Average number of injection	not considered	PGE$_1$ 72% Papaverine/phentolamine 63%
Average number of injection > 50	not considered	PGE$_1$ 13% Papaverine/phentolamine 26%

Although papaverine has been the first substance to be used worldwide for cavernosal injection therapy of erectile dysfunction, the numbers of cases published in the literature are distinctly smaller than those with papaverine/phentolamine or PGE$_1$. This is partly due to the fact that papaverine induced inflammatory, and consequently fibrotic alterations of considerably more marked degree than PGE$_1$ in animal experiments [1, 32]. Animal experiments, moreover, demonstrated the hepatotoxicity of papaverine [10]. Both local fibrotic alterations and the possibility of hepatotoxicity as suggested by an increase in liver transaminase values were described repeatedly as results of intracavernosal injection therapy with papaverine, so that the use of papaverine alone, which requires much higher dosages than a combination solution, is today generally considered obsolete.

Perspectives for Intracavernosal Injection Therapy

At present, alprostadil (PGE_1) is a drug used worldwide that combines high efficacy, a low risk of priapism, and – after long-term use – less than 10% rate of local complications in the form of fibrotic alterations. This has caused two pharmaceutical companies, independently of each other, to develop the substance so it can be approved worldwide; in some countries, it has already been approved for the indication of erectile dysfunction under the names of Caverject (Pharmacia/Upjohn) or Virilan/EDEX (Schwarz Pharma), and in Germany market approval has been applied for.

As already mentioned, at a dosage of 20 µg alprostadil shows a responder rate of about 70%. In our own patient series of 450 non-responders to 20 µg PGE_1, a dose increase to 40 µg led to sufficiently rigid erections suitable for sexual intercourse in only 20% (Fig. 1). This means that an overall PGE_1 nonresponder rate of 25% is to be expected even if the dose is raised to 40 µg, i.e., one fourth of patients cannot benefit from injection therapy.

The combination therapy with papaverine/phentolamine/PGE_1 (triple drug) led to an increase in responder rates to about 85% in the USA (references in [28]), so that only 15% of all patients may be fundamentally untreatable by injection therapy. Considering the fact that this therapy uses a solution of three different components and that the efficacy and the safety of each component have to be proven, the official approval of such a combination preparation does not seem to be achievable for a pharmaceutical company; the triple-drug therapy will therefore always be up to the individual physician and an associated pharmacist – with all the legal consequences that may result, should there be complications.

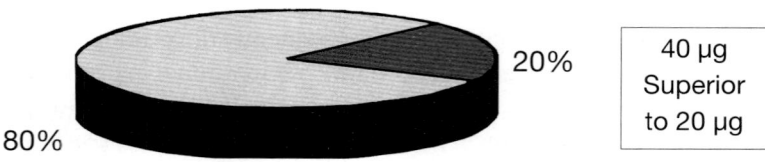

20%

40 µg
Superior
to 20 µg

80%

40 µg
Equieffective
with 20 µg

Fig. 1.   Results of tests with 40 µg vs. 20 µg PGE_1 in 450 patients. The higher dose was superior in 91 patients (20%), while in 359 patients (80%) the effect was equal. (From [28])

Another disadvantage of PGE$_1$ is the induction of painful erections in about 10% of patients, a condition that can lead to a decrease in the sensation of pleasure during sexual intercourse and – in exceptional cases – to the patient´s being altogether unable to have intercourse.

Not to be neglected is the present price for alprostadil, which, given the discussion on cost reduction in the public health sector that has been going on for years, is a problem that should not be underestimated for the large-scale use of PGE$_1$ intracavernosal injection therapy, although a great number of patients would obviously benefit from this treatment. There is thus still reason to search for new substances that are more effective, have fewer side-effects, and are less expensive than currently available therapies.

Perspectives for New Vasoactive Substances

Phosphodiesterase Inhibitors

Basic research by Stief et al. [36] has shown that the phosphodiesterase inhibitors III–V are present in human cavernous tissue and that the phosphodiesterase-III-inhibitor in the form of milrinone and quazinone, effects the most marked relaxation of the cavernosal muscles. First trials in subjects showed that the intracavernosal injection of milrinone (Corotrop) resulted in erections. It remains to be seen whether these results can be confirmed in larger patient series and, in particular, by other authors, the latter condition being all the more important as the linsidomine results published by the same team could not be confirmed by other scientists [2, 21, 26].

Potassium Channel Openers

So-called potassium channel openers lead to hyperpolarization of the muscle cell, which inhibits the extracellular calcium influx and thus results in relaxation. Contrary to other substances such as PGE$_1$ and papaverine, potassium channel openers, without acting via the 3´,5´-cAMP or the 3´,5´-cGMP mechanism, eventually have the same result, i.e., intracellular calcium depletion. It is therefore conceivable that such direct potassium channel openers could be effective in case of biochemical defects with respect to $3',5'$-cAMP and $3',5'$-cGMP production when PGE$_1$ and papaverine are not effective.

Giraldi et al. [14], for instance, performed in vitro trials to examine the potassium channel openers pinacidil, minoxidil, and three other components manufactured by Pharmacia/Upjohn and found that all the components examined relaxed precontracted cavernous tissue. Hedlund et al. [16] demonstrated similar effects for nicorandil, which is supposed to lead to the release of NO, in addition to acting directly on potassium channels.

Trigo-Rocha et al. [37] induced erections in both dogs and monkeys after intracavernosal injection of the potassium channel openers pinacidil and cromakalim. It remains to be seen whether this substance group, which certainly has interesting biochemical properties, will produce equally promising results in trials with human subjects.

Calcium Channel Blockers

Fovaeus et al. [12] demonstrated in vitro as early as 1987 that the calcium antagonists verapamil, nifedipine, and diltiazem were capable of reducing the contraction induced by norepinephrine by up to 90%. The intracavernosal injection of diltiazem, verapamil or felodipine in rats resulted in dose-dependent erections, with felodipine, a new calcium antagonist, proving to be three to four times more efficacious than the two other drugs [9]. It remains to be seen whether this substance group, whose biochemical action is also very interesting, can be used for intracavernosal injection therapy in man.

Other substances such as **adenosine, histamine,** and **sulpiride,** a dopamine antagonist, were injected into a small number of patients and resulted in tumescence or erection in some of them. Not least because of the possible potential of these substances to cause side-effects, they seem to be rather unsuitable for approval to be used in intracavernosal injection therapy, so we will not elaborate on these trials here.

The conclusive statement is therefore that intracavernosal injection therapy as such represents the principal progress made in the therapy of erectile dysfunction during the past 10 years, and that alprostadil, the standard substance worldwide, is a drug easy to use in everyday practice. Whether another substance will be come an alternative to PGE$_1$ or even supersede it within the 5–10 years to come remains open, but this is doubtful on the basis of what is known today in this area.

References

1. Aboseif SR, Breza J, Bosch RJCH, Benard F, Stief CG, Stackl W, Lue TF, Tanagho EA (1989) Local and systemic effects of chronic intracavernous injection of papaverine, prostaglandin E$_1$ and saline in primates. J Urol 142: 403
2. van Ahlen H, Schmidt C, von Heyden B, Hertle L (1995) Intracavernöser Stoffwechsel unter SIN-1. Urologe A34 Suppl 1: S13
3. Andersson KE, Holmquist F, Wagner G (1991) Pharmacology of drugs used for treatment of erectile dysfunction and priapism. Int J Impotence Res 3: 155–172
4. Aronson WJ, Busch PA, Buga GM, Ignarro LJ, Rajfer J (1991) The mediator of human corpus cavernosum relaxation is nitric oxide. J Urol 145 No. 4: 341A
5. Blum MD, Bahnson RR, Porter TN, Carter MF (1985) Effect of local alpha-adrenergic blockade on human penile erection. J Urol 134: 479–481
6. Brindley GS (1983) Cavernosal alpha-blockade: a new treatment for investigating and treating erectile impotence. Br J Psychiatry 143: 332–337
7. Brock G, Breza J, Lue TF (1993) Inracavernous sodium nitroprusside: inappropriate impotence treatment. J Urol 150: 864–867
8. Buvat J, Buvat-Herbaut M, Lemaire A, Marcolin G (1991) Reduced rate of fibrotic nodules in the cavernous bodies following auto-intracavernous injections of moxisylyte compared to papaverine. Int J Impotence Res 3: 123–128
9. Cho CK, Suh JK, Chang TG, Kim YS, Park TC, Choi HK (1995) Effect of calcium channel blockers on penile erection in vivo. J Urol 151 No. 5: 321–A373
10. Davila JC, Reddy CG, Davis PJ, Acosta D (1990) Toxicity assessment of papaverine hydrochloride and papaverine-derived metabolites in primary cultures of rat hepatocytes. In vitro Cell Dev Bio 26: 515–524
11. van Driel MF, van de Wiel HBM, Weymar Schulz WCM, Mensink HJA (1992) The history of papaverine in erectile dysfunction. Int J Impotence Res 4: 59–63
12. Fovaeus M, Andersson KE, Hedlund H (1987) Effects of some calcium channel blockers on isolated human penile erectile tissues. J Urol 138: 1267–1272
13. Gerstenberg TC, Metz P, Ottesen B, Fahrenkrug J (1992) Intracavernous self-injection with vasoactive intestinal polypeptide and phentolamine in the management of erectile failure. J Urol 147: 1277–1279
14. Giraldi A, Zhao W, Gondre M, Murray F, Christ GJ (1995) Differential relaxation of human corpus cavernosum smooth muscle by potassium (K) channel openers: evidence that relaxation is both agonist dependent and altered by diabetes mellitus. Int J Impotence Res 7 Suppl 1: 010
15. Hedlund H, Andersson KE (1985) Contraction and relaxation induced by some prostanoids in isolated human penile erectile tissue and cavernous artery. J Urol 134: 1245
16. Hedlund P, Homquist F, Hedlund H, Andersson KE (1994) Effects of Nicorandil on human isolated corpus cavernosum and cavernous artery. J Urol 151: 1107–1113
17. Imagawa A, Kimura K, Kawanishi Y, Tamura M (1989) Effect of moxisylyte hydrochloride on isolated human penile corpus cavernosum tissue. Life Sci 44: 619–623
18. Juenemann KP, Lue TF, Fournier JRGR, Tanagho EA (1986) Hemodynamics of papaverine- and phentolamine-induced penile erection. J Urol 136: 158–161
19. Juenemann KP, Ehmke H, Kummer W, Greschner M, Persson-Juenemann Ch, Alken P (1994) Nitric oxide synthase in coexistence with vasoactive intestinal polypeptide in nerve terminals of human corpus cavernosum. Int J Impotence Res 6 Suppl 1: A3

20. Juenemann KP, Schmidt P, Hatzinger M, Alken P (1995) Pharmakokinetische Untersuchungen von Prostaglandin E_1, 15-Keto-PGE$_0$ und PGE$_0$ nach intracavernöser Injektion bei Patienten mit erektiler Dysfunktion. Urologe A 34 Suppl 1: S13

21. Knispel HH, Wegner HEH, Miller K (1995) Value of nitric oxide donor linsidomine chlorhydrate (SIN-1), in the diagnosis and treatment of erectile dysfunction. Int J Impotence Res 7 Suppl 1: D26

22. Linet O (1994) PGE$_1$ toxicology, safety and efficacy. Read at international symposium on basic and clinical pharmacology of penile smooth muscle. Madrid, December 2–3, 1994

23. Martinez-Pineiro L, Tello JL, Dorrego JA, Cisneros J, Cuervo E, Martinez-Pineiro JA (1994) Preliminary results of a comparative study with intracavernous sodium nitroprusside and prostaglandin E_1 in the diagnosis and treatment of penile erectile dysfunction. J Urol 151 No. 5: 455A

24. Porst H (1988) Stellenwert von Prostaglandin E_1 (PGE$_1$) in der Diagnostik der erektilen Dysfunktion im Vergleich zu Papaverin und Papaverin/Phentolamin bei 61 Patienten mit ED. Urologe A 27: 22–26

25. Porst H, van Ahlen H (1989) Pharmakoninduzierte Priapismen – Ein Erfahrungsbericht über 101 Fälle. Urologe A 28: 84–87

26. Porst H (1993) Prostaglandin E_1 and the nitric oxide donor linsidomine for erectile failure: a diagnostic comparative study of 40 patients. J Urol 149: 1280–1283

27. Porst H, Buvat J, Hauri D, Krotovsky GS, Meuleman EJH, Michal V, Wagner G, Wespes E (1994) Self-injection therapy with prostaglandin E_1: long-term results of an international multicenter study according to the GCP standard. Int J Impotence Res Suppl 1, 6: D108

28. Porst H (1996) Review Article. The rationale for prostaglandin E_1 in erectile failure: a survey of worldwide experience. J Urol 155: 802–815

29. Roy AC, Adaikan PG, Sen DK, Ratnam SS (1989) Prostaglandin 15-hydroxydehydrogenase activity in human penile corpora cavernosa and its significance in prostaglandin-mediated penile erection. Brit J Urol 64: 180

30. Schwarzer UJ, Hofmann R, Pickl U, Hartung R (1992) Calcitonin-gene-related-peptide for therapy of erectile impotence. Int J Impotence Res 4: 219–222

31. Stackl W, Hasun R, Marberger M (1988) Intracavernous injection of prostaglandin E_1 in impotent men. J Urol 140: 66–68

32. Stackl W, Loupal G, Holzmann A (1988) Intracavernous injection of vasoactive drugs in the rabbit. Urol Res 16: 455–458

33. Stief CG, Benard F, Bosch RJCH, Aboseif SR, Lue TF, Tanagho EA (1990) A possible role for calcitonin-gene-related peptide in the regulation of the smooth muscle tone of the bladder and penis. J Urol 143: 392–397

34. Stief CG, Wetterauer U, Schaebsdau FH, Jonas U (1991) Calcitonin-gene-related peptide: a possible role in human penile erection and its therapeutic application in impotent patients: J Urol 146: 1010–1014

35. Stief CG, Holmquist F, Allhoff EP, Andersson KE, Jonas U (1991) Preliminary report on the effect of the nitric oxide donor SIN-1 on human cavernous tissue in vivo. World J Urol 9: 237

36. Stief CG, Ückert S, Truss MC, Becker AJ, Taher A, Jonas U (1995) Cyclic nucleotide phosphodiesterase (PDE) isoenzymes in human cavernous smooth muscle: characterization and functional effects of PDE-inhibitors in vitro and in vivo. Int J Impotence Res 7 Suppl 1: 03

37. Trigo-Rocha F, Donatucci CF, Hsu GL, Nunes L, Lue TF, Tanagho EA (1995) The effect of intracavernous injection of potassium channel openers in monkeys and dogs. Int J Impotence Res 7: 41–48
38. Virag R (1982) Intracavernous injection of papaverine for erectile failure. Lancet 2:938
39. Wagner G, Gerstenberg T (1987) Intracavernosal injection of vasoactive intestinal polypeptide (VIP) does not induce erection in man per se. World J Urol 5: 171–177
40. Wagner G, Lacy S, Lewis R, Zorgniotti AW (1994) Buccal phentolamine – a pilot trial for male erectile dysfunction at three separate clinics. Int J Impotence Res 6 Suppl 1: D78
41. Wespes E, Rondeux C, Schulman CC (1989) Effect of phentolamine on venous return in human erection. Br J Urol 63: 95–97
42. Zorgniotti AW, Lefleur RS (1985) Autoinjection of the corpus cavernosum with a vasoactive drug combination for vasculogenic impotence. J Urol 133: 39–41

Intraindividual Comparative Studies on Efficacy, Safety, and Side-Effects of Different Vasoactive Drugs in Erectile Dysfunction

JACQUES BUVAT AND ANTOINE LEMAIRE

Intracavernosal injections (IC) of papaverine originated a major break-through in the diagnosis and the treatment of erectile dysfunction (ED) in the early 1980s [37]. However several limits of this procedure soon emerged, regarding safety and efficacy.

Prolonged erections proved to occur in 3% to 19%, in average 9.5%, of patients during the diagnostic work-up or the titration periods, and in 8.7% of patients during the auto-injections treatment [3,16]. This adverse event can lead to definitive iatrogenic impotence due to the development of diffuse corporeal fibrosis. Moreover corporeal fibrotic nodules and albugineal plaques were reported to also occur in patients having not previously presented prolonged erection, sometimes resulting in penile curvature or reduction or even loss of erectile response to treatment [3,16] In 2 prospective studies, the rate of fibrotic nodules and plaques reached 57% and 31% after one year [20,23]. Lastly the papaverine efficacy was limited since it induced adequate rigidity in a maximum of 66% of the patients [16].

Many new drugs or combination of drugs were proposed to overcome these limits and improve the safety and efficacy of the ICI. We will mainly review here the results of the studies based on intra-individual comparisons, that is to say consisting of a cross-over design, each patient being tested with both the compared drugs. The very large variability of the individual responses to intracavernosal injections in the different etiological categories of ED patients, and even in normal males, makes it difficult to select really comparable groups for parallel group studies. Only the intra-individual comparative studies can give full objective evidence on the advantages and disadvantages of different drugs, especially if those studies are double blind.

Some of the new drugs or combinations proposed to improve the ICI results mainly aimed to improve safety: Moxisylyte, which we used since

1985 [4], was the first. Then Vasoactive-Intestinal-Polypeptide (VIP) proved to be disappointing when used alone [7,19], but to give interesting results when combined with phentolamine (Vasopotin, [14]). The nitric oxide donor Linsidomine was proposed by Stief [34] at the same time. The latter 2 drugs will be presented after prostaglandin E1 (PGE_1) since intra-individual comparative studies of these drugs were done only against PGE_1 and not against papaverine. Other drugs or mixtures mainly aimed to improve efficacy, although many of them proved to simultaneously improve safety: the mixture of papaverine with phentolamine was the first. PGE_1 was introduced in 1986 by Ishii et al. (in [16]). Then Stief et al. in 1990 proposed the combination of Calcitonin-Gene-Related-Peptide (CGRP) with PGE_1 [33] and Goldstein et al. proposed the triple drug mixture (PGE_1 + papaverine + phentolamine) [15].

Office and Laboratory Comparative Studies

Papaverine + Phentolamine

The results of 3 studies reporting intra-individual comparisons of this combination with papaverine alone, involving a total of 326 patients, are compiled in Table 1. The mixture significantly increased the effectiveness of the injections, with a rate of full rigidity growing from 32.8% up to 58.3%. But it did not solve the problem of the prolonged erections (5.2% compared to 3.1% with papaverine alone).

Table 1.   Compilation of 3 intra-individual comparisons of papaverine alone with papaverine + phentolamine

	Full rigidity	Prolonged erection
No patients	326	326
Papaverine	107 (32.8%)	10 (3.1%)
Papaverine + phentolamine	192 (58.3%)	17 (5.2%)
p (Chi Square)	< 0.001 (2.06)	ns (0.17)

Based on Wetterauer et al. 1988: 15 ED patients, up to 90 mg papaverine versus 45 mg papaverine + 1.5 mg phentolamine; Keogh et al. 1989: 40 ED patients, up to 40 mg papaverine vs. 20 mg papaverine + 0.5 mg phentolamine; Porst 1989: 249 ED patients: up to 50 mg papaverine vs. 50 mg papaverine + 2 mg phentolamine.

Moxisylyte

We started using this alpha-1 blocking agent intracavernously 1985. In 1989, we reported on an escalating dose study comparing Moxisylyte to papaverine in 50 patients tested in the supine position [4] (Table 2). The Moxisylyte potency proved to be considerably less than that of papaverine since the rate of erectile responses consistent with vaginal intromission (partly + fully rigid responses) was of only 18% compared to 48% with papaverine. Conversely Moxisylyte induced much less prolonged erections (2% compared to 12% with papaverine). Its weak potency, however, made its usefulness in the management of ED doubtful.

However, in another intra-individual comparative study, Moxisylyte proved to work at home much better than in the office [4] (Table 3). Ninety one patients had 2 injections of the same dose in our office. Fol-

Table 2. Intra-individual comparison of Moxisylyte with papaverine in 50 unselected ED patients

Drug	No patients	Partial rigidity	Full rigidity	Prolonged erection
Papaverine	50	10 (20%)	14 (28%)	6 (12%)
Moxisylyte	50	4 (8%)	5 (10%)	1 (2%)

Papaverine: 40 mg, then 80 mg if no full rigidity with 40. Moxisylyte: 10 mg, then 20 mg, then 30 mg if no full rigidity at the previous steps. Adapted after Buvat et al. 1989 [4].

Table 3. Effect of the same dose of Moxisylyte in the physician´s office and at home

Response in the office	All the cases	Success at home	Failure at home
All the cases	91	42 (46%)	49 (54%)
No or poor rigidity	68 (75%)	24 (35%)	44 (65%)
Adequate rigidity	23 (25%)	18 (78%)	5 (22%)

10 or 20 mg according to the cases; adapted after Buvat et al. 1989 [4]

lowing the first one they were observed for 1 h in the office. Following the second one, they were immediately sent at home where they had scheduled to attempt intercourse. Although only 25% developed a rigidity apparently adequate for intercourse in the office, 46% succeeded at home, including 35% of those having presented either no rigidity, or only a poor rigidity in the office. This demonstrated that Moxisylyte, was able to facilitate the erection induced by erotic stimuli produced in privacy.

We confirmed this facilitating effect in our laboratory. A double-blind study with a cross-over design compared the effects of an intra-cavernosal injection of 10 mg Moxisylyte with those of a placebo injection on the erectile response to different types of sexual stimulations [11]. Tumescence and rigidity were recorded following the injection (10 min), then during the 7 min following the application of a 3 min long vibration on the penis, and lastly during a 10 min long visual sexual stimulation. Following Moxisylyte, every erectile parameter was significantly greater at any time. Vibration, which can be considered as an experimental model of tactile stimulation, resulted in a significantly greater increase in erection following Moxisylyte than following placebo. Lastly visual sexual stimulation, which can be considered as an experimental model of psychic stimulation, also resulted in a greater increase of erection following Moxisylyte, though this time the difference was not significant.

Prostaglandin E1

PGE1 versus Papaverine Alone

Nine studies with intra-individual comparison, including 3 double blind studies, are compiled in Table 4. They compared 20 µg PGE_1 (15 µg in 1 study) with doses of 30 to 60 mg of papaverine. When only the double blind studies are considered (117 patients), the only significant difference concerned the greater efficacy with PGE_1. When all the 9 studies were put together, not only the greater efficacy of PGE_1 was confirmed (rigidity adequate for intercourse in 71% of the 571 tested patients as compared to only 43% following papaverine), but the rate of prolonged erections was also significantly lower with PGE_1 (respectively 0.5% vs. 4%), as it was also found a lower rate in the patients having reported pain due to the injection (respectively 17% vs. 37%).

Table 4.   Compilation of 9 intra-individual comparisons of papaverine alone (30 to 60 mg) with PGE$_1$ (20 µg, except 15 µg in 1)

	3 double-blind studies			All 9 studies		
	Adequate rigidity	Prolonged erection	Pain	Adequate rigidity	Prolonged erection	Pain
No patients	117	117	117	571	571	249
PGE$_1$	71 (61%)	0	33 (28%)	404 (71%)	3 (0.5%)	42 (17%)
Papaverine	47 (40%)	0	39 (33%)	247 (43%)	23 (4%)	93 (37%)
p (Chi Square)	< 0.001 (3.42)	ns	ns (0.39)	< 0.001 (6.33)	< 0.001 (6.89)	< 0.001 (2.94)

Three double-blind studies: Sarosdy et al. 1989, 15 patients, 30 then 60 mg of papaverine vs. 10 then 20 µg PGE$_1$; Kattan et al. 1991, 50 patients, 60 mg vs. 20 µg; Mahmoud et a.. 1992, 52 patients, 30 mg vs. 20 µg. Six open studies: Porst 1989, 249 patients, Xavier et Searp 1990, 22 patients, Chiang et al. 1990, 50 patients, Tamura et al. 1990, 39 patients, Lin et al. 1991, 34 patients, Wang et al. 1994, 60 patients. The data regarding pain are missing in 3 studies [24, 28, 35].

For many people, the question was more important, however, whether PGE$_1$ gave better results than the papaverine-phentolamine mixture, which was the reference intracavernosal drug in many countries in the late 80´s.

PGE$_1$ versus Papaverine + Phentolamine

Seven studies with intra-individual comparison of 10 to 20 µg of PGE$_1$ with 15 + 0.5 to 60 + 2 mg of papaverine + phentolamine are compiled in Table 5. They involve 640 ED-patients, and include 2 double-blind studies. Again, PGE$_1$ is significantly more effective, although the difference is smaller than to papaverine alone (rigidity adequate for vaginal intromission in 76% of the patients receiving PGE$_1$ compared to 67% of patients receiving the papaverine/phentolamine mixture). In 2 double-blind studies, involving a total of only 37 patients, the corresponding rates were 97% compared to 84%.

Despite this higher efficacy, the prolonged erection rate is significantly lower with PGE$_1$, and the difference is rather greater than with papaver-

Table 5. Comparison of 7 intra-individual comparisons of PGE_1 (10 to 20 µg) with the mixture of papaverine + phentolamine (15 + 0.5 to 60 + 2 mg)

	Adequate rigidity	Prolonged erection	Pain
No patients	412	640	391
PGE_1	307 (76%)	7 (1%)	139 (36%)
Papav. + phentol.	278 (67%)	44 (7%)	125 (32%)
p (Chi Square)	< 0.05 (0.026)	< 0.001 (8.83)	ns (0.29)

Includes 2 double-blind studies (Waldhauser et Schramek, 1988, 12 patients; Lee et al. 1989, 25 patients) and 5 open studies (Berger et Hartsell 1988, 27 patients; Floth et Schramek 1991, 49 patients; MacMahon 1991, 228 patients; Porst 1989, 249 patients; Wetterauer 1990, 50 patients). The data regarding adequate rigidity are missing in the MacMahon study [25] as well as the data regarding pain in the Porst study [28].

ine alone (1% compared to 7% with the combination). However, there was no difference according to pain, which occurred in about one third of the patients with both drugs.

The intra-individual comparison of different doses of PGE_1, papaverine alone, and papaverine + phentolamine, by Porst et Biederman (1993) (Table 6), clearly points the better safety of PGE_1 with respect to prolonged erections. Their rate was of only 1% compared to 13% with

Table 6. Duration of the prolonged erections following PGE_1, papaverine, and papaverine-phentolamine (intra-individual comparison in 101 patients, escalating dose). The numbers into brackets indicate the number of patients having presented a prolonged erection/the total number of patients tested. (Porst et Biederman 1993)

Erection Duration	PGE_1 (10 µg)	PGE_1 (20 µg)	Papav. (25 mg)	Papav. (50 mg)	Papav. + Phentol. (50 + 2 mg)
> 3 h	1% (1/84)	– (0/71)	6% (5/84)	4% (3/83)	13% (10/76)
> 4 h	–	–	3.5% (3/84)	2.5% (2/83)	4% (3/76)
> 6 h	–	–	3.5% (3/84)	–	2.6% (2/76)

papaverine + phentolamine in the same patients. No erection lasted more than 4 hours with PGE$_1$ compared to 3.5–4% with papaverine or the mixture, including priapisms in 3% and 2%. That confirms the results of numerous open studies which emphasize the spontaneous cessation of most of the prolonged erections following PGE$_1$, in contrast to the noticeable rate of priapisms following papaverine or the mixture. Another intra-individual comparison by Weiske (1988) still supports this important advantage of PGE$_1$. Fifteen impotent patients having all presented with a priapism following papaverine + phentolamine injections were tested with escalating doses of 5 to 20 µg of alprostadil-alfadex. An erection adequate for intromission could be obtained in all (8 required 20 µg PGE$_1$). A prolonged erection occurred in only 5 (33%, 180 to 500 mn) requiring to be treated in 3 patients (20%, metaraminol in all, puncture in only 1). That shows that although PGE$_1$ gives less risk of priapism, this complication can also occur with this drug, and thus strict precautions should also be taken.

Although pain is reported by about the same percent of patients following PGE$_1$ and papaverine, the 2 drugs induce very different sensations as is illustrated by other data of the intra-individual comparison (Table 7) by Porst and Biederman [30]. A burning sensation during the first minute following the injection is specific for papaverine (28% of the patients). It occurs in only 1% of the patients following PGE$_1$. Conversely, a sensation of tension in the penis, is specific for PGE$_1$ (11% of the patients). In addition, only after PGE$_1$, 8.5% report a sensation of testicular pressure.

Table 7.   Differences in the painful sensations following PGE$_1$, papaverine, and papaverine + phentolamine (intra-individual comparison with escalating dose in 101 patients). (Porst et Biederman 1993). More injections were done with PGE$_1$ and papaverine than with papaverine + phentolamine because only 1 dose of the mixture was tested

Drug (doses)	No injections	all painful injections	Burning at injection	Painful tension during erection	Testicular pressure
PGE$_1$ (5 to 20 µg)	177	67 (38%)	2 (1%)	20 (11%)	15 (8.5%)
Papaverine (25 and 50 mg)	167	64 (38%)	46 (28%)	–	1 (0.6%)
Papaverine + phentolamine (50 + 2 mg)	76	22 (29%)	14 (18%)	–	–

PGE₁ versus Papaverine and Papaverine-Phentolamine: Diagnostic Applications

In a comparative study, we precised the diagnostic values of the 80 mg papaverine test and the 20 µg PGE_1 test in 26 psychogenic and 46 vasculogenic (both arterial and venogenic dysfunctions) impotent patients [6]. Because of its greater potency, PGE_1 proved to give slightly less false negative responses in the psychogenic cases (no rigidity at all in 15% compared to 23% with papaverine, full rigidity in 62% compared to 58%). It probably better suppresses the stress inhibition of the erections. Also due to its greater potency, it gave more false positive responses in the vasculogenic patients (no rigidity at all in only 41% compared to 81% following papaverine, full rigidity in 12% compared to 8% with papaverine). Finally the PGE_1 test loses in specificity what it gains in sensitivity. With respect to the detection of the vascular causes, it does not perform much better than papaverine. The PGE_1 test should, however, be prefered because of its safety. In our psychogenic groups, the rates of prolonged erection and of priapism amounted to 10% and 0% respectively with PGE_1, compared to 40% and 7.7% with papaverine, stressing the necessity of first testing lower doses when using papaverine.

Another interesting aspect of the PGE_1 diagnostic test is shown on Table 8. PGE_1, papaverine and papaverine + phentolamine were all tested in the same patients during different sessions of pulse-doppler testing of the penile arteries. Following each tested dose of PGE_1, the dorsal and

Table 8.   Results of pharmaco-doppler testing following PGE_1, papaverine, or papaverine + phentolamine (intra-individual comparison in 101 patients, Porst and Biederman 1993)

Drug	Dose	No injections	Dorsal arteries normal	severely abnormal	Deep arteries normal	severely abnormal
Papaverine	25 mg	84	44.4%	23.8%	46%	20.6%
Papaverine	50 mg	83	36.6%	26.4%	42.7%	20.7%
Papav. + phentol.	50 + 2 mg	76	39.3%	27.3%	42.6%	22.7%
PGE₁	10 µg	84	53.5%	16.6%	55.9%	15.5%
PGE₁	20 µg	71	47.9%	23.2%	54.9%	16.2%
PGE₁	5 µg	22	50%	18.4%	52.2%	13.6%

deep arteries seemed to be normal in a higher percentage of the same patients, and severely abnormal in a lower percentage. Thus PGE₁ should be preferred for this test as it seems to give less falsely abnormal results, again suggesting a better suppression of the stress inhibitory effect on the erectile process. In addition, 2 others studies with intra-individual comparison have pointed another advantage of PGE₁ or the pharmaco-doppler testing: more time is needed to attain full erection following PGE₁ (about 15 min versus 5 min with papaverine or the mixture [24, 46]. Thus more time is left to perform doppler, while following papaverine, in many cases only 1 or 2 arteries can be studied before the test becomes unreliable due to the high intracavernosal pressure.

Calcitonin Gene-Related Peptide (CGRP) and CGRP + PGE₁

CGRP was one of the first drugs proposed to rescue the failures of PGE₁. Stief tested it in open studies [33]. CGRP seemed too weak to work by itself, but it seemed to potentiate the effects of PGE₁ when combined with it. The only study with intra-individual comparison regarding CGRP was conducted by Schwarzer et al. (1992). Sixteen patients with veno-occlusive dysfunction resistant to both papaverine (80 mg), papaverine + phentolamine (60 + 2 mg) and PGE₁ (40 µg) received injections of the combination of CGRP + PGE₁ according to an escalating dose design, up to 5 + 15 µg. The combination proved to be superior to the previously tested drugs in about one third of the cases (full rigidity in 3, and partial, but adequate for intromission, in 2 more), without resulting in significant side effects.

Linsidomine

This nitric oxide donor was again proposed by Stief [34] on the basis of open studies. The results of 4 studies with intra-individual comparison with PGE₁, including 1 double-blind study, are compiled in Table 9. PGE₁ proved to be very significantly more potent than Linsidomine. The later obtained full rigidity in only 15% of the patients and a rigidity adequate for vaginal intromission in 33%. Its only significant advantage was a lower percentage of pain (1%). In the most recent study, Wegner et al. [40] also tested the combination of an alpha-blocking agent (Urapidil)

Table 9.   Compilation of 4 intra-individual comparisons of linsidomine (1 mg) and PGE$_1$ (5 to 20 μg)

	Full rigidity	Adequate rigidity	Pain
No patients	149	116	76
Linsidomine	22 (15%)	38 (33%)	1 (1%)
PGE$_1$	75 (53%)	79 (68%)	9 (12%)
p (Chi Square)	< 0.001 (5.66)	< 0.001 (7.29)	< 0.01 (0.008)

One double-blind study (Wegner et al. 1995, 40 patients, 20 μg PGE$_1$), 3 open studies (Lemaire et al. 1992, 36 patients, 10 μg PGE$_1$; Porst 1993, 40 patients 20 μg PGE$_1$, Weiske 1994, 33 patients, 5 to 20 μg PGE$_1$). No data was provided regarding adequate rigidity in 1 study [42] and regarding pain in 2 [29, 42].

with Linsidomine. The efficacy of the mixture was much better, but it was associated with an unacceptable rate of severe side effects like hypotension, nausea and vomiting.

Two of the preceding studies compared the effects of Linsidomine (1 mg) with those of PGE$_1$ (either 10 μg [22], or 20 μg [29]) on the results of pharmaco-doppler tests done in the same patients. Peak flow velocity proved to be significantly higher following PGE$_1$ injections in both studies (46.7 vs. 29.5 cm/s with 20 μg, 28.9 vs. 25.2 cm/s with 10 μg, $p < 0.05$). Linsidomine does not seem to have any advantage over PGE$_1$ for pharmaco-doppler testing.

Vasoactive Intestinal Polypeptide + Phentolamine (Vasopotin)

In our experience [7] and in others [19] vasoactive intestinal polypeptide proved to be disappointing when used alone, but to give interesting results when combined with other agents, especially phentolamine [7, 14, 19]. This mixture is available under the brand name Vasopotin. We reported the only study with intra-individual comparison of Vasopotin [8]. This association was compared with Linsidomine, Moxisylyte and PGE$_1$ in the same 13 patients (Table 10). PGE$_1$, at the dose of only 10 μg, proved to be, by far, the most potent, followed by

Table 10.   Intra-individual comparison of Linsidomine, Moxisylyte, PGE$_1$ and vaso-active-intestinal-polypeptide + phentolamine (Vasopotin) in 13 patients (adapted after Buvat et al. 1994) [8]

Drug (dose)	No rigidity	Partial rigidity	Full rigidity	Prolonged erection
Moxisylyte (10 or 20 mg)	8 (61%)	4 (31%)	1 (8%)	–
Linsidomine (1 mg)	5 (38%)	5 (38%)	3 (23%)	1 (90 min)
Vasopotin (30 mg + 1 mg)	5 (38%)	3 (23%)	5 (38%)	1 (270 min)
PGE$_1$ (10 µg)	3 (23%)	1 (8%)	9 (69%)	1 (420 min)

Vasopotin, Linsidomine, and lastly Moxisylyte. Only one patient presented prolonged erections, each time spontaneously subsiding. They occur following 3 drugs, confirming the range of the potencies 420 min following PGE$_1$, 270 min following Vasopotin, 90 min following Linsidomine, < 60 min following Moxisylyte. The other side effects were pain (only with PGE$_1$), and flushes (mainly with Vasopotin, also some with Linsidomine). Our study confirms that, for the moment, PGE$_1$ is the most potent of the monosubstance drugs available. Moxisylyte is the less potent, and Vasopotin could be an interesting option in the case of an intense pain following PGE$_1$. In this study, one spinal cord injured man resistant to 10 µg PGE$_1$ obtained fully rigid erections following the injection of Vasopotin.

PGE$_1$ Combinations

PGE$_1$ + Papaverine

Two studies with intra-individual comparison [1, 13] demonstrated a synergistic effect of papaverine and PGE$_1$, and the possibility of rescuing the failures of both papaverine + phentolamine and PGE$_1$ by combining papaverine and PGE$_1$. Lower doses of papaverine proved to be effective in this combination, and thus less fibrosis should be expected.

In the Allen et al. double-blind study [1], a Rigiscan assessment in 7 patients found that the mean duration of erection was of 26 min when PGE_1 was added to papaverine, compared to 6 min when phentolamine was combined with the same dose of papaverine.

PGE_1 + Phentolamine

Padma-Nathan et al. (1990) found in an intra-individual double blind comparison a superiority of PGE_1 + phentolamine over papaverine + phentolamine or PGE_1 alone [27]. When questioned regarding their preference following the double blind home trials, 82% of the 48 patients and 91% of their partners preferred the PGE_1 + phentolamine mixture due to a "more natural erection", enhanced by sexual stimulation, and more often an erection readily reestablished even 20–30 min following ejaculation if sexually restimulated (42%). Three of the 6 patients in whom PGE_1 + phentolamine failed responded to the triple-mixture.

PGE1 + Papaverine + Phentolamine (Triple Drug Mixture)

This combination was introduced in 1990 by Goldstein et al. [15] and became very popular in USA until the approval of PGE_1. Different formulas have been proposed. We found by using the mixture of 10 µg PGE_1 with 8 mg of papaverine and 0.2 mg of phentolamine per ml that 2 ml induced enough rigidity for intercourse in 20/36 impotent patients (55%) resistant to 20 to 40 µg of PGE_1 alone [10]. By restricting the use of the triple mixture to those patients resistant to PGE_1, we never saw any prolonged erection, and, in the long time auto-injection use, rather few fibrosis. Other studies with intra-individual comparison reported adequate rigidity in 20/32 patients (62%) resistant to papaverine + phentolamine [15] and in 3/6 patients resistant to PGE_1 alone and to PGE_1 + phentolamine [27].

The most objective data with respect to the triple drug mixture was reported by MacMahon (1991) in an intra-individual comparative study [25]. He compared in 228 impotent patients PGE_1 with papaverine + phentolamine (30 + 0.5 mg/ml) and papaverine + phentolamine + PGE_1 (20 mg +0.6 mg + 5 µg/ml) at dosages titrated according to the etiology of ED. After each injection, the patients received visual sexual stimulation and the response was assessed with real time Rigiscan. No difference, and thus no interest in the triple drug mixture appeared in the neurogenic, the psychogenic, and the mildly arteriogenic patients in whom all the 3 drugs were effective. On the contrary, a clearly significant advantage of the triple drug mixture was observed in the patients with severe arterial disease and mild venous leakage, alone or combined with arterial disease. In both these 3 categories only the triple drug mixture induced adequate rigidity, although its mean duration with 10 min was short.

Regarding the side-effects, although the efficacy of the triple drug mixture was equal or superior to those of papaverine + phentolamine and PGE_1 alone, no pain was reported with the triple drug mixture compared to a transient pain in 124 patients (54%) following papaverine + phentolamine and a persistent pain in 54 (24%) with PGE_1 alone. Few priapisms (> 5 h erections) occurred after the triple drug mixture (2/228: 0.8%), compared to PGE_1 alone (3/228: 1.3%), which was significantly less than following papaverine + phentolamine (18/228: 7.9%, p < 0.01).

Auto-Injection: Comparative Studies

No intra-individual comparative studies have been reported in this field. We will however cite some "intracenter" comparative studies. Although obviously less objective, they have some interesting aspects because the patients were treated by the same physicians, during the same period of time, and with the same methodology of training and follow-up.

Moxisylyte versus Papaverine

We compared the rates of the complications observed following auto-ICI of these drugs in our center [5] (Table 11). The 2 series of patients were comparable concerning their mean ages, number of injections, and duration of follow-up. More prolonged erections (> 4 h) occurred in the papaverine group, though the difference was not significant. All required treatment on the contrary of the only one which occurred in the Moxisylyte group. But the most interesting observation was a significantly lower rate of fibrosis, especially of fibrotic nodules, following the Moxisylyte auto-ICI (1% compared to 32% in the papaverine group). In addition, the Moxisylyte injections were never painful.

Table 11. Complications of the auto-injections of Moxisylyte and PGE$_1$. (Adapted after Buvat et al. 1991 [5])

Drug (no patients)	Prolonged erections	Nodules, fibrosis	Pain	Dizziness
Papaverine (n = 34)	3 (9%)	11 (32%)	25 (59%)	2 (6%)
Moxisylyte (n = 72)	1 (1.3%)	1 (1.3%)	– –	3 (4%)
p value	ns	< 0.001	–	ns

Nicergoline versus Papaverine

A study conducted by Tulli et al. (1989) had already confirmed a tendency towards less fibrotic lesions following auto-ICI of alpha-blocking agents compared with papaverine [36]. In 3 groups of 20 ED patients each, the rate of cavernosal fibrosis was 0% with nicergoline alone, 30% with papaverine, and 5% with a mixture of both drugs allowing to reduce the papaverine dosage.

Moxisylyte versus PGE$_1$

We compared in a retrospective study the first 130 patients included from the beginning in our Moxisylyte auto-ICI program to the first 130 ones included in our PGE$_1$ auto-ICI program [9].

The mean duration of the follow-up was comparable in the 2 groups (respectively 14.8 and 14.6 months per patient) but the mean number of ICI was 20% higher in the PGE$_1$ group (73 ICI per patient, 5 per month, compared to 53 per patient and 3.8 per month in the Moxisylyte group). The efficacy of PGE$_1$ proved to be significantly superior to that of Moxisylyte: good results (satisfying intercourse following > 75% of the ICI) in 92/130 (71%) compared to 65/130 (50%) after Moxisylyte; fair results in respectively 12% and 18%; poor or nil results of the ICI in 22 (17%) compared to 41 (32%) (p < 0.01). The 68% rate of acceptable results with Moxisylyte again demonstrates that this drug works better at home than in an office. When we splitted the patients according to the main etiological categories, the rate of the good results proved to be significantly higher with PGE_1 only in the arteriogenic group (27/28: 96% vs. 11/24, 48%, p < 0.001), but not in the psychogenic (79% vs. 56%) and neurogenic (83% vs. 71%) groups. Moxisylyte was effective in no case with veno-occlusive dysfunction, while PGE_1 induced adequate rigidity in 4/13 patients.

The main observed side effects are listed on table 12. Significantly less patients of the Moxisylyte group presented prolonged erections > 2 h, and no one resulted in a priapism (only 1 patient, compared to 8, including a priapism in 2, in the PGE_1 group). Almost no pain was reported by the Moxisylyte patients, while this side effect concerned 10% of the PGE_1 patients (although mild in all). Few fibrotic nodules and plaques were found (same rate in both groups).

Table 12.   Main side effects of the auto-injections of Moxisylyte and PGE_1. (Adapted after Buvat et al. 1994 [9])

Drug (treated patients)	Erection > 2 h	Erection > 6 h	Local pain	Diffuse pain	Fibrosis
Moxisylyte (n = 130)	1 (0.7%)	–	1 (0.7%)	–	2 (1.5%)
PGE_1 (n = 130)	11 (8%)	2 (1.5%)	6 (5%)	6 (5%)	3 (2.3%)
p	< 0.01–	–	ns	–	ns

In conclusion, PGE_1 proved to be significantly more effective, especially in the arteriogenic patients, but less well tolerated, inducing more pain and more prolonged erections (preferably in the neurogenic and the psychogenic patients). However, despite its better tolerance, the frequency of use, and the continuation rate of Moxisylyte were lower. For the latter parameter, the difference was highly significant at each time. Especially after 36 months, only 20% of the Moxisylyte patients were still continuing the auto-ICI, compared to 40% of the PGE_1 patients. Therefore it may be supposed that the use of Moxisylyte is less satisfying than that of PGE_1.

Conclusions

Today 3 drugs or mixtures are officially approved for the ICI: papaverine + phentolamine in some countries, PGE$_1$ in most, and Moxisylyte in France. It is probably risky for a physician to use the other ones, at least as first choice drugs, even if the cost of the officially approved drugs considerably limits their use. When classified according to their safety, Moxisylyte is undoubtedly the safest, and PGE$_1$ is clearly safer than papaverine-phentolamine. When classified according to their potency, PGE$_1$ is clearly the most potent, Moxisylyte being a rather weak drug, however successful at home in over 50% of the patients. The question may be raised of which preference should be given for the choice of drug, when each of the 3 drugs is available as in France. For many years, we were promoting Moxisylyte, because the only alternative was papaverine which should now be only rarely used (only in the people who are reliable and really cannot afford safer drugs). Now PGE$_1$ is available, and in our experience, fits as first choice agent in almost all the cases. There are only 3 conditions in which Moxisylyte may be preferred: when the patient will be taught and followed by a little experienced physician, like in France where many sexologists and some general practitioners are beginning to use ICI. Moxisylyte has then the chief advantage of its safety. Another indication is the obviousness of a supersensitivity to the ICI, for example in some neurogenic and psychogenic patients, or the unreliability of the patient, reinforcing the risk of priapism. The last indication for Moxisylyte are those patients with significant pain related to PGE$_1$, persisting despite the repetition of the injections, eventually at a lower dosage, what is indeed not frequent. In that case papaverine-phentolamine could also be used. Lastly it has to be emphasized that the triple drug mixture rescues about 50% of the PGE$_1$ failures, without any prolonged erection in this selected population, and with a rather low rate of fibrosis, occurring anyway in patients without any other alternative than a penile prosthesis implantation.

References

1. Allen RP, Engel RM, Smolev J, Brendler CB (1992) Objective double blind evaluation of erectile function with intracorporeal papaverine in combination with phentolamine and/or prostaglandin. E1. J Urol 148: 1181–1183

2. Berger RE, Hartsell C (1988) Comparison of patient-administered intracorporeal injections of Papaverine 30 mg plus Phentolamine 0.5 mg versus 16.6 μg of PGE₁. 6th International Symposium for corpus cavernosum revasularization, Boston, p 155

3. Buvat J, Buvat-Herbaut M, Lemaire A, Marcolin G (1989) Applications diagnostiques et thérapeutiques des injections intracaverneuses de drogues vasoactives dans l´impuissance. Journal d´Urologie 95: 33–39, et 89–96

4. Buvat J, Lemaire A, Buvat-Herbaut M, Marcolin G (1989) Safety of intracavernous injections using an alpha-blocking agent. J Urol 141: 1364–1367

5. Buvat J, Buvat-Herbaut M, Lemaire A, Marcolin G (1991) Reduced rate of fibrotic nodules in the cavernous bodies following auto-intracavernous injections of Moxisylyte compared to Papaverine. Int J Impotence Res 3: 123–128

6. Buvat J, Buvat-Herbaut M, Lemaire A, Marcolin G, Dehaene JL (1991) Diagnostic value of intracavernous injections of 20 μg of Prostaglandin E1 in impotence. Int J Impotence Res 3: 105–111

7. Buvat J, Lemaire A, Buvat-Herbaut M, Marcolin G (1992). Réponse érectile à une association de Vasoactive Intestinal Polypeptide et de Phentolamine chez 15 impuissants Compte-rendus du congrès de la Société d´Andrologie de Langue Francaise (SALF): 25

8. Buvat J, Lemaire A, Buvat-Herbaut M, Marcolin G (1994) Comparison of the erectile responses to Linsidomine, Moxisylyte, Prostaglandin E1 and Vasopotin injected in the same patients. Int J Impotence Res 6, Suppl 1: D157

9. Buvat J, Lemaire A, Marcolin G, Buvat-Herbaut M (1994) Comparison of the 2 second generation drugs for intracavernosal injections Moxisylyte and Prostaglandin E1. Int J Impotence Res 6, Suppl 1: P39

10. Buvat J, Marcolin G, Buvat-Herbaut M (1994) Auto-injection therapy with a triple association (papaverine + phentolamine + prostaglandin E1) is successful and safe in 50% of the impotent patients resistant to PGE₁. Int J Impotence Res 6, Suppl 1: D122

11. Buvat-Herbaut M, Buvat J, Lemaire A, Marcolin G (1990) Evidence of a facilitating effect of Moxisylyte, an alpha-blocking agent, on the erectile response to sexual stimulation: a double blind controlled study. Int J Impotence Res: 301–302

12. Chiang HS, Wen TC, Wu CC, Chiang WH (1990) Prostaglandin E1 versus Papaverine for diagnosis of erectile dysfunction. Int J Impotence Res 2: 127–130

13. Floth A, Schramek P (1991) Intracavernous injection of Prostaglandin E1 in combination with Papaverine: enhanced effectiveness in comparison with Papaverine plus Phentolamine and Prostaglandin E1 alone. J Urol 145: 56–59

14. Gerstenberg TC, Metz P, Ottesen B, Fahrenkrug J (1992) Intracavernous self-injection with Vasoactive Intestinal Polypeptide and phentolamine in the management of erectile failure. J Urol 147: 1277–1279

15. Goldstein I, Borges FD, Fitch WP, Kaufman J, Damron K, Morens J, Payton T, Yingst J, Krane RJ (1990) Rescuing the failed papaverine/phentolamine erection: a proposed synergistic action of papaverine, phentolamine and prostaglandin E1. J Urol 143: 304A

16. Jünemann KP, Alken P (1989) Pharmacotherapy of erectile dysfunction: a review. Int J Impotence Res 1: 71–93

17. Kattan S, Collins JP, Mohr D (1991). Double-blind cross-over study comparing Prostaglandin E1 and Papaverine in patients with vasculogenic impotence. Urology 37: 516–518

18. Keogh EJ, Watters GR, Earle CM, Carati CJ, Wisniewski ZS, Tulloch AGS, Lord DJ (1989) Treatment of impotence by intrapenile injections. A comparison of Papaverine versus Papaverine and Phentolamine: a double-blind, crossover trial. J Urol 142: 726

19. Kiely EA, Bloom SR, Williams G (1989) Penile response to intracavernosal Vasoactive-Intestinal-Polypeptide alone and in combination with other vasoactive agents. Brit J Urol 64: 191–194

20. Lakin MM, Montague DK, Medendorp SV, Tesar L, Schover LR (1990) Intracavernous injection therapy: analysis of results and complications. J Urol 143: 1138–1141

21. Lee LM, Stevenson WD, Szasz G (1989) Prostaglandin E1 versus Phentolamine/Papaverine for the treatment of erectile impotence: a double-blind comparison. J Urol 141: 549–550

22. Lemaire A, Buvat J, Buvat-Herbaut M, Marcolin G (1994) Erectile response to intracavernous injections of Linsidomine in 38 impotent patients. Int J Impotence Res 6, Suppl 1: D148

23. Levine SB, Althof SE, Turner LA, Risen CB, Bodner DR, Kursh ED, Resnick MI (1989) Side effects of self-administration of intracavernous Papaverine and Phentolamine for the treatment of impotence. J Urol 141: 54–57

24. Liu LC, Wu CC, Chiang CP, Huang CH, Chou YH, Tan LB (1991). Comparison of the effects of Papaverine versus Prostaglandin E1 on penile blood flow by color duplex sonography. Eur Urol 19: 49–53

25. MacMahon CG (1991) An comparison of the response to the intracavernosal injection of a combination of Papaverine and Phentolamine, Prostaglandin E1 and a combination of all three agents in the management of impotence. Int J Impotence Res 3: 113–121

26. Mahmoud KZ, El Dakhli MR, Fahmi IM, Abdel-Aziz AB (1992) Comparative value of Prostaglandin E1 and Papaverine in treatment of erectile failure: double-blind crossover study among Egyptian patients. J Urol 147: 623–626

27. Padma-Nathan H (1990) The efficacy and synergy of polypharmacotherapy in primary and salvage therapy of vasculogenic erectile dysfunction. Int J Impotence Res 2: 257–258

28. Porst H (1989) Prostaglandin E1 bei erektiler Dysfunktion. Urologe A 28: 94–98

29. Porst H (1993) Prostaglandin E1 and the nitric oxyde donor Linsidomine for erectile failure: a diagnostic comparative study of 40 patients. J Urol 149: 1280–1283

30. Porst H, Biedermann V (1993) Open comparative study on the intracavernous injection of Papaverine (or Papaverine + Phentolamine) versus Prostavasin for erectile dysfunction. Schwarz-Pharma clinical research report F8299

31. Sarosdy MF, Hudnall CH. Erickson DR, Hardin TC, Novocki DE (1989) A prospective double-blind trial of intracorporeal Papaverine versus Prostaglandin E1 in the treatment of impotence. J Urol 141: 551–553

32. Schwarzer JU, Hofmann R, Pickl U, Hartung R (1992) Calcitonin-gene-related-peptide for therapy of erectile impotence. Int J Impotence Res 4: 219–222

33. Stief CG, Thon WF, Wetterauer U, Schaebsdau F, Jonas U (1990) Calcitonin-gene-related peptide. A possible neurotransmitter for human penile erection and its therapeutical application in impotent patients. Int J Impotence Res 2: 22–23

34. Stief CG, Holmquist F, Krah H, Djamilian M, Andersson KE, Jonas U (1992) Preliminary results with nitric oxyde donor SIN-1 in the treatment of human erectile dysfunction. J Urol 147: 265

35. Tamura M, Hashine K, Kimura K, Kawanishi Y, Imagawa A (1990) Comparison of the effect of Papaverine hydrochloride and Prostaglandin E1 on human corpus cavernosum. Int J Impotence Res 2: 141–145

36. Tulli RE, Degni M, Pinto AFC (1989) Fibrosis of the cavernous bodies following intracavernous auto-injection of vasoactive drugs. Int J Impotence Res 1: 49–54

37. Virag R (1982) Intracavernous injections of Papaverine for erectile failure. Letter to the editor. Lancet 2: 938

38. Waldhauser M, Schramek P (1988) Efficiency and side effects of Prostaglandin E1 in the treatment of erectile dysfunction. J Urol 140: 525–527

39. Wang CJ, Wu CC, Huang CH, Chiang CP (1994) A comparative study with intracavernosal injection of prostaglandin E1 versus papaverine for the diagnostic assessment of erectile impotence. Int J Impotence Res 6, Suppl 1: D146

40. Wegner HEH, Knispel HH, Klän R, Miller K (1995) Efficacy of Linsidomine chlorhydrate, a direct nitric oxyde donor, in the treatment of human erectile dysfunction: results of a double-blind cross over trial. Int J Impotence Res 7: 233–237

41. Weiske WH (1988) Prolonged erection by vasoactive drugs: its avoidance with PGE₁. Proceedings of the Sixth Biennal International Symposium for Corpus Cavernosum Revascularization, Boston, p 89

42. Weiske WH (1994) Efficacy of PGE₁ and SIN-1 testing under Rigiscan real-time monitoring. Int J Impotence Res 6, Suppl 1: D109

43. Wetterauer U, Weiske WH, Stief CG, Zentgraf M (1988) Intra-individual comparison of the efficacy of the intracavernously injected single agents papaverine and phentolamine with the combination of both. Proceedings of the sixth Biennal International Symposium for Corpus Cavernosum Revascularization, Boston, p 86

44. Wetterauer U (1990) Intra-individual comparison of papaverine-phentolamine combination versus prostaglandin E1 in intracavernous injection therapy for erectile dysfunction. Int J Impotence Res 2: 238–239

45. Xavier A, Searp PP (1990) Prostaglandin E1 versus Papaverine. A comparative study in 22 patients with erectile dysfunction. Int J Impotence 2: 127–128

46. Yasumoto R, Asakawa M, Horii A, Terada T, Yoshimura R, Sawamura A, Kamizuru M, Kawashima H, Nishio S, Maekawa M (1987) Comparison of vasoactive drugs for patients with erectile dysfunction. Proceedings of the first Asia-Pacific meeting on Impotence, November 5–6, Hong-Kong

47. Zorgniotti AW, Lefleur RS (1985) Auto-injection of the corpus cavernosum with a vasoactive drug combination for vasculogenic impotence. J Urol 133: 39

Comparison of Self-Injection Modalities with and without Injection Devices in Erectile Dysfunction

Edoardo S. Pescatori

Introduction

Thirteen years after the introduction of intracavernosal injection with vasoactive agents as treatment of erectile dysfunction [1] it clearly appears that this approach constitutes the treatment of choice for the majority of patients affected by erectile impairment. Reasons for such a success include: treatment effectiveness, physiologic-like erections, minimal invasivity, absence of systemic side effects, reasonably low risks of local side effects, possibility of withdrawal for treatment with no preclusion to other therapeutic options.

More than a decade of clinical investigations nonetheless pointed out the larger limit of this approach: a surprising high drop-out rate from treatment, even in presence of functional erections at the office intracavernosal injection test. Several are the possible reasons for not entering, and for dropping from the intracavernosal injection program. They include: poor manual dexterity, morbid obesity, concern over side effects, dissatisfaction with artificial erection, return of spontaneous erections during the self-injection program, cost of medication [2, 3]. In particular, more than 30% of candidates have been reported to refuse to try intracavernosal injections because of psychogenic inhibition to self-injection ("needlephobia") [4]; another 20% drops during the teaching phase for reasons including needlephobia, artificiality, bother of injection maneuvers and partner resistance [4]. Finally, 24–50% of the patients entering the self-injection program drop out during follow-up [4, 5], for one or more of the above listed reasons.

The first report of a self-injection device as alternative to the standard syringe for patients in intracavernosal treatment for erectile dysfunction appeared in the literature in 1988 [6]. From then on several devices have been proposed, all with the common purpose to allow an easier drug administration, therefore decreasing manual difficulties of intracavernosal pharmacotherapy, with the overall goal of lowering the drop-out rate of this treatment.

This paper intends to review the recommended procedures for a correct manual injection and to deal subsequently with self-injection devices.

Manual Injection: Proper Technique

Patients willing to enter a program of self-injection for erectile dysfunction routinely undergo one or more teaching sessions that also cover recommendations concerning the proper technique of manual injection. It should be stressed that many of the given directions lack a solid scientific support, being more often the result of "good sense" thinking.

One of the few available studies on the effect of repeated injections on the cavernosal tissue showed on primates consistent findings of a localized area of mild fibrosis at the site of repeated needle puncture, regardless of the agent injected. In that study pigtail monkeys were injected twice a week, on the same site, with a 27G needle; manual compression at the injection site was exerted for one minute [7]. The use of ultrathin (29–30G) needles appears advisable since in this study the injection itself caused trauma in the corpus cavernosum. Notably, both the major companies that supply alprostadil for intracavernosal use provide their product with a 30G needle. Furthermore, it is common clinical experience that patients do feel discomfort using a 27G needle for intracavernosal injection, while reporting the injection with a 30G needle as painless.

Patients are then instructed to a straight insertion of the needle in the correct area, with an appropiate angle, aiming to the center of the corpus cavernosum. Following, they learn to deliver the drug slowly to avoid possible trauma to the cavernosal tissue. Patients are especially taught to stop the delivery, if they should feel resistance or pain. In such a case the needle tip could in fact be in the tunica albuginea, in the septum or in a trabecula.

Lastly, patients should compress the injection site between index and thumb for 3 minutes (5 minutes if they are on anticoagulants).

Self-Injection Devices: Classification and Safety Considerations

Several self-injection devices have been recently proposed as an aid to home intracavernosal self-injection treatment for erectile dysfunction. Originally similar devices became popular among insulin-dependent diabetic patients for daily subcutaneous administrations of insulin; they are preferred over the direct injection because of simplicity of use and lack of pain at the injection site [8]. In the candidates to self-injection treatment such devices have the purpose to allow an easier drug administration, decreasing technical problems of intracavernosal pharmaco-theraphy, with the overall goal of increasing the acceptability of this treatment.

A classification of self-injection devices, according to their mechanical impact on the cavernosal tissue, has recently been proposed [9]. This classification identifies three device categories: self-injection pens, autoinsertors and autoinjectors.

Self-Injection Pens. These devices still allow manual needle insertion and manual drug delivery [5, 6, 10]. Originally devised for insulin-dependent diabetic patients, they have been the first self-injection devices to be proposed for the intracavernosal treatment in impotent patients [6]. These pens host a cartridge, pre-filled with the vasoactive drug. Their advantage over syringes chiefly consists in the possibility to comfortably carry around a device that simply requires to uncap its needle and, after needle insertion, to press the pen knob. This avoids the bother of carrying around both drug and syringe, possible maneuvers of on-site drug reconstitution, and drawing the drug from a vial.

Autoinsertors. They provide automatic needle insertion but still allow for manual drug delivery (11, and InjecAid – Osbon, USA). They consist of an injector that can accept a standard, pre-loaded disposable syringe. Such devices, widely used by insulin-dependent diabetic patients, have recently been proposed also for intracavernosal pharmacotherapy [11]. They are provided with a safety lock mechanism to prevent accidental firing, and with the possibility to preset the depth of needle. The advantage of automatic needle insertion is the possibility to overcome problems of both needlephobia and poor manual dexterity, as in patients with neurological deficits or hand tremor.

Autoinjectors. They are spring-loaded guns that host a pre-filled dispos-able syringe or cartridge and, upon firing, provide both automatic nee-dle insertion and automatic drug delivery [12–15]. As for autoinsertors, common features include a safety lock mechanism to prevent accidental firing, and the possibility to preset the depth of needle penetration. While the first described autoinjector [12] was somewhat bulky and noisy upon firing, the more recent ones [13, 14 and Autoject 2 – Owen Mumford, Eng-land, Fig. 2) are handy to carry and less noisy. The first disposable device of this group has recently been investigated in a clinical trial [15].

Two are the main safety concerns with the use of autoinjectors. The first is an increased risk of extra-corporal drug delivery. Commonly, in fact, users of the classic insulin syringe learn to feel the "right resistance" while delivering the drug to the corpora. Furthermore, they are taught not to force the injection, should they feel some unusual resistance, because in such a case the needle could be out of the corpora, in the septum, in a trabecula or in the tunica albuginea. Such a patient-con-trol during injection is lost with an automatic drug delivery. The sec-ond concern relates to the potential of some devices for a high delivery pressure. It has been reported that an autoinjector may deliver a pres-sure 15 times higher than the pressure values reached by manual injec-tion, and statistically higher also than the pressures obtained by manual injection performed by operator maximal manual strenght [9]. Theo-retically, such pressures could mechanically damage the trabeculae of the cavernosal tissue. In fact, although the maximal pressures developed by an autoinjector do not exceed 20 mm Hg, i.e. well below the intra-cavernosal pressure arising within the corpora during erection, it must also be considered that autoinjector injection takes place in the flaccid state with the cavernosal trabeculae in the contract, which is a less com-pliant state than during erection. Furthermore, during the erectile proc-ess the intracavernosal pressure gradually and uniformly increases throughout the corpora, whereas with autoinjector drug delivery there is a sudden discharge of energy in the cavernosal area with an expected pressure gradient that does not occur during the physiologic erection.

Discussion

The introduction of intracavernosal vasoactive pharmacotherapy pro-vided the currently most used treatment for erectile dysfunction. It soon appeared, nonetheless, that the overall procedures connected to the manual self-injection cause a strong resistance in a significant number of potential users of such a treatment. Ancillary strategies are therefore needed to render the intracavernosal delivery of vasoactive drugs more acceptable.

Alternative delivery routes are under investigation; topical creams presently do not appear to be extremely effective, while the first trials of intraurethral administration of alprostadil pellets are promising [15].

In the effort to improve the acceptability of the direct intracavernous injection, several self-injection devices have been proposed. They are handy tools that host the vasoactive compounds ready for use and that are comfortably carried with the patient, allowing a self-injection procedure easier and simpler than with the standard syringe. According to the type of mechanical impact on the cavernosal tissue, they are classi-

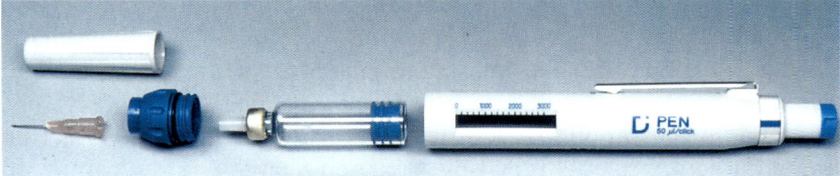

Fig. 1.   Self-injectra pen (D PEN)

COMBINATION INSULIN INJECTOR AND BLOOD LANCET DEVICE

Instaject®

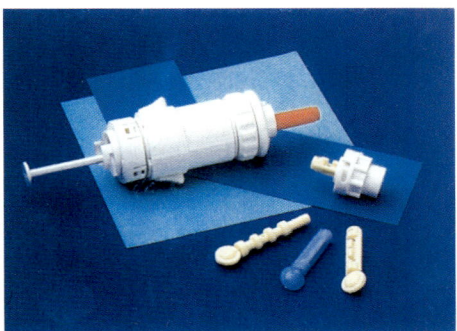

- For use with **most sizes and brands** of disposable insulin syringes.

- Can be adjusted for **depth of needle penetration**.

- **Small** enough to fit in the palm of your hand.

- Fits all **square-bodied lancets** (i.e. Surelet, Surelite, Monolet, Trends, Autoclix, Autolancet and EZ-let).

- Made of **shatterproof polycarbonate**

Fig. 2.   Auto-inserta (Instaject)

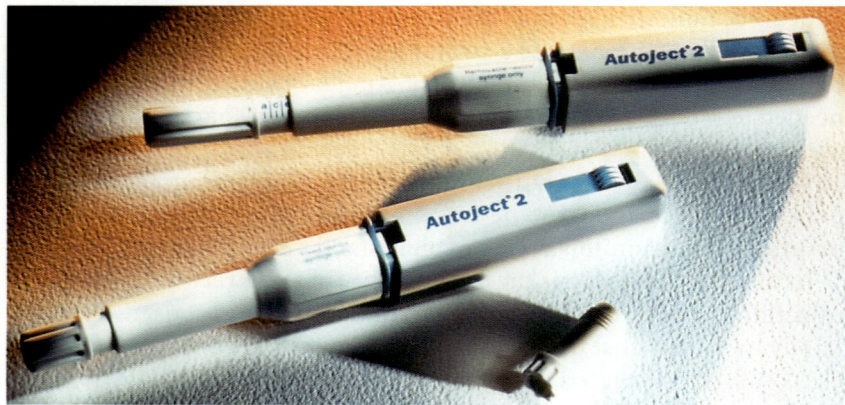

Fig. 3.   Auto-injecta (Autoject 2)

fied as: *self-injection pens,* that still allow for manual needle insertion and manual drug delivery (Fig. 1.), *autoinsertors,* allowing for automatic needle insertion but still providing manual drug delivery (Fig. 2.), and *autoinjectors,* spring-loaded guns hosting a pre-filled disposable syringe or cartridge that, upon firing, provide both automatic needle insertion and automatic drug delivery (Fig. 3.). Their characteristics, compared to manual injection, are summarized in Table 1.

Table 1.   Comparison of control possibilities during self-injection among manual injection and different self-injection devices

	Manual injection	Self-injection Self-injection pens	Auto insertors	Devices Auto-injectors
Correct injection site	yes	yes	yes	yes
Straigth needle insertion with correct angle	yes	yes	less controlled	less controlled
Slow drug delivery	yes	yes	yes	device dependent
Stop delivery if resistance or pain	yes	yes	yes	no

Specific advantages are offered by the three different classes of devices. Self-injection pens are safe and are reportedly effective in reducing the drop-out rate in the self-injection treatment. Autoinsertors additionally address the problems of both psychogenic inhibition to self-injection because of needle fear, and of poor manual dexterity. Auto-injectors provide the advantages of a fully automatic operation; theoretical risks for potential damage to the cavernosal tissue include both the possibility of extracorporal drug delivery and of high delivered pressures.

References

1. Virag R (1982) Intracavernous injection of papaverine for erectile failure. Lancet 2: 938
2. Barada JH, McKimmy RM (1994) Vasoactive pharmacotherapy. In: Bennett AH (ed) Impotence. Diagnosis and Treatment of Erectile Dysfunction. W. B. Saunders Co., Philadelphia, pp 22–50
3. Althof SE, Turner LA, Levine SB, Risen C, Kursh ED, Bodner D, Resnick MI (1989) Why do so many people drop out from auto-injection therapy for impotence? J Sex Marital Ther 15: 121–129
4. van Driel MP, Mooibroek JJ, van de Wiel HBM, Mensink HGA (1991) Intracavernous pharmacotherapy: psychological, sexological and medical aspects. Int J Impot Res 3: 95–104
5. Thon WF, Seidl E, Kramer AE, Jonas U (1990) Andropen – preset self-injection pen for intracavernous auto-injection therapy in erectile impotence. World J Urol 8: 87–89
6. Kromann-Andersen B (1988) Intracavernosal pharmacotherapy with injection pen. Lancet 1: 54
7. Aboseif SR, Breza J, Bosch RJLH, Bernard F, Stief CG, Stackl W, Lue TF, Tanagho E (1989) Local and systemic effects of chronic intracavernous injection papaverine, prostaglandin E1, and saline in primates. J Urol 142: 403–408
8. Resman Z, Metelko Z, Skrabalo Z (1985) The application of insulin using the jet injector DG-77. Acta Diabetol Lat 22: 119–125
9. Pescatori ES, Calpista A, Artibani W, Pagano F, Calabro´ A (1996) Self-injection devices for intracavernosal pharmacotherapy: operational classification and safety considerations. Int J Impot Res (accepted for publication)
10. Montorsi F, Guazzoni G, Bergamaschi F, Orlandini A, Da Pozzo L, Barbieri L, Rigatti P (1993) Intracavernous vasoactive pharmacotherapy: the impact of a new self-injection device. J Urol 150: 1829–1832
11. Chen J, Greenstein A, Kaver I, Braf Z (1994) Use of automatic insulin injector for intracorporeal injection in erectile dysfunction. J Urol 152: 461–462
12. Virag R, Shoukry K, Floresco J, Nollet P, Greco E (1991) Intracavernous self-injection of vasoactive drugs in the treatment of impotence: 8-year experience with 615 cases. J Urol 145: 287–293

13. Gilbert HW, Gingell JC (1992) The autoinjector device: an aid to intracavernous pharmacotherapy. Br J Urol 70: 211–212
14. Greco E, Polonio Balbi P (1994) Selfinject: a fully automatic injector for intracavernous injections. A clinical study. Int J Impot Res 6 (Suppl. 1): P 116
15. Gerstenberg T (1995) A novel auto-injector for the administration of vasopotin – A new treatment for erectile dysfunction. Int J Impot Res 7 (Suppl 1): D 28
16. Padma-Nathan H, Bennett A, Gesundheit N, Hellstrom W, Henry D, Lue TF, Morley J, Peterson C, Prendergast JJ, Tam P, Teresi A, Place V, the VIVUS-MUSE Study Group (1995) Treatment of erectile dysfunction by the medicated urethral system for erection (MUSE). J Urol 153: 472A

After a Decade of Venous Surgery –
Is there a Place for it in 1996?

Ronald W. Lewis

Etiological Considerations

In 1992, I composed a talk called "Fact or Fiction" regarding vascular impotence. In that presentation, I prepared slides with various points that needed to be questioned. One of the statements was "Veno-occlusive dysfunction is a major single entity cause of impotency". I posed that statement for reflection. We were beginning to discover, at that time, that although veno-occlusion is an extremely important part of the male erectile cycle it is not truly a venous disorder responsible for veno-occlusive dysfunction. The faulty veno-occlusion is, in fact, a reflection of an underlying healthy cavernosa tissue with a structurally intact trabecular system, an intact arterial in-flow system, and an uncompromised elastic tunica albuginea.

Three other statements included in that talk were the following:

1. Maintenance flow rate is the best and only diagnostic tool to determine veno-occlusive disorders;
2. The second phase of cavernosometry/cavernosonography (DICC) is a good diagnostic tool to determine veno-occlusive disorders; and
3. Veno-occlusive surgery is highly successful.

We will look at each of these statements as we try to answer the main question of this talk.

There are several points which should be discussed first. A veno-occlusive disorder can present as total erectile failure in which there is inability to obtain adequate rigidity for vaginal penetration; or can simply present as erectile impairment where there are strong rigid erections that last for a very short time. Veno-occlusive disorders can also be a source of primary erectile dysfunction, which is rare and might represent some congenital abnormal venous drainage from the penis, or, as is more commonly present, as a secondary erectile dysfunction.

Many different disorders may account for abnormal venous drainage from the corpora cavernosa. There may be rare congenital abnormal veins or A/V fistula. Abnormal development of draining veins can be secondary to diseases of the tunica albuginea of the corpora, such as Peyronie´s or associated with urethral stricture involving severe fibrosis of the corpus spongiosum. Recently, there have been some papers, discussed below, that report lack of elasticity and abnormal collagen deposition in the tunica albuginea do not allow for adequate venous occlusion. Persistent shunts secondary to treatment for priapism, such as transglanular shunts between the corpora cavernosa and the corpus spongiosum, may also account for a rare case of veno-occlusive disorder. It has even been suggested in the literature that in veno-occlusive disorders, the deep dorsal vein of the penis may lack valves and thus produce incompetent veins. This is not really reasonable. The most popular reason or explanation for veno-occlusive disorder today is inadequate relaxation of the corpora cavernosa so that not enough pressure can be generated and maintained to occlude the subtunical veins which prevents subsequent drainage through the emissary veins into the veins on the surface of the tunica albuginea.

In understanding the modern concepts of physiology of veno-occlusive dysfunction, it is now known that veno-occlusion in the erectile cycle is dependent upon good arterial inflow, intact sinus smooth muscle with the ability to relax, and intact, elastic tunica albuginea. The rationale for veno-occlusive surgery for the treatment of impotence is either directed at treating congenital venous disease or to treat developmental or iatrogenic causes. Basically, there is still some reason to believe that there may be patients who have a partial structural abnormality of the corpora cavernosal tissue that might benefit from the elimination of draining veins on the surface of the tunica albuginea. When this disease becomes moderate or severe, removing these venous channels will probably not produce a successful result.

Surgery for veno-occlusive sexual dysfunction results in only a 50% success rate. (See Table 1 for data from the literature) Excellent return of rigidity varies from 12.5% in a small series from Rossman et al. [11] to 60% reported after a 12 month follow-up in report from Weidner et al. [6]. Some of the long term follow-up, as outlined in the table including my own series, report only a 25% to 30% success rate at two years. There is another group of patients apparently helped by the surgery who are unable to obtain erections with pharmacological injection agents prior to venous

Table 1. Results of surgery for veno-occlusive sexual dysfunction

Study (Years of Study) (n)	Patients	Excellent	Improved	Immediate success/later failure	Failures	Average follow-up months
Lewis-Tulane Series (1981–1987)[1]	49	12 (24%)	12 (24%)	8 (16%)	17 (35%)	15
Wespes et al. (1982–1986)[2]	67[a]	31 (46%)	16 (24%)		20 (30%)	24
Donatucci and Lue (1986–1988)[3]	100	44 (44%)	24 (24%)		32 (32%)	(12–50)
Bondil et al. (1981–1988)[4]	60	25 (42%)[b]			35 (58%)	22
Lunglmayr et al. (1984–1986)[5]	29	9 (31%)[b]			10 (34.5%)	to 24
Weidner et al.[6] (1985–1987)	51	28 (55%)		8 (16%)	15 (29%)	12
(1988–1989)	40	24 (60%)		11 (27.5%)	5 (12.5%)	12
Gilbert et al. (1985–1990)[7]	134	26 (19.4%)	47 (35.1%)		61 (45.5%)	12.9
Lewis-Mayo Series[5] (1987–1988)	28	7 (25%)	4 (14%)	8 (29%)	9 (23%)	48
(1988–1989)	32	9 (28%)	13 (41%)	5 (15.5%)	5 (15.5%)	24
Knoll et al. (1987–1989)[9]	41	19 (46%)	Unknown	Unknown	22 (54%)	28
Kropman et al. (1987–1989)[10]	20	6 (30%)	4 (20%)	8 (40%)	2 (10%)	15
Rossman et al. (1985–1988)[11]	16	2 (12.5%)	2 (12.5%)	10 (62.5%)	2 (12.5%)	Unknown
Claes and Baert (1987–1989)[12]	72	30 (41.7%)	23 (31.9%)		19 (26.4%)	> 12
Montague et al. (1988–1990)[13]	18	11 (61%)		6 (33%)	1 (6%)	24
Freedman et al. (1986–1991)[14]	46	11 (24%)	8 (17%)	23 (50%)	4 (9%)	31–33
Stief et al. (1989–1992)[15]	77	31 (40.3%)[d]	9 (10.3%)		38 (49.4%)	6

[a] 67 patient questionnaire responses to 105 letters sent
[b] Series reported as excellent or improved as a group not in each individual category
[c] 17 of 39 are now able to achieve erection with pharmacologic agent injection
[d] 1 of 31 when followed for extended period (18.5 months) needed pharmacotherapy to obtain an erection

surgery, but are able to obtain rigid erections with cavernosal injections after venous surgery. These make up approximately 25% to 30% of patients who respond to the surgery. Failures, which can include immediate success with erectile dysfunction recurring within a year and patients who are not improved at all, range from 40% to 50% of the cases.

The criteria for recommending surgery for veno-occlusive disorder consists of the following:

1. A patient complaint of short duration erections or tumescence only with sexual stimulation,
2. failure to maintain or obtain an erection with the use of intracavernous injections on multiple trials with different agents with sexual stimulation,
3. normal cavernous arteries as evaluated by color duplex Doppler studies or the second phase of DICC,
4. determination of faulty veno-occlusive mechanism as determined by maintenance flow on infusion pump cavernosometry or gravity cavernosometry,
5. localization of the site of venous leakage from the corpora cavernosa on pharmacocavernosography,
6. no medical contraindications for surgery, and
7. selection of this therapy by the patient after presentation of alternative therapy choices despite the fact of long term success rates of 40% to 50%.

We are left with four reasons for venous surgery to fail which comprises the remainder of the discussion in this presentation. First, there may be faulty diagnostic tools that may account for some of the 40% to 50% failure rate. Second, some venous outlets may be missed and third, after removing the draining veins, collateral veins, still remain which may enlarge and thus produce a recurrent venous runoff as occurs with venous surgery in many other regions of the body such as varicose veins of the lower extremities. Lastly, a most important probable reason for failure, which should be a major area of research emphasis in 1996, is the presence of corpora cavernosa tissue and/or tunica disease. Veno-occlusion is dependent on the lack of disease affecting sinus smooth muscle or changes in the elastic nature of the tunica albuginea or disorders of these tissues. There are a few initial studies conducted in 1996 that we will examine that may allow the surgeon to diagnose probable failure prior to venous surgery. If we become able to evaluate these disease states, we might eliminate the patients who will probably fail veno-occlusive surgery thus allowing us to select patients who benefit from surgery. There may be a crucial level of sinus smooth muscle disease which, when surpassed, surgery eliminating the draining veins on the surface of the tunica albuginea will not help under any circumstance.

Diagnostic Tools

The diagnosis of venogenic impotence is made by pharmacocavern-osometry. It is my opinion that the infusion pump maintenance flow rates (after smooth muscle relaxation by intracavernosal injection) and plateau pressures reached on gravity studies are the most important diagnostic tools. Pharmacocavernosography is the anatomical study performed to aid the surgeon in knowing which veins have to be elimi-nated by surgery. The second phase of dynamic infusion cavernoso-metry and cavernosography (DICC) which describes the amount of crop in pressure from 150 mm/Hg (in a steady state) over a period of 30 sec-onds, is not in my opinion a good diagnostic study. In a presentation at the International Society of Impotence Research meeting in Boston, we reported that this test will diagnose all patients with veno-occlusive dis-order but will also have a high number of false positives in patients without veno-occlusive dysfunction. In addition, a study reported by Eric Meuleman [16] looked at various reported diagnostic tests used to establish a veno-occlusive disorder using a very sophisticated statisti-cal analysis in two groups of patients. One group obtained a rigid erec-tion with an injection of vasoactive agent and the other group obtained no rigid erection from two such injections. The two most statistically valid tests for the evaluation of the veno-occlusive disorder included the steady state intracavernosal pressure on gravity cavernosometry and infusion pump maintenance flow rates after smooth muscle relaxation obtained by intracavernosal injection. The mean steady state intra-cavernosal pressure of the patients who obtained rigid erections was 87 ± 19 cm of water with the median of 102 (range of 56 to 120). Those patients who did not obtain a rigid erection with the two injections had a mean of 50 ± 36 cm of water (± standard deviation) with a median of 58 (range of 10 to 100). The difference between the two groups was sig-nificant (P value was less than 0.001). The mean maintenance flow rate in those patients who obtained a rigid erection from injection was 14 ± 13 ml/min (± standard deviation) with a median of 10 (range of 0 to 40). In those patients who did not obtain an erection, the mean maintenance flow rate after injection was 50 ± 22 ml/min with a median of 50 (range of 15 to 200). The P value comparing differences between these two groups was less than 0.001. When I looked at a number of patients in my clinic using the same criteria as Meuleman, there was a very, very strong correlation between those patients who obtained a steady state under gravity cavernosometry of 60 cm of water or greater and those who had a maintenance flow rate of less than 30 ml per second. The correlation was also apparent between those patients who did not reach 60 cm of water and had maintenance flow rates greater than 30 ml per second.

In previous publications reviewed by me [17], maintenance flow greater than 50 ml per min was certainly indicative of venous leak. Maintenance flow between 20 and 50 ml/min were suspicious for venous leak and maintenance flow less than 20 ml/min did not indicate significant leak. This was substantiated as veno-occlusive disorder by rapid runoff of the contrast into dilated deep dorsal penile veins or other channels subsequently draining the internal and external pudendal veins when pharmacocavernosography was performed at the rate necessary to obtain 100 mm Hg, when possible. There was also ghost-like appearance of or rapid contrast washout from the corpora cavernosa in such a study. Pescatori and his associates also suggest that normal flow to maintain erection with infusion pump after adequate smooth muscle relaxation is only 0.5 to 3 ml per minute [18]. This paper also cautioned that a good response to smooth muscle relaxant does not indicate a normal arterial inflow system but does clearly establish a good veno-occlusive mechanism.

Technical Considerations

Two other reasons for venous surgery failure are missing some venous outlets at the time of surgery and collaterals subsequently arising after venous surgery. Neither of these two technical complications are unusual for venous surgery when performed elsewhere in the body. Pharmacocavernosography is necessary to establish preoperatively what veins should be addressed at the time of surgery. The drainage of the corpora cavernosa involves three systems – the superficial, the intermediate and the deep drainage systems. Superficial venous drainage into the external pudendal veins and subsequently into the saphenous veins occurs when there are collaterals between the intermediate system or direct drainage from the distal penis into the superficial system. The intermediate drainage system is traditionally described as the major drainage system of the corpora cavernosa and consists of a single dorsal midline or multiple deep dorsal penile vein(s) fed by direct emissaries along the shaft of the penis or the circumflex veins into which the emissary veins of the corpora drain. The deep dorsal vein usually terminates as one branch to join the retropubic plexus and/or drains subsequently into the internal pudendal system. The deep drainage system consists of crural veins which usually drain into the internal pudendal vein and rarely communicates with the retropubic plexus. The more medial of the crural veins, termed by Tom Lue "cavernosal veins", drain into the internal pudendal vein frequently communicating to the periprostatic (retropubic) plexus. Table 2 lists the sites of common venous drainage [19, 20,

Table 2. Site of venous leakage in veno-occlusive dysfunction

Study number Site of leakage	1[a]		2[b]		3[c]	
	Pt (no.)	%	Pt (no.)	%	Pt (no.)	%
Superficial system only	6	6	—	—	—	—
Intermediate system only	8	9	8	18	6	17
Deep system only	16	17	—	—	9	25
Cavernous veins only	15	16				
Crural veins only	1	1				
Superficial and intermediate systems	11	12	6*	13	8	22
Deep dorsal vein and cavernous veins	7	7	—	—	—	—
Deep dorsal vein, cavernous veins, and glans/spongiosum	—	—	17	37	—	—
Deep system and spongiosum	—	—	—	—	2	5.5
All three systems	24	25	1	2	2	5.5
Total patients	96		46		36	

* = Leakage through deep dorsal vein and glans/spongiosum
[a] = Reference 19
[b] = Reference 20
[c] = Reference 21

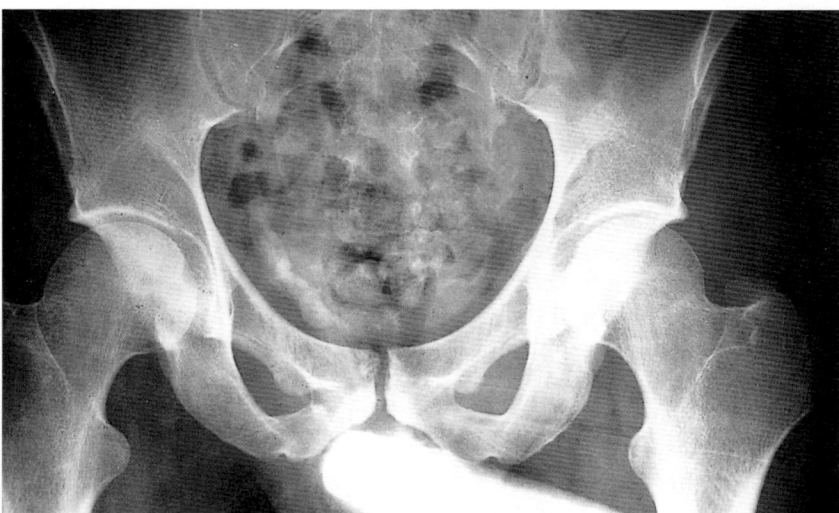

Fig. 1. Cavernosogram that shows no significant venous leak

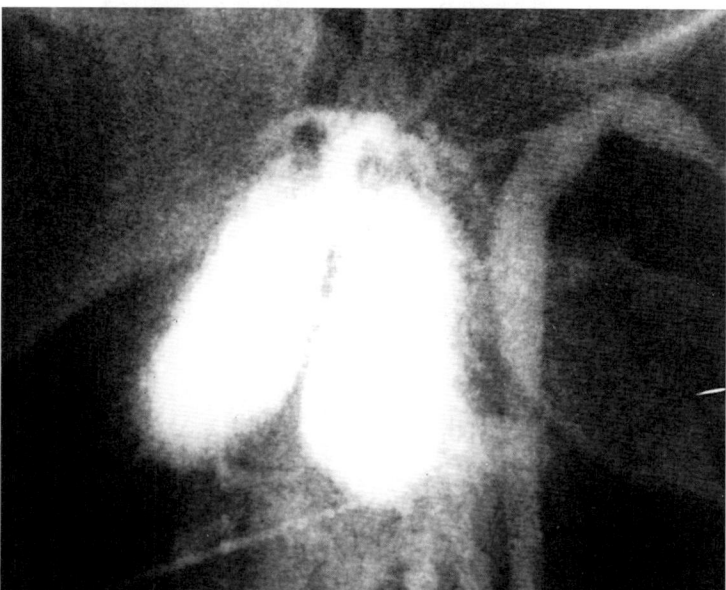

Fig. 2. Cavernosogram that shows a rare defect in the tunica albuginea that drains into the superficial system on the left side of the penis. This subsequently drains into the left saphenous vein by the external pudendal vein. This patient has a circumcision incision and a ligation of the defect in the tunica albuginea with a ligation of the superficial vein. At 5 years of follow-up, he had regained potency

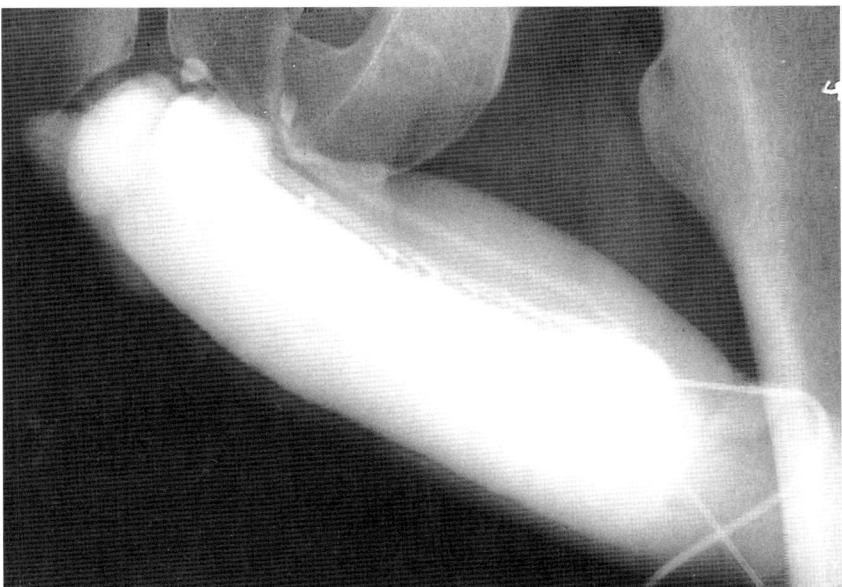

Fig. 3. This cavernosogram shows primary drainage into the deep dorsal vein with evidence of direct circumflex and emissary drainage into that vein. This also shows a communication to the superficial system just below the glans that drains into the left external pudendal vein and subsequently into the saphenous system

21]. Figures 1–5 show different degrees of venous leakage. In Fig. 5, the leakage is so massive that it is doubtful if venous dissection surgery will allow the elimination of all the draining veins.

The steps of venous surgery are outlined in Figs. 6 and 7. Several points should be made here. I prefer supine positioning of the patient and do not feel that the dorsal lithotomy position is necessary. The peripenile anterior scrotal incision should curve gently around the base of the penis allowing the penis to be inverted through this incision see Fig. 6). I place a 19–21 gauge needle into the base of one of the corpora at this point and sew it in place with a chromic suture since it can be dislodged during the dissection. After the injection of a vasoactive agent, an indigo carmine colored saline is injected ten minutes later to help visualize draining veins. As the penis is inverted into the wound, any communication from the corpora cavernosa or intermediate system to the superficial system can be divided and ligated. All ligatures placed on the penile shaft should be absorbable. The fundiform and suspensory ligaments must be completely taken down to the infrapubic region

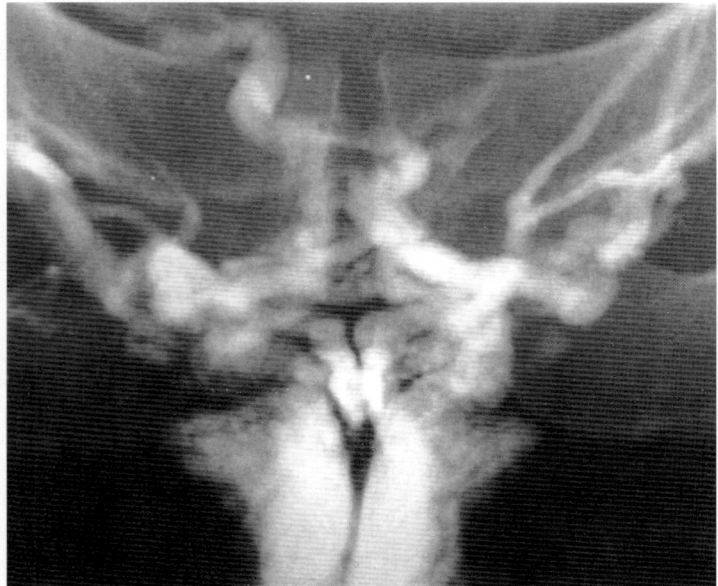

Fig. 4. This cavernosography shows drainage into what Tom Lue call the "cavernosal veins" which are the medial crural veins. There is massive drainage into the retropubic venous plexus and both bilateral internal pudendal systems

Fig. 5. Cavernosogram which shows massive venous drainage including superficial, deep and deep dorsal vein. This patient has such massive venous leakage, it is doubtful that venous surgery would result in any improvement

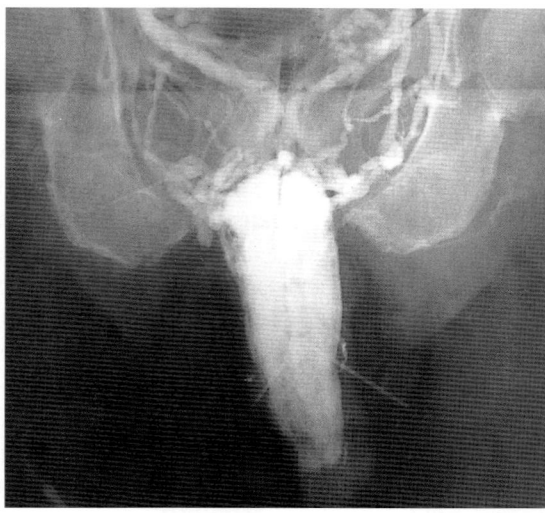

Fig. 6. This shows the preferred penile incision for venous surgery

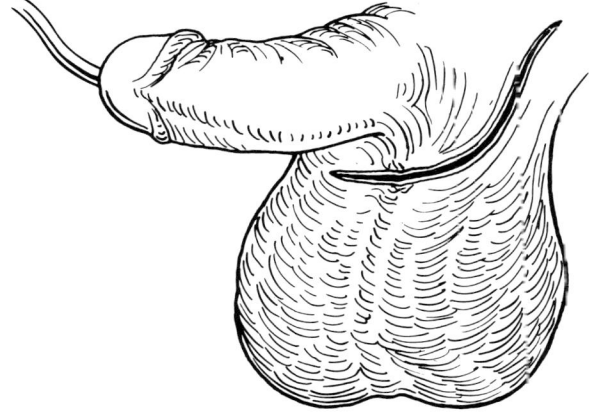

in order to be able to completely dissect the deep dorsal vein of the penis. Intraoperative Doppler probes may be beneficial if there is a question whether a vessel is a vein or an artery. Once the deep dorsal vein is dissected from its middle sulcus by opening Buck´s fascia while taking great care to stay in the midline, communicators (including circumflex veins) and direct emissaries are carefully ligated. Sometimes a suture ligature is needed to completely occlude the vessel as it emerges from the tunica albugenia of the corpora cavernosa. Communicators of the circumflex system that join the spongiosum system are carefully ligated on each lateral side of the penis as well. I usually reform the suspensory ligament after complete deep dorsal vein dissection by fixation of the deep midline dorsal penis to the infrapubic periostium of the pubic bone. A drain is placed for 24–48 hours that exits from a separate stab wound. My preference is a fenestrated tubular drain. I find a lighted suction device is useful for illumination of the infrapubic region during dissection of these vessels. The crural veins can be occluded to some degree by lateral exposure from this incision. Crural plication by perineal exposure for a more accurate dissection and ligation of crural vessels may be necessary under some circumstances. I only use this as a secondary procedure. After closure of the wound with an absorbable suture, I loosely wrap the penis with self adherent elastic dressing and leave a urethral catheter in overnight. The dressing and catheter are both removed the following day. As mentioned above, the drain will be left 1–2 days depending upon the amount of drainage. The resumption of sexual activity usually begins about six weeks after surgery.

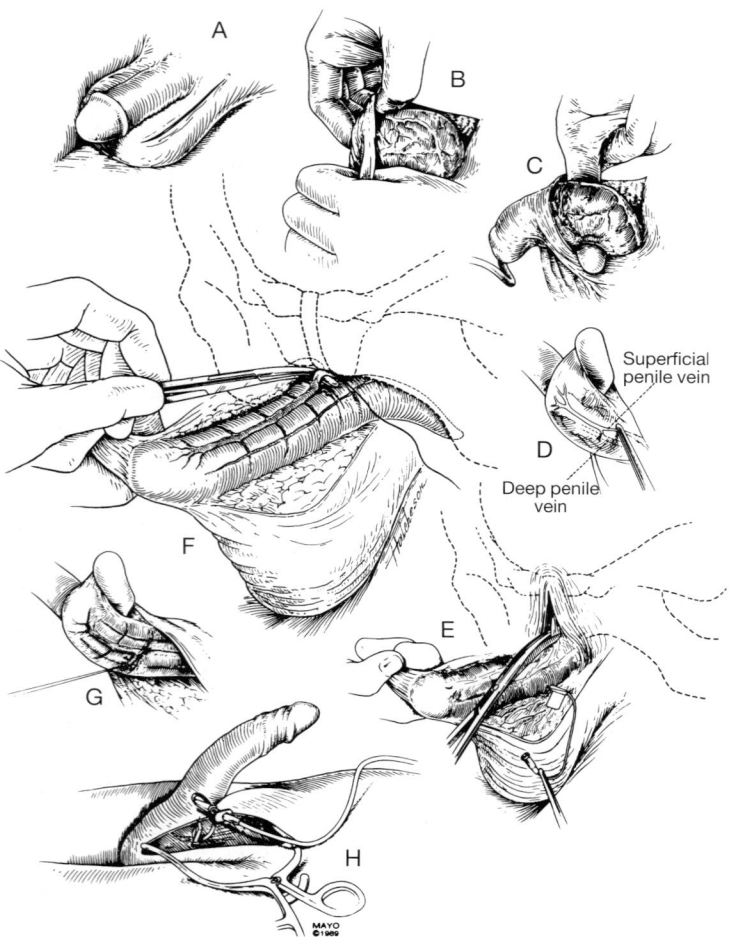

Fig. 7a–h. This shows the steps in venous surgery. **a** This shows a penile incision but Figure 6 is the preferred incision. **b, c** The entire penis can be inverted through this peripenile incision. **d** As this is done, there are connections identified between the superficial and the deep venous system that can be ligated. **e** The fundiform and suspensory ligament of the penis is completely taken down in the infrapubic region. **f** The deep dorsal vein is ligated in the infrapubic region. This is difficult to show in a drawing and is diagrammatic. **g** The Buck´s fascia is opened over the deep dorsal vein and dissected toward the glans. Direct emissary veins draining into this vein as well as circumflex veins are individually isolated and ligated. **h** Following the surgery, smooth muscle relaxant is injected into the corpora. Ten minutes later, a control cavernosometry is obtained to compare with the preoperative cavernosometry to ensure that an adequate venous dissection has been performed

Simultaneous Existence of Other Corporeal Cavernosal Disorders

Recently, Dr. A. Nehra won second prize at the American Urological Association´s annual meeting for clinical research [22]. He stated in his paper that venous leak is really a result of trabecular structural alterations and impaired tissue compliance. He feels surgery does not address underlying pathophysiology. This may be true to some extent but I wish to propose other ideas regarding venous surgery.

In previous papers I described results obtained in two different years of performing venous surgery [17]. The outcome between patients with surgery in 1987–88 was not as good compared to those who were operated on between 1988–89. I feel one of the reasons for the difference in the results was the more sophisticated diagnosis of concomitant arterial disease by using color duplex Doppler [23]. Color duplex Doppler of the penile arteries is a highly sophisticated method of evaluating arterial function. In the presence of moderate to severe arterial disease, venous surgery will usually fail. Also, an important concept recently introduced by presentations from Dr. Goldstein´s group in Boston is complete corpora cavernosal smooth sinus muscle relaxation must be obtained during pharmacocavernosometry and color duplex Doppler ultrasonography [24, 25]. If a patient obtains an erection similar to the best erection he is able to obtain on his own and bilateral arterial systolic velocities are greater than 30 cm/s, the patient probably does not have significant arterial disease. If the patient has high end diastolic velocities or if the end diastolic velocities do not approach zero or a negative value and the patient does not obtain a rigid erection with good systolic velocities, this indicates a veno-occlusive disorder. In the Nehra et al. report given at the AUA, it was necessary to give four injections of an agent (containing 5.9 mg of papaverine, 0.2 mg of phentolamine, and 2 micrograms of prostaglandin E-1) in two patients to achieve the best erection. Three injections were done in 8 patients and two injections in 38 patients. Only 8 of this series (14%) obtained an erection similar to the best erection obtained at home with the first injection [25].

Wespes and his co-workers have recently published a very significant paper that addresses the issue of performance of venous surgery in the presence of corporal cavernosal smooth muscle disease. It is a premise that the closure of the draining veins of the penis is dependent upon complete relaxation of this tissue. Therefore, it could be asked if there is a crucial level of sinus smooth muscle disease which contraindicates venous surgery. Wespes presented a study of 23 patients who had veno-occlusive surgery. Twelve of these responded to surgery in a 1–2 year follow-up (successes) and eleven who did not respond to surgery (failures) [26]. He performed an immunohistochemical staining using an Desmin anti-desmin technique. He found that the mean percentage of smooth muscle in those who failed the surgery to be 22.4% (range 18–29) and 31.3% (range 29–34) in those who successfully responded to surgery. This suggests that venous surgery might be useful for some patients who have minimal smooth muscle disease. Another paper by Gentile and his associates studied ultrastructural and histochemical changes in patients with Peyronie´s disease and veno-occlusive disorder [27]. Tunica albuginea and corpora cavernosa samples were obtained in 6 patients with Peyronie´s disease, 7 patients with veno-occlusive disorder and 5 control patients. Hypercellular fibroblasts (showing activation) were compressed between heterogenous disorganized extracellular collagen fibers in the tunica albuginea in the diseased specimens in both Peyronie´s and veno-occlusive disorders but not in controls. Cavernosal tissue in all groups did not show any difference. There was also an increased Type I–III collagen ratio in the diseased conditions. Type V collagen was found only in diseased tunical tissue. Antibodies to platelet derived growth factors (AA and BB) were found only in the diseased tunica fibroblasts. There was also an increase in amorphous tissue in the diseased tunica albuginea. Controls showed none of these changes. It was the conclusion of that group that this data negates the ability of venous surgery to be effective. I suggest an alternative. If some of the veno-occlusion is due to inelastic tunica albuginea which does not allow for proper occlusion of the emissary veins, why not consider surgery that eliminates the veins on the surface of the tunica albuginea into which these emissary veins drain. Certainly, this area of veno-occlusive surgery should be more fully addressed. Some of the experimental work suggests that all of the answers are not yet in.

Conclusions

Venous surgery has only 40%–50% long term success. It should be offered to patient with this understanding. Only those patients fulfilling all criteria for venous occlusive disorder with performance of pharmacocavernosometry and pharmacavernosography should be considered candidates for surgery. Patients with poor or borderline arterial flow shown on color duplex Doppler ultrasonography should not be offered venous surgery alone. They might benefit from revascularization surgery if proper arteriography shows focal lesions. Patients with combined arterial and venous disease might be candidates for vein ligation and arterial revascularization to the deep dorsal vein. Patients with massive venous leak or severe Peyronie's disease may not benefit from venoocclusive surgery. Complications from the surgery are minor although some penile shortening does occur. Scar contraction may also occur which produces some angulation of the penis with erection. Major complications are rare. There are a group of patients who will not obtain a full, rigid erection after surgery but might be converted to injection therapy. This may account for as many as 20% of patients who would benefit from the surgery. These patients should be carefully tried on home injection with multiple doses before performance of venous surgery. It is my opinion that venous surgery is not entirely without merit, and there probably is a small group of patients who will benefit from this intervention.

References

1. Lewis RW, Puyau FA, Bell DP (1986) Another surgical approach for vasculogenic impotence. J Urol 136: 1210–1212
2. Wespes E, Delacour L, Prejzerowicz L et al. (1988) Long-term follow-up of operations for venous leakage. In: Proceedings of Sixth International Symposium for Corpus Cavernosum Revascularization and Third Binennial World Meeting on Impotence. International Society of Impotence Research, Boston, p 193
3. Donatucci CF, Lue TF (1992) Venous surgery: Are we kidding ourselves? In: Lue TF (ed) World Book of Impotence. Smith-Gordon and Co, London, pp 221–227
4. Bondil P, Schauvliege T, Nguyen Qui JO (1988) Venocavernous leakages: Consideration in 60 operated cases. In: Proceedings of Sixth Biennial Corpus Cavernosum Revascularization and Third Biennial World Meeting on Impotence. International Society of Impotence Research, Boston, p 189
5. Lunglmayr G, Nachtigall M, Grindl K (1988) Long-term results of deep dorsal penile vein transsection in venous impotence. Eur Urol 15: 209–212
6. Weidner W, Weiske WH, Rudnick J et al. (1992) Venous surgery in veno-occlusive dysfunction: Long-time results after deep dorsal vein resection. Urol Int 49: 24–28
7. Gilbert P, Sparwasser C, Beckert R et al. (1992) Venous surgery in erectile dysfunction: The role of dorsal-penile-vein ligation and spongiosolysis for impotence. Urol Int 49: 40–47

8. Lewis RW (1992) Venous ligation for venogenic impotence. In: Whitehead ED, Nagler HM (ed) Management of Impotence and Infertility. Lippincott JB, Philadelphia, pp 73–92

9. Knoll LD, Furlow WL, Benson RC (1992) Penile venous ligation surgery for the management of cavernosal venous leakage. Urol Int 49: 33–39

10. Kropman RF, Nijeholt AABL, Giespers AGM et al. (1990) Results of deep penile vein resection in impotence caused by venous leakage. Int J Impotence Res 2: 29–34

11. Rossman B, Mieza M, Melman A (1990) Penile vein ligation for corporeal incompetence: An evaluation of short-term and long-term results. J Urol 144: 679–682

12. Claes H, Baert L (1991) Cavernosometry and penile vein resection in corporeal incompetence: An evaluation of short-term and long-term results. Int J Impotence Res 3: 129

13. Montague DK, Angermeier KW, Lakin M et al. (1993) Penile venous ligation in 18 patients with 1 to 3 years of follow-up. J Urol 149: 306–307

14. Freedman AL, Neto FC, Rajfer J (1993) Long-term results of penile vein ligation for impotence from venous leakage. J Urol 149: 1301–1303

15. Stief CG, Djamilian M, Truss MC et al. (1994) Prognostic factors for the postoperative outcome of penile venous surgery for venogenic erectile dysfunction. J Urol 151: 880–883

16. Meuleman EJH, Wijkstra H, Doesburg WH et al. (1991) Comparison of the diagnostic value of gravity-and pump-cavernosometry in the evaluation of the cavernous veno-occlusive mechanism. J Urol 146: 1266–1271

17. Lewis RW (1993) Venous surgery in the patient with erectile dysfunction. Atlas of the Urol Clin NA 1: 21–38

18. Pescatori ES, Hatzichristou DG, Hamburi S et al. (1994) A positive intracavernous injection test implies normal veno-occlusive but not necessarily normal arterial function: A hemodynamic study. J Urol 151: 1209–1216

19. Aboseif SR, Breza J, Lue TF et al. (1989) Penile venous drainage in erectile dysfunction: Anatomical, radiological and functional considerations. Br J Urol 64: 183–190

20. Shabsigh R, Fishman IJ, Toombs BD et al. (1991) Venous leaks: Anatomical and physiological observations. J Urol 146: 1261–1265

21. Fuchs A, Mehringer CM, Rajfer J (1989) Anatomy of penile venous drainage in potent and impotent men during cavernosography. J Urol 141: 1353–1356

22. Nehra A, Moreland R, Saenz de Tejada I et al. (1995) What is venous leak and why is there limited success with venous leak surgery in patients with vasculogenic impotence associated with vascular risk factors? A correlation of clinical, histological, molecular, and engineering aspects of corporeal veno-occlusion. J Urol 153: 471A (Abstract 972)

23. King BF, Lewis RW, McKusik MA (1994) Radiological evaluation of impotence. In: Bennet AH (ed) Impotence-Diagnosis and Management of Erectile Dysfunction. Saunders, Philadelphia, pp 52–91

24. Udelson D, Hatzichristou DG, Saenz de Tejada I et al. A new methodology of pharmacocavernosography which enables hemodynamic analysis under conditions of known corporeal smooth muscle relaxation. J Urol 141: 320A (Abstract 370)

25. Nehra A, Hakim LS, Abobakr RA et al. (1995) A new method of performing duplex Doppler ultrasonography: The effect of re-dosing of vasoactive agents on hemodynamic parameters. J Urol 153: 332A (Abstract 415)

26. Wespes E, deBoes PM, Saltar AA et al. (1994) Objective criteria in the long-term evaluation of penile venous surgery. J Urol 152: 888–990
27. Gentile V, Modesti A, LaPera G et al. (1996) Ultrastructural and immunohistochemical characterization of tunica albuginea in Peyronie's disease and veno-occlusive dysfunction. J Androl 17: 92–103

Critical Evaluation of Methods for Arterial Revascularization of the Penis

K.-P. JÜNEMANN

Two methods of surgical therapy that differ completely, i.e., with respect to both the surgical and the pathophysiological approach, are available for vascular reconstruction in vasculogenic erection disorders.
1. Penile venous surgery (ligation, excision, plication of the crura of both cavernous bodies)
2. Arterial revascularization

The latter means a special challenge, because the necessity of microsurgery makes it very demanding under surgical aspects, on the one hand, and because reconstructive vascular surgery is, at present, the only causal approach to treat vascular impotence.

Contrary to the venous surgery performed first as early as the turn of the century [16, 26], vascular reconstruction in the penis gained increasing attention only in the late 1970s as a result of Michal´s [17, 18] and Virag´s [24, 25] publications. The clinical use of penile revascularization surgery was widened and its importance increased, in particular in the German-speaking countries, not least as a result of the modification introduced by Hauri [7]. The controversial hemodynamic mechanism set off in the erectile tissue by a revascularizing intervention [21, 23, 27] on the one hand, and the very mixed and irregular long-term results, on the other hand, have led researchers to develop and try a great number of surgical modifications (Table 1). All techniques have in common that the inferior epigastric artery has prevailed as the arterial donor vessel.

Irrespective of the different modifications, three basic principles of penile revascularization can be distinguished and account for the majority of revascularization procedures today (Table 2). In Virag´s technique [25], the exposed inferior epigastric artery is drawn down to the penis and joined with the deep dorsal vein of the penis in an end-to-side

Table 1. Techniques of penile revascularization

Reference	Anastomosis between the inferior epigastric artery and the:
Michal I [17]	Cavernous body
Michal II [18]	Dorsal penile artery
Virag I–VI [24, 25]	Deep dorsal vein of penis (six modifications)
Crespo [3]	Cavernous artery (deep penile artery)
Hauri [7]	Dorsal penile artery + arteriovenous shunt with deep dorsal vein of penis
Furlow-Fisher modification [4]	Isolated segment of deep dorsal vein of penis
Konnak/Ohl [13]	Deep penile artery
Löbelenz/Jünemann [15]	Deep dorsal vein of penis + two arteriovenous shunts with proximal and distal segments of one dorsal penile artery (triple anastomosis)
Austoni [2]	Dorsal penile artery, orthograde and retrograde

Table 2. Basic principles of penile revascularization (from [11])

The donor vessel is the inferior epigastric artery
Anastomosis with:

1. Venous arterialization
   - deep dorsal vein of penis
2. Formation of arteriovenous shunt
   - deep dorsal vein of penis + dorsal penile artery
3. Formation of arterioarterial shunt
   - dorsal penile artery
   - deep penile artery

anastomosis (Fig. 1). Hauri [7], on the other hand, was the first to describe a triple shunt between the inferior epigastric artery and the deep dorsal vein of the penis, which had previously been anastomosed side-to-side with one of the two dorsal penile arteries (Fig. 2). Depending upon the author, the long-term results of the two surgical procedures as to the rates of spontaneous erections range between 73% [24] and 81% [8]. Such good results were not achieved by other authors [1, 5, 9, 15, 22, 27] or by us [12], even when various modifications were used. It became apparent, on the contrary, that the initially good results were markedly

Fig. 1. Revascularization technique according to Virag. Anastomosis between inferior epigastric artery and deep dorsal vein of penis (end-to-side). (From [15])

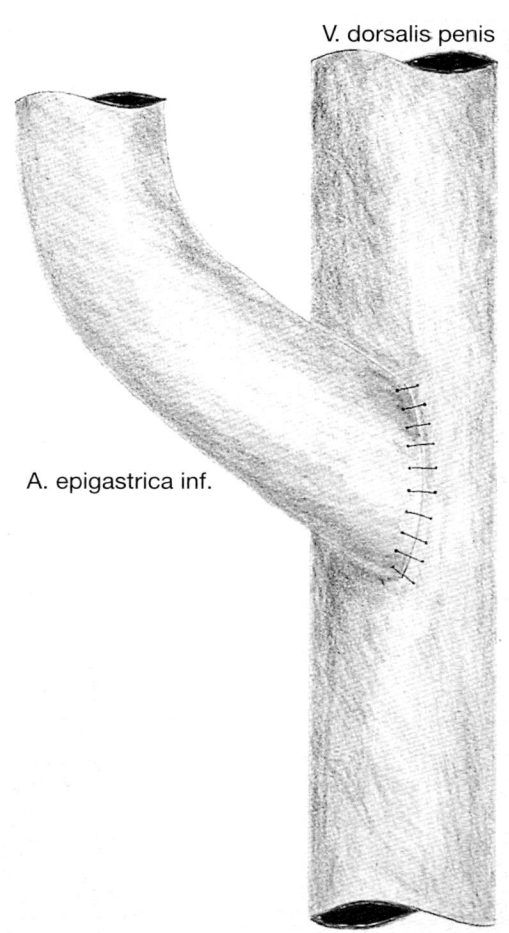

V. dorsalis penis

A. epigastrica inf.

with long follow-up (average 72%, 33–100%) [14, 20], this is also the case for the data and experience gained with venous surgery.

The postoperative decrease in responders is not caused by an occlusion of the anastomosis [12, 22], since the rates of spontaneous erections were markedly below the demonstrated bypass patency rates of up to 91% (our own patients [12]; see above).

The complications reported are typical balanic hyperemia in up to 25% of cases [20] and bypass aneurysms in up to 20%; in our own patients, however, we have never seen the latter event, so we think that it

Fig. 2. Threefold anastomosis
according to Hauri. (From [10])

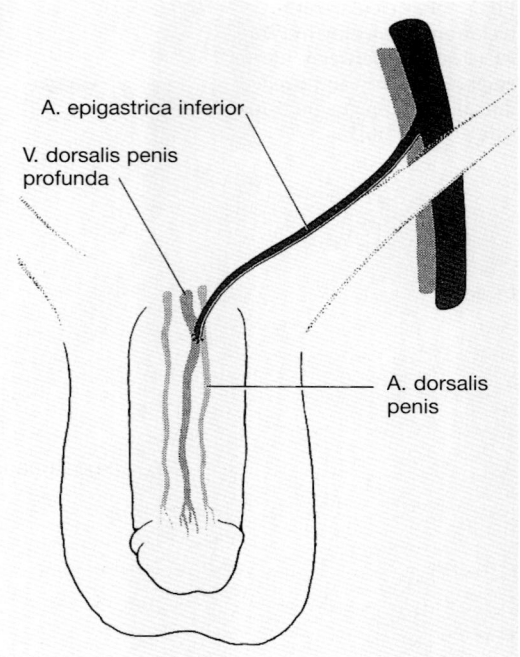

A. epigastrica inferior

V. dorsalis penis
profunda

A. dorsalis
penis

is due to an insufficient anastomotic technique (insufficient intima approximation), all the more so as references in the literature are scarce.

The question now arises as to which patients profit from penile revascularization. Zumbé [27] reported that among his patients those classified as nonresponders to SICI showed better results regarding the rate of spontaneous erections than those who did respond to the administration of a vasoactive substance (55% vs. 48%). Jünemann and co-workers [12] obtained similar results on the rate of spontaneous erections of nonresponders to SICI (53%).

Which other possibilities of patient selection are available at present? Hatzichristou and Goldstein [6] based their selection criteria on various factors: on the one hand, they found hemodynamic aspects that greatly influenced the surgical success (Table 3a); on the other hand, distinct contraindications for vascular reconstruction (Table 3b) were found in patients whose erection disorders were known, or could be demonstrated, to possess a neurogenic component.

Table 3. Selection criteria for penile revascularization (from [6])

a   Hemodynamic

- Delayed response to the intracorporeal administration of a vasoactive substance
- Gradient of systolic occlusion pressure between brachial and cavernous artery ≥ 35 mm Hg
- Flow-to-maintain between 0 and 3 ml/min
- Fall of intracorporeal pressure from 150 mm Hg to less than 45 mm Hg within 30 s results in exclusion.

b   General

- Exclusion of blunt pelvic or perineal trauma
- Exclusion of neurologic cause
- No diabetes mellitus
- No systemic arteriosclerosis
- No veno-occlusive insufficiency
- Arterial insufficiency established hemodynamically and arteriographically

Zumbé [27] and our own group [12] have further derived prognostic factors that were used to develop clear selection criteria (Table 4). When the above-mentioned hemodynamic and risk factors and the selection criteria derived from them are taken into account, long-term results of between 50 and 53.3% can be obtained.

Although preliminary prognostic factors are now available, revascularization surgery should still be reserved for centers that follow Sharlip´s principle [19] that surgery should be executed only if regular

Table 4. Selection criteria (from [11])

According to Zumbé and co-workers [27]	According to Jünemann and co-workers [12]
Nonresponders to SICI	Nonresponders to SICI
Patient´s age < 55 years	< 49 years: surgery indicated 50 to 59 years: surgery dependent on the patient and risk factors
No diabetes mellitus Exclusion of cavernous insufficiency	Less than two risk factors; no diabetes mellitus, no serious hypolipo-proteinemia, nonsmoker
Stenosis of internal pudendal artery (segments 1 and 2) established	

after-care for the patient can be guaranteed. As long as we do not know the mechanism of action and can rely only on few and still insufficient prognostic factors, no wide spread use is advisable, although reconstructive revascularization can help certain individual patients to achieve a normal erection and can therefore provide causal healing.

References

1. Alefelder J, Kutta A, Schürholz T, Wistuba S, Engelmann U (1994) Langzeitergebnisse mikrochirurgischer Penisrevaskularisationen zweier urologischer Zentren. Akt Urol 25: 93–97
2. Austoni E, Colombo F, Mantovani F (1992) Arteriogenic impotence: Long-term follow-up in 68 patients treated by end-to-end epigastro-dorsal ortho and antiflow double anastomosis. In: Giuliani L, Puppo P (eds) Urology 1992. Monduzzi Editore S.p.A., Bologna, Italy, p 805
3. Crespo E. Soltanik E, Bove D, Farrell G (1982) Treatment of vasculogenic sexual impotence by revascularizing cavernous and/or dorsal arteries using microvascular techniques. Urology 20: 271–275
4. Furlow WL, Fisher J, Knoll DL (1988) Penile revascularization experience with deep dorsal vein arterialization – the Furlow-Fisher modification with 27 patients. In: Proceedings of the Sixth Biennial International Symposium for Corpus Cavernosum Revascularization and Third Biennial World Meeting on Impotence. International Society for Impotence Research (ISIR), Boston, p 139
5. Furlow WL, Fischer J, Knoll DL, Benson RC (1990) Current status of penile revascularization with deep dorsal vein arterialisation: experience with 95 patients. Int J Impotence Res 2/S2: 348–349
6. Hatzichristou D, Goldstein I (1993) Penile microvascular arterial bypass surgery. Atlas Urol Clin North Am 1: 39–60
7. Hauri D (1984) Therapiemöglichkeiten bei der vaskulär bedingten erektilen Impotenz. Akt Urol 15: 350–354
8. Hauri D (1989) Operative Möglichkeiten in der Therapie der erektilen Dysfunktion. Urologe A 5: 260–265
9. L´Hermite J, Hubert J, Maute F (1990) Revascularization of the penis in arteriogenic impotence. 10 years´ experience. J Urol Paris 96(2): 102–106
10. Jünemann KP (1992) Erektionsstörungen. In: Alken, Walz (eds) Urologie. VCH-Verlag Weinheim, Kap. 12, pp 305–315
11. Jünemann KP (1996) Impotenzchirurgie. Revaskularisationstherapie. In: Schreiter, Bartsch (eds) Plastisch-rekonstruktive Chirurgie in der Urologie. Thieme Verlag, Stuttgart, Kap. 9A, in Druck
12. Jünemann KP, Hatzinger M, Schmidt P, Persson-Jünemann Ch, Alken P (1995) Two years´ follow-up on penile revascularization in pharmacotesting nonresponders. J Urol 153 Suppl: 369A: 564. 90th Annual AUA Meeting, Las Vegas, USA, April 23–28, 1995

13. Konnak JW, Ohl DA (1989) Microsurgical penile revascularization using the central corporeal penile artery. J Urol 142: 305–308
14. Lewis RW (1992) Arteriovenous surgeries: Do they make any sense? In: Lue TF (ed) World book of impotence. Smith-Gordon, London, pp 199–205
15. Löbelenz M, Jünemann KP, Siegsmund M, Rassweiler J, Alken P (1991) Penisrevaskularisation bei SKAT-Non-respondern in einer modifizierten mikrochirurgischen Technik. Akt Urol 22: 151–156
16. Lydston GF (1908) The surgical treatment of impotency. Am J Clin Med 15: 1571–1573
17. Michal V, Kramar R, Pospichal J (1973) Direct arterial anastomosis to the cavernous body in the treatment of erectile impotence. Rozhal Chir 52: 587
18. Michal V, Kramar R, Pospichal J (1977) Arterial epigastrica venous anastomosis for the treatment of sexual impotence. World J Surg 1: 515
19. Sharlip ID (1991) The incredible results of penile vascular surgery. Int J Impotence Res 3: 1–6
20. Sohn M, Barada JH (1994) Ergebnisse der penilen Gefäßchirurgie bei erektiler Impotenz. Akt Urol 25: 133–142
21. Sohn M, Wein B, Bohndorf K, Handt S, Jakse G (1991) Dynamic magnetic resonance imaging (MRI) with paramagnetic contrast agents: a new concept for evaluation of erectile impotence. Int J of Impotence Res 3: 37
22. Sohn MH, Sikora RR, Wein B, Jakse G (1992) Objective invasive follow-up after penile revascularization: The end of the quest? Int J Impotence Res 4 [Suppl 2]
23. Sohn MH, Wein B, Handt S, Bohndorf K, Jakse G (1992) Gadolinium-enhanced dynamic MRI of the penis: a new diagnostic tool in erectile dysfunction. Int J Impotence Res 4 [Suppl 2]
24. Virag R (1986) Surgical treatment of impotence: Indications and late results on 300 cases. In: Proceedings of the Fifth Conference on Vasculogenic Impotence and Corpus Cavernosum Revascularization. Second World Meeting on Impotence. Prague: International Society for Impotence Research (ISIR). 7.1
25. Virag R, Zwang G, Dermange H, Legman M (1981) Vasculogenic impotence: A review of 92 cases with 54 surgical operations. Vasc Surg 15: 9
26. Wooten JS (1903) Ligation of the dorsal vein of the penis as a cure for atonic impotence. Texas Med J 18: 325–328
27. Zumbé J, Grozinger K, von Pokrzywnitzki W (1995) Selektionskriterien zur penilen Revaskularisation bei arteriell bedingter erektiler Dysfunktion. Akt Urol 26: 114–118

Enhancement Phalloplasty with Girth Augmentation by Autologous Fat Transfer: A Further Report of 700 Cases

Sheldon O. Burman and Thomas P. Kelly

It is possible by surgical means to enhance the length and girth of the pendulous penis. Previously [7], we reported our experience with our first 162 patients. The purpose of this paper is to document our experience since June 2, 1992, with around 700 enhancement phalloplasty procedures.

Masters and Johnson [10] note that "the size of the male organ both in the flaccid and erect state has been presumed by many cultures to reflect directly the sexual prowess of the individual male." Widely diverse cultures, ancient and modern, have linked penis size to virility, dominance, and power. Even among the affluent and well-educated, penis size often equates to manliness. Few men, including those presumably indifferent to penis size, would wish to have a smaller penis. If a man´s perception is that his penis is too small, it will matter little to him when his surgeon assures him that he is "normal" or "average." Feelings of inadequacy and low self-esteem often influence, even dominate, his personal and occupational relationships.

The nature of the operation and its exploitation by surgeons promising unrealistic results have understandably provoked the opposition of surgeons whose training is traditionally directed toward improving physical function or correcting pathology. The argument is advanced that if a man´s penis is already normal there can be no justification for his wanting to be larger. Feelings of inadequacy and poor self-esteem are not "manly" and are matters more appropriate to the psychiatrist´s couch than to the operating room. Yet plastic surgeons routinely deal with issues of image and self-esteem [1]. There may also be the unspoken suspicion that a man overly concerned with the size of his penis is probably homosexual. In fact, the vast majority of our phalloplasty patients are heterosexual. Most candidates are aware that they have penises of normal or average dimensions. Interestingly, most patients have never suffered disparaging remarks from their sexual partners.

Their desire is to improve their locker-room appearance. Many of our patients are body builders and weight lifters who are committed to obtaining a highly developed, idealized vision of themselves. Such men often are not satisfied with an average or normal penis. Other patients have suffered youthful ridicule and humiliation from other males over undersized penises. Our first patient had attempted suicide twice before he and his parents consulted us in June 1992. Such patients may become reclusive and avoid relationships and situations where their bodies become exposed. These patients are often the most grateful for even modest gains. Many men come seeking the operation who are obsessed with the most minute details of their physical appearance.

Questioning will often reveal deep-seated feelings of inadequacy. Our experience is that no matter the results, these patients will be dissatisfied. No matter how perfect you make their penis, it will never be perfect enough. Such patients should not undergo surgery. Dissatisfied patients can be vociferous, vituperative, violent, and vindictive.

Various studies [3, 8, 11, 12] have indicated that the average erect penis is between 13.8–16.6 cm. Caucasians and Blacks are comparable in the erect state. In the flaccid state Blacks appear to average about a centimeter longer. Asians are smaller, a fact taken into account by manufac-

Fig. 1.   True congential micropenis

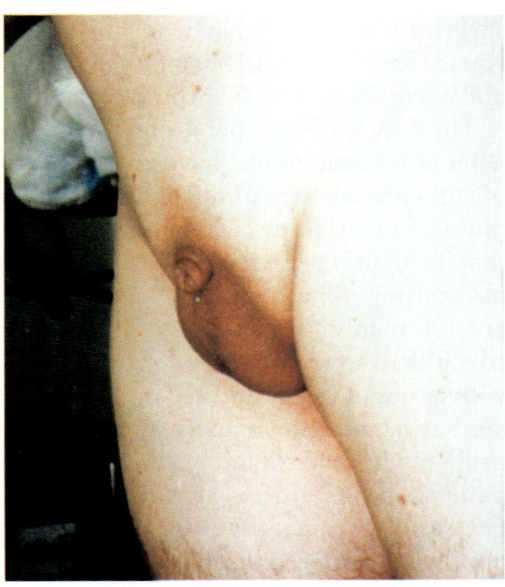

turers of penile prostheses and condoms. Patients with abnormally small penises, including true micropenis, can be helped significantly. Micropenis is defined as a penis size less than 2 standard deviations from the mean. For adults, this is stretched or erect penis length of 9.3 cm. The so-called concealed, buried, or retracted penis is a consequence of too much skin having been removed during circumcision and/or the presence of an overhanging hypertrophic suprapubic fat pad (Fig. 1).

History

The earliest references to penile lengthening techniques are found in the pediatric urology literature [28, 29, 30, 33]. These variously describe resection of the suspensory ligament, release of restricting bands of Scarpa´s fascia, suprapubic lipectomy and tethering the dermis at the base of the penis to the pubic periosteum or proximal tunica albuginea. Our own independent recognition of the possibilities for penile lengthening stems from the mid-1980s when, upon dividing the suspensory ligament during insertion of penile prostheses, we noted an apparent increase in the length of the pendulous penis. Likewise, following ligament transection during proximal ligation of their deep dorsal vein for venous leak, several patients volunteered the information that their penises appeared longer. Subrini [5] reported a mean gain of 3 cm in 49 patients after release of the suspensory ligament. Furlow [4] also described length increases in prosthesis patients after dividing the suspensory ligament.

Incisions

Advancement of the penis requires some sort of lengthening incision. At the base of the penis all incisions except the transverse cut across skin creases and, while necessary for function, are more or less undesirable for appearance. We have at various times tried M-incisions, single Z-plasties, multiple Z-plasties, and inverted V–Y advancement techniques. We have found the V–Y advancement technique to be preferable. It is simplest and provides adequate length.

Ligamentous Attachments (Fig. 2, 3)

The pendulous penis is attached to the pubic bone by dense areolar tissue and the fundiform (superficial) and suspensory (deep) ligaments. The fundiform is the extension downward of Scarpa´s and Camper´s fasciae from the rectus fascia just above the pubic symphysis to the dorsal and lateral penis [8]. The suspensory ligament is a three-dimensional triangular sheet of dense fibrous tissue stretching from the linea alba and upper portion of the symphysis pubis and arcuate pubic ligament to the center of the penis where it fans out laterally from the dorsum [1]. Added support of the penis is provided by the dense attachments of the crura bilaterally to the ischiopubic rami.

Fig. 2. Cross-section of penile shaft showing normal anatomy

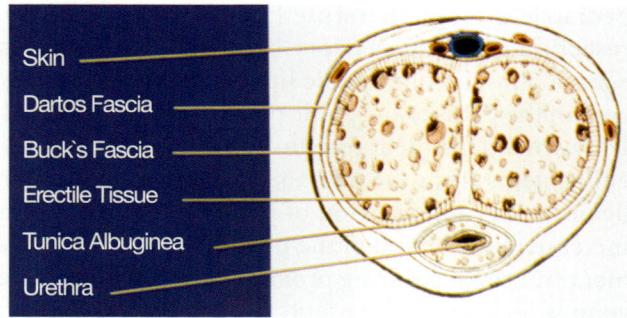

Skin

Dartos Fascia

Buck's Fascia

Erectile Tissue

Tunica Albuginea

Urethra

Fig. 3. Left: Location of structures divided for length enhancement

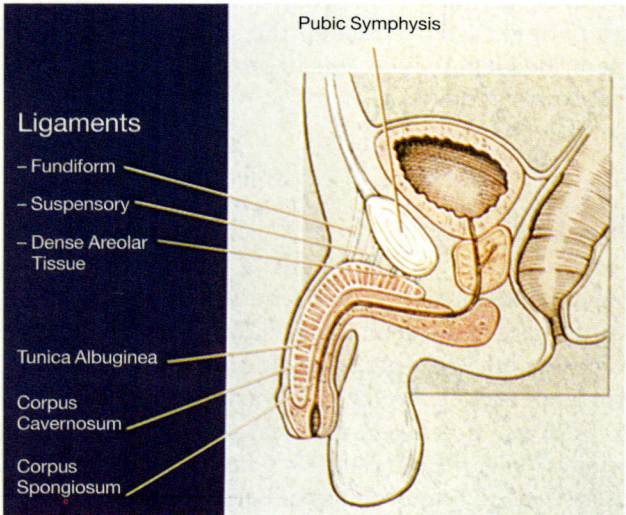

Pubic Symphysis

Ligaments

– Fundiform

– Suspensory

– Dense Areolar
  Tissue

Tunica Albuginea

Corpus
Cavernosum

Corpus
Spongiosum

The Suprapubic Fat Pad

Illouz [25, 26, 27] suggested that certain zones of the body are target sites for the abnormal accumulation of "privileged" fat. In males these sites include the suprapubic region [30], which remains resistant to the severest dietary restriction or intensive exercise. If this area should regress during famine, when caloric intake resumes this area rapidly and preferentially reaccumulates fat. In obese men, a normal penis will often be buried beneath the overhanging suprapubic panniculus. Suprapubic lipectomy is necessary to achieve optimal penile lengthening. In our experience direct scissors lipectomy is preferred to suction lipectomy. Fat thus removed from this suprapubic area is unlikely to reaccumulate.

Girth Enhancement

According to Reed [9], penile girth enhancement using modern techniques was first performed by Samitier in 1989. The two techniques available for girth enhancement are dermal fat grafts (DFG) and autologous fat transfer (AFT). Our experience has been chiefly with AFT.

Dermal Fat Grafts (Fig. 4–6)

Dermal fat grafts are composite grafts, consisting of de-epithelialized dermis and fat. Donor sites generally are from the inguinal creases anteriorly or from the medial buttock-thigh creases posteriorly. Depending on the size of the penis each donor graft is around 14 cm long and 6–12 cm wide, depending on whether one or two grafts are taken. After the grafts are removed, the incisions are undermined and closed with buried sutures, taking care to avoid dog ears. To maximize concealment the incision closure should be kept within the crease. The epidermis of the graft is stripped off the dermis and the graft thinned to about 1.5 cm. The penis is degloved and the grafts fixed fat side down onto the dartos fascia. Some surgeons use two or more grafts placed side by side; others prefer a single large graft wrapped circumferentially around the shaft, usually stopping short of the urethra. With dermal-fat grafts almost no girth shrinkage occurs although there may be some shrink-

Fig. 4.   Thigh-buttock
dermal fat graft donor
sites marked

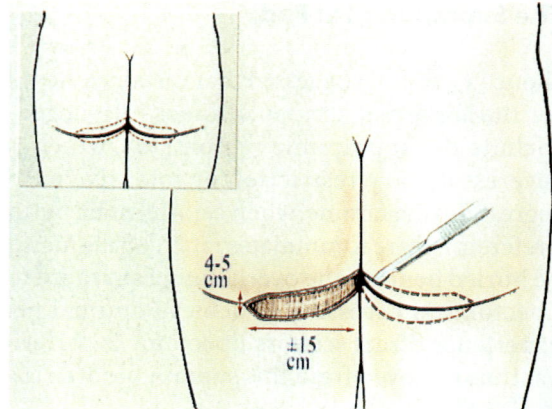

Fig. 5.   Left: Cirumcision-
type incision for distal
graft fixation
Right and lower: Diagrams
show grafts sewn in place

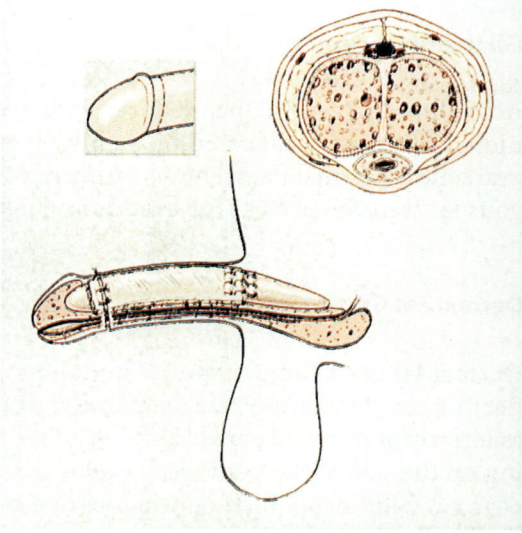

age of length. The graft may dislodge and become bunched up underneath the proximal or distal ends. If grafts are laid side by side, longitudinal grooves may develop. The large scars created at the donor sites
may be troubling, especially to devotees of the beach or the gym. Patients
may complain of incisional discomfort when they sit down. The operation itself takes most surgeons about three hours.

Fig. 6.   Insert: Incision
edges undermined and
closure begun
Right: Closure complete

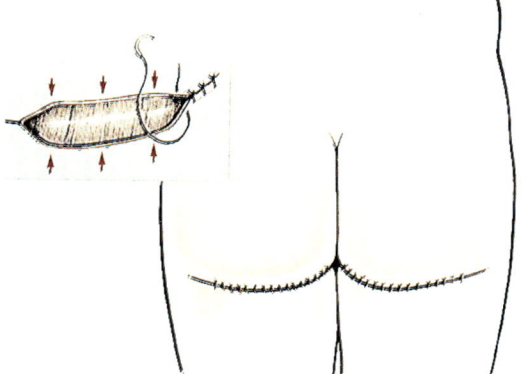

Autologous Fat Transfer

The usefulness of injected autologous fat for cosmetic purposes has long
been vigorously debated by plastic surgeons, without consensus. In 1990
Carraway [16] proposed the use of aspirated fat for facial contouring.
Ellenbogen [17], in an invited comment, likened fat transfer to the
emperor´s new clothes in Grimm´s fairy tale. What is abundantly clear,
however, is that much of the injected fat is rather promptly reabsorbed.
Peer [23, 37] reported that reabsorption of 50% or more of autologous
transferred fat could confidently be anticipated. Chajchir and Benzaquen
[20] reported satisfactory results in most of their patients but noted that
they routinely transplant 50% more fat in anticipation of partial
resorption. A committee of the American Society of Plastic and Reconstructive Surgery in 1987 [2] concluded that after one year 30% of injected fat could be expected to survive. "Therefore, overcorrection is
necessary when performing fat transplants." Fredericks [24] raised the
possibility that the survival of transplanted fat may depend on the
recipient site.

   Although it is unclear why autologous transferred fat survives better in some cases than in others, certain fundamental principles promoting graft survival are well known. When donor tissue, whether fat, a
heart or a kidney, is removed from its native site, it becomes deprived
of its nutrient blood supply. Its need for oxygen and nutrient substrate

remains, but most tissues can survive by anaerobic metabolism for a limited time. Fat should transfer well since even under ideal conditions it has a relatively poor blood supply, and presumably can tolerate a higher degree of oxygen deprivation. After donor tissue is transplanted to a recipient site, there is an outpouring of nutrient-rich plasma at that site [12, 13]. Out of this fluid the transplanted tissue absorbs dissolved oxygen and nutrients. Within a few days, endothelial proliferation begins, and there is a purposeful, directional ingrowth of blood vessels from the recipient sites into the donor tissues. Thick grafts take poorly because tissue death occurs before the ingrowing blood vessels can reach the interior. Thin grafts take well because the bulk of the graft can be revascularized in a timely fashion. In the same way, large quantities of injected fat survive poorly; smaller amounts survive relatively well.

AFT takes about one hour, two hours less than DFG. There are no unsightly or uncomfortable scars. There are no longitudinal ridges. There is no loss of penile length. On the other hand reabsorption of fat is variable and sometimes uneven. There may be contour irregularities and residual nodules which sometimes do not respond to pressure. We have done a second procedure in about 12% of our patients. With AFT, unlike DFGs, if additional girth is desired later, it can readily be done.

Factors which may contribute to survival of autologous fat are:

1. Selecting patients with bountiful donor fat. Thin or muscular patients with little body fat require vigorous aspiration which may damage the fat cells and impair their "take." Harvested fat is often dry, stringy, and admixed with fibrous connective tissue.
2. Infiltrating the donor site with buffered (pH 7.4) physiologic solution before harvesting fat.
3. Aspirating gently.
4. Cleaning donor fat of detritus.
5. Chilling fat until implantation.
6. Dissecting gently and bluntly in recipient subcutaneous dartos tissue of penis, avoiding damage to blood vessels and lymphatics.
7. Injecting smaller (30–60 cc) rather than larger amounts of fat, depending on penis size.
8. Avoiding bleeding or infection at recipient site.
9. Immobilizing the penis for 10 days postoperatively.
10. Avoiding trauma to the penis for 6 weeks, including intercourse and masturbation.
11. Refraining from cigarette smoking.

Circumcision

All uncircumcised patients are urged to undergo circumcision at least 6 weeks before phalloplasty. Simultaneous circumcision has been associated with an undesirable incidence of wound dehiscence, delayed healing, edema, and increased postoperative discomfort.

The Weight Device

After the ligaments are divided and the penis slides forward, healing begins with the formation of scar tissue. As the scar tissue matures, it contracts and tends to draw the penis back towards its original position. Before the weight device (American Bodycrafters, Huntington Beach, CA) became available every patient lost some part of the inch and a half he gained by this operation. Filling this space with liposuctioned fat does not prevent retraction and reattaching the penis seems to defeat the purpose of the operation. Using Goretex or other foreign material is unappealing because of the increased risk of infection. Injecting the area repeatedly with triamcinolone has proven ineffective. With proper use of the weight device, loss of new length is no longer a problem.

Material and Methods

Proper patient selection is the first essential of enhancement phalloplasty. The surgeon himself must evaluate the emotional stability, expectations and motivation of the patient. If there is any question, psychological consultation can be helpful. Candidates exhibiting serious doubts or reluctance, or who cling to unrealistic expectations, or who view penis enlargement as the panacea for all their problems, should not undergo surgery. No one should be persuaded or "talked into" surgery. The vast majority of stable, psychologically healthy men with realistic expectations, who have had the benefit of full, frank and complete disclosure, will be pleased with their results.

Several categories of patients seek phalloplasty:
1. Those with true penile hypoplasia;
2. those with marginally small or low normal penises with poor self-esteem;

3. those who have suffered ridicule or humiliation;
4. those who desire enhanced sensation during intercourse;
5. those whose ability to practice their occupations – actors, models, dancers – might be enhanced;
6. body builders and weight lifters whose penile size is not commensurate with their idealized vision of themselves;
7. those, like other males having cosmetic surgery, who simply seek to improve their appearance.

Since July 6, 1992, we have performed 738 phalloplasties on 640 patients. Ninety eight of these were additional procedures, 36 for residual nodules and/or for asymmetric or excessive fat resorption. After initial successful girth enhancement, 62 patients elected to have a second or third girth enlargement. Twelve patients had girth only and 14 had length only. Twelve patients had initially been operated upon elsewhere. Six patients who had undergone lengthening before the weight device became available and who had developed excessive scar tissue, underwent a second lengthening procedure after we had the weight device. At least 6 of our patients, and probably more, have gone elsewhere for a revision. Five patients underwent simultaneous enhancement phalloplasty and insertion of a penile prosthesis.

Most patients were in their third and fourth decade. The youngest was 18 and the oldest 61.

On the initial contact, a receptionist delivers basic information including cost and answers questions. The candidate completes a detailed questionnaire regarding his medical, psychological, social, family and sexual history. Patients who smoke are encouraged to refrain from the time of the initial interview until 8 weeks after surgery. At the preoperative meeting with his surgeon, the patient undergoes a physical examination. Flaccid and erect measurements are recorded for length and girth and photographs taken. As circumstances permit, the erect measurement is done either after an injection of 7.5–22.5 mg of Papaverine or else with stretched length. The two methods of length measurement have been found to conform to within 0.65 cm. We invite the patients to ask questions. In the past year it has become our practice to ask the patient what he understands about the operation and what he expects its outcome to be. We strongly recommend this practice. It is by far the best way to correct misconceptions which the patient would otherwise carry with him into the operating room. We describe in detail the length and girth enhancement procedures. We show the patient how to use the weight device. He is told how to care for himself postoperatively. Finally, the patient reads and signs an extensive informed consent. He also reads and signs the position statement of the Society for the Study of Impotence of the American Urological Association which contains strong cautionary language. All patients receive a complete blood count, urinalysis and a standard chemscreen. Patients over 40 receive an electrocardiogram.

Operative Technique

How We Do It

The patient shaves his abdomen, genitalia and upper thighs before entering the operating room. General, spinal, or epidural anesthesia is used depending on the anesthesiologist´s and the patient´s preference and where the fat is to be harvested. Intravenous Gentamicin and Vancomycin are started 20 min before surgery. Before liposuction, the abdominal wall, flanks and pubic area down to the inferior pubic notch are infiltrated with a liter of buffered sterile normal saline containing 2 cc of 1/1000 epinephrine and 30 cc of Lidocaine (Fig. 7).

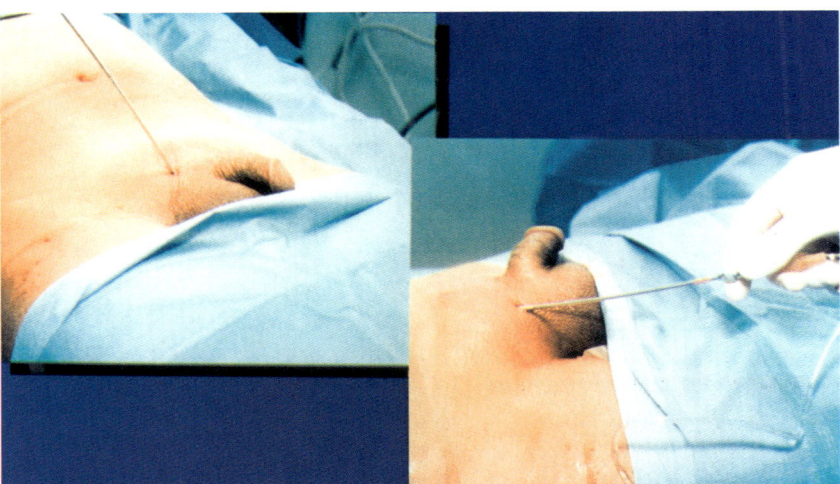

Fig. 7.   Subcutaneous spaces of abdomen, supra- and infra-pubic areas being infiltrated with saline – lidocaine, epinephrine, before fat harvest

A vertical line is drawn from the middle of the base of the penis to-ward the umbilicus to ensure symmetrical flap design. An inverted V to Y advancement flap is made on the lower abdomen at the base of the penis within the pubic escutcheon (Fig. 8–10). Each leg of the V is usu-ally about 4 cm long and the distance between the two legs at the base is about 5 cm. The base of the incision is placed 2 cm above the base of the penis to avoid creating "cheeks." The resulting skin advancement is about 2.5 centimeters. Some surgeons prefer a Z-plasty; we have found that an inverted V to Y provides equal advancement and takes less time.

Fig. 8.   Right: Incision for advancement flap

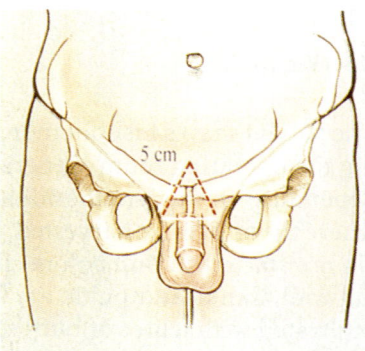

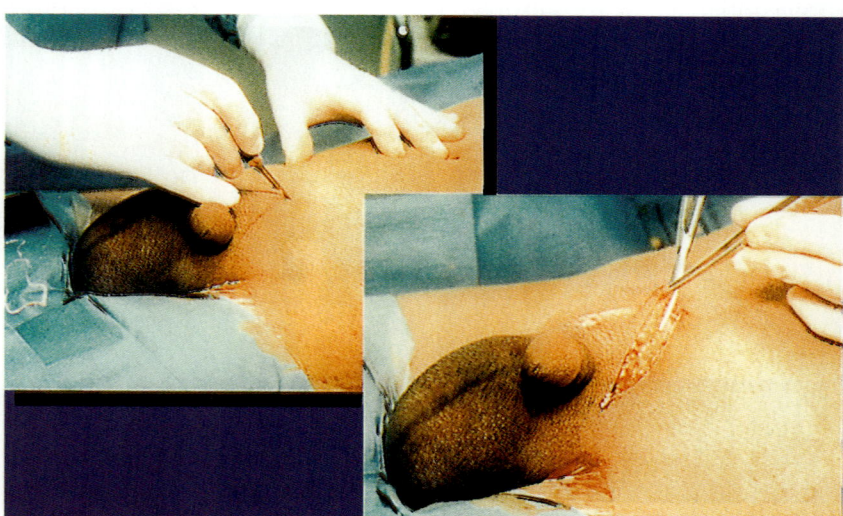

Fig. 9.   Advancement flap begun

Fig. 10.   Dissection of fundiform (superficial) ligament begun

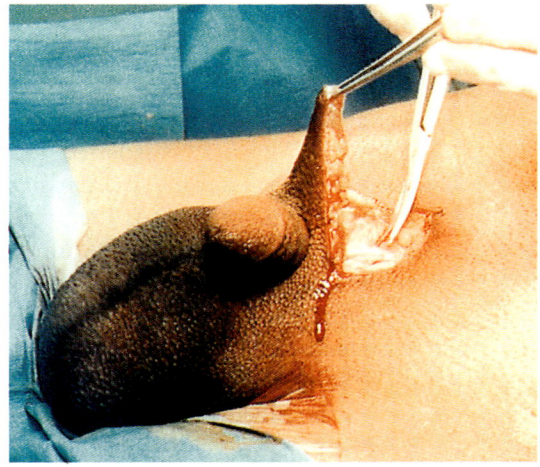

The dissection is carried down to the symphysis pubis. The second assistant retracts the penis caudad, "bowstringing" the attachments of the penis to the pubis. Richardson retractors are placed to protect the spermatic cords bilaterally and by exerting gentle lateral traction, the lateral extensions of Scarpa´s fascia are identified. The fundiform ligament and its lateral extensions are divided flush with the periosteum. (Fig. 11). The surgeon places a laparotomy pad over the dorsum of the penis and with his noncutting hand exerts pressure caudad against the dorsum of the

Fig. 11.   Ligaments divided. Penile advancement achieved

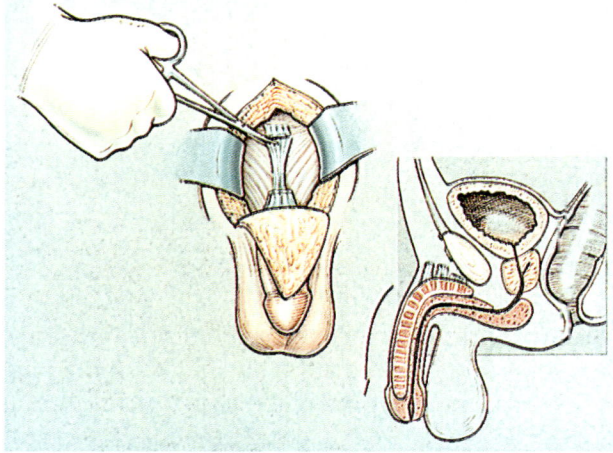

penis. Behind the surgeon´s hand, and safe from the scissors, is the neu-rovascular bundle in the midline, covered by Buck´s fascia. Failure to maintain backward pressure against the penis allows the deep dorsal vein to enter the field and puts it at risk. Using blunt and sharp dissec-tion the suspensory ligament is isolated and cut with all lateral exten-sions, flush on the periosteum. The dense areolar tissue beneath the suspensory ligament is freed from the pubic periosteum by blunt dis-section, and carried medially and laterally for about 1.5 cm. When the free edges of the inferior symphysis and pubic rami can be palpated, the dissection is complete. The deep dorsal penile vein and its trifurcation can be seen beneath the inferior pubic notch. Great care must be taken not to cut these veins; if bleeding occurs, exposure may not be adequate for ligation, and the bleeding may be too much for the cautery. In this difficult circumstance hemostasis can reliably be achieved by wrapping large squares of gelfoam in a sheet of Oxycel, soaking this in thrombin, coating it with Avitene, wedging the plug into the space and maintain-ing pressure for 15 min. Ordinary hemostasis such as oozing from the periosteum is easily accomplished with the cautery. Meticulous hemo-stasis is essential to prevent postoperative problems. Hematoma beneath the flap or blood dripping down and causing scrotal swelling is distress-ing and delays resumption of normal activities. Before closing, we ask the anesthesiologist to lighten the level of anesthesia, to raise the patient´s blood pressure to preoperative levels, in order to identify even slight oozing. Scissors lipectomy of the "V" flap and the suprapubic fat pad is performed. The flap is handled gently. We avoid putting sutures into the tip or squeezing the tip with the forceps. It should not be thinned excessively nor deprived of its blood supply. A dry laparotomy sponge is tucked into the infrapubic space while we proceed to girth enhance-ment. Attention is now directed to harvesting the fat.

Girth Enhancement:

Harvesting: Abdomen (Fig. 12–14)

Liposuction is performed through the opening provided by creating the flap. The right-handed surgeon stands on the patient´s right side. A number 6 cannula is used and the suction machine (Wells Johnson Co., Tucson, AZ) is set well below maximum. Depending on the size of the

Fig. 12, 13. Suprapubic and abdominal fat harvest begun

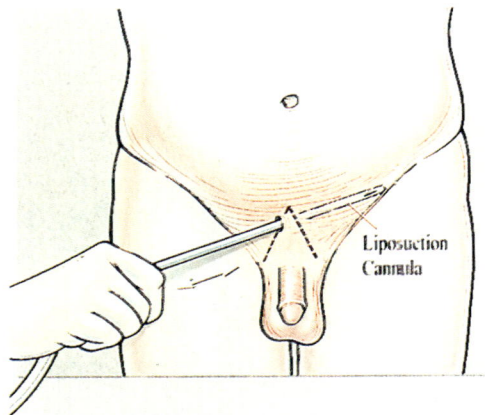

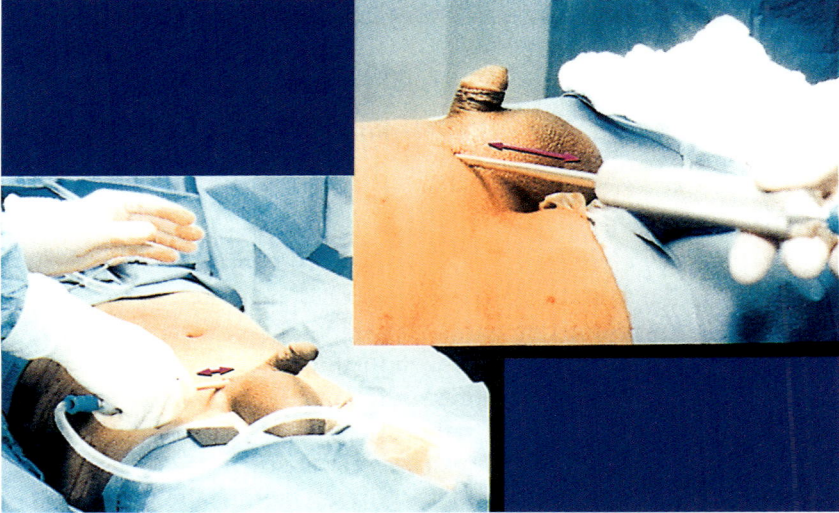

Fig. 13

penis and the patient´s wishes, between 30 and 60 cc of fat are harvested. The earliest aspirations are the least traumatized, contain the least detritus and are the most desirable. An endometrial curettage-type fat trap is used, with a funnel-shaped filter (Milex Corp., Chicago). Aspirated fat is scraped off the filter with a scalpel handle onto four folded sheets of sterile filter paper and gently pushed back and forth over the paper´s surface so that saline, blood and tissue juice will be absorbed and detritus identified and separated. We do not wash the fat. The clean,

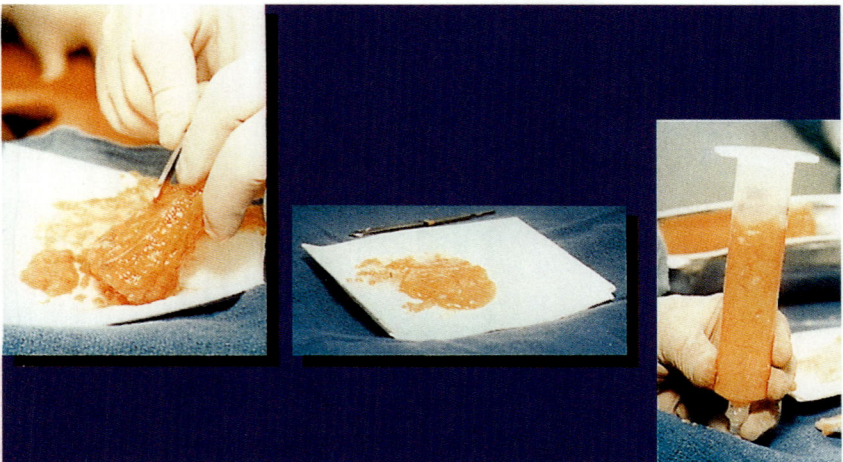

Fig. 14.   Left: Harvested fat scraped from tissue trap. Central: Sterile filter paper used to absorb fluid. Right: Fat stored in 30 cc syringes in ice slush, until injection

moist fat is stored in 30 cc syringe cylinders which stand upright in a metal beaker containing sterile ice.

Harvesting: Buttocks

When the patient´s abdominal donor site lacks insufficient fat, we usually defer surgery until he gains 4.5–6.8 kg, or else perform a DFT. Occasionally, we will harvest fat from the buttocks. Even in spare, lean young men with concave buttocks, the buttocks almost always yield 60 cc of at least fair quality fat. In these cases, the patient receives an epidural or spinal anesthesia so he can assist in the turning process. If general anesthesia is used, intubation is required. One-half liter of the saline/epinephrine/lidocaine solution is infused into each buttock, flank and medial thigh. Liposuction is carried out through a one mm. inferolateral incision in each buttock. The incision is closed with a single 2-0 chromic catgut suture, covered by a Steri-strip and the patient is turned supine again.

Fat Injection (Fig. 15–17)

A 16F Foley catheter is inserted to avoid urethral injury. The right-handed surgeon moves to the patient´s left side. The assistant pulls the

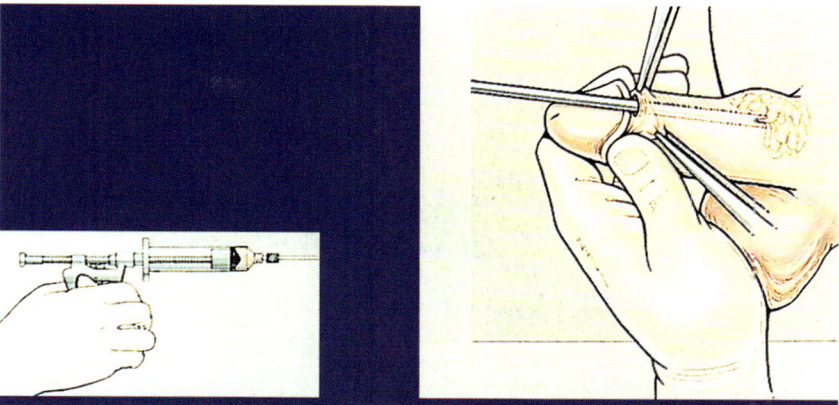

Fig. 15

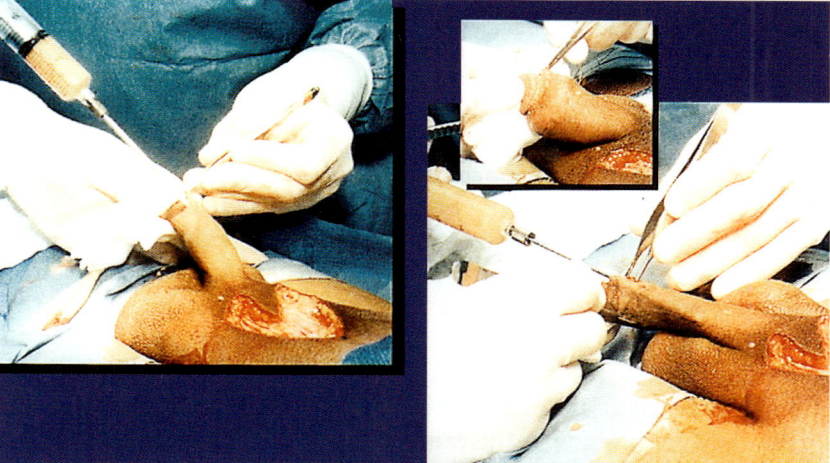

Fig. 15, 16.   Fat injected into subcutaneous space of penile shaft

penis caudad and using Adson-Brown forceps he and the surgeon grasp a thin fold of loose skin in the coronal sulcus. A 2-port 13-cm fat injection cannula (Wells Johnson, Tucson, AZ) is bluntly thrust through the skin fold into the subcutaneous dartos fascia on the dorsal midline of the shaft. The subcutaneous space on the penile shaft normally is trabeculated into compartments by the dartos fascia, lymphatics and blood vessels. To inject fat smoothly and uniformly and minimize clumping, these compartments must be made to communicate freely.

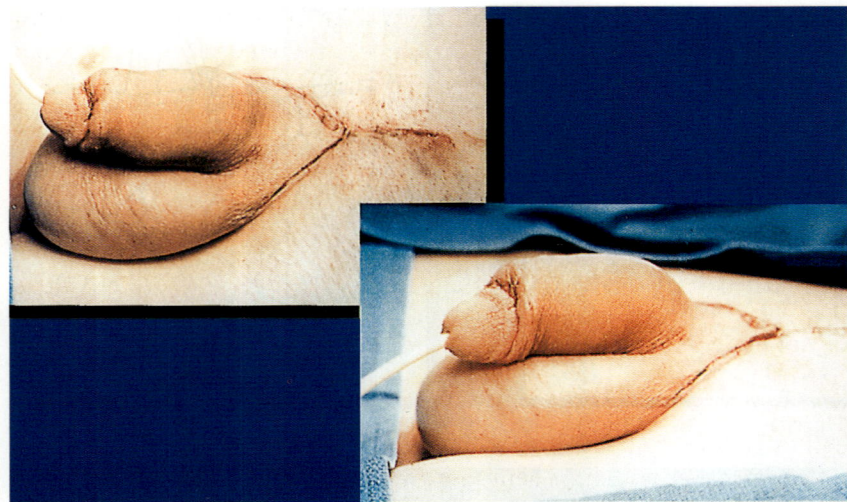

Fig. 17. Fat injection completed. Smooth symmetrical girth enhancement achieved. About 50% of the fat remains permanently

Through a single penetration, using a back and forth motion from the coronal sulcus to the base, the blunt cannula is repeatedly thrust and withdrawn everywhere except over the urethra. This dissection must be carefully done. This is not the place to hurry. The cannula will harmlessly slide off vessels and lymphatics without injuring them. After free communication has been established throughout, the fat is injected. A grease-gun type injection syringe (Byron Medical, Tucson, AZ) with one of the cylinders containing the fat is attached to the cannula, and the fat is injected beginning with the cannula tip at the base of the penis and withdrawing it toward the entry point. If adequate dissection has been accomplished and all spaces communicate, usually only one injection site is needed. Sometimes, more laterally, a second, or rarely, a third entry is needed. How much fat to inject is determined by the patient´s wishes, the availability of quality fat, the looseness of the skin, the overall size of the penis, especially the glans, and the certain knowledge that excess fat will clump and degenerate. Some surgeons use a rubber band around the base of the penis to avoid perforating Buck´s fascia posteriorly with the cannula.

Injected fat tends to collect at the base and in the frenular area where the skin is loosest. It can be manually molded into a more symmetrical cylinder and held in place with a dressing. Before edema starts to occur the penis is sprayed with a liquid adhesive and then wrapped snugly but not tightly with a sterile gauze (Kling) dressing, which helps to mold the fat and hold it in place until it "takes." A sterile Coban is applied. The penis wrap is not an afterthought. It is an important part of the operation. If the dressing is too loose, it will slide off; if too tight, nocturnal erections will be uncomfortable and ischemia and even necrosis may occur.

Closure (Fig. 18–20)

Before starting the closure we again inspect the infrapubic space for hemostasis. Using 2-0 Vicryl interrupted sutures, the remnants of the fascia and areolar tissue just beneath the pubis are brought together in the midline. Several bites are taken attaching the deepest layer of the dermis and Buck´s fascia at the base of the penis to the proximal tunica albuginea. This pulls the skin at the base of the penis backward, defining the penile-scrotal crease and adding apparent length to the shaft. Beginning

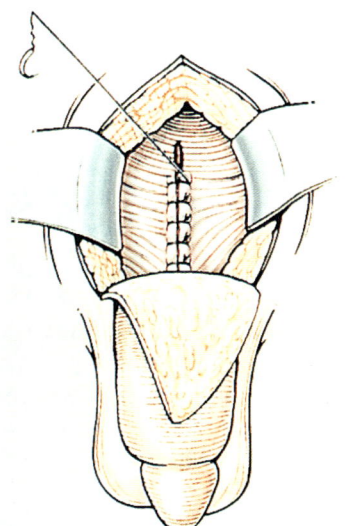

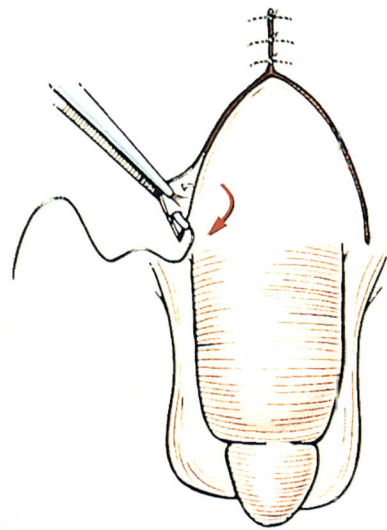

Fig. 18.   Closure begun

Fig. 19.   V-Y incision closed in 3 layers.
Subcuticular skin structures

Fig. 20.   Closure completed

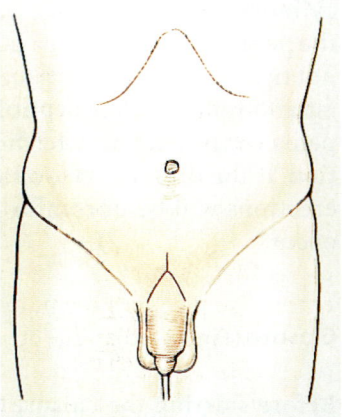

at the apex of the "V," the incision is closed from side to side in layers with 3-0 Vicryl until some resistance is felt. The "V"-shaped flap is then sutured into the remaining tissue defect with 3-0 Vicryl sutures. At the confluence of the three lines of closure, the blood supply is precarious at best. It is well to avoid placing sutures in the very tip and the flap must be handled tenderly. If the tip of the flap is redundant, it is excised and discarded. The skin is closed with subcuticular 3-0 Vicryl. Meticulous attention must be paid to the closure. It will be subjected to the most minute scrutiny by the patient. No drain is used. A dry sterile dressing is applied. The catheter is removed. An abdominal binder is applied.

Postoperative Care

On the day after surgery we remove the wrap and inspect the penis. Any asymmetry or clumps can easily be smoothed out with gentle molding. We then rewrap the penis. The patient receives Ciprofloxacin 500 mg twice daily for one week. The abdominal binder comes off in a week, the penile and incision dressings in 10 days. The patient refrains from abdominal stretching maneuvers and intercourse for 6 weeks. For the first few nights the patient deals with uncomfortable erections by keeping two ice bags beside his bed which he uses when necessary. Diazepam 10 mg taken at bedtime will usually control nocturnal erections. Three to four weeks after the operation he begins using the weight device.

Results (Fig. 21, 22)

During the first 6–8 weeks after surgery, about half of all injected fat is reabsorbed. As reabsorption takes place about 15% of patients report asymmetry or a residual lump. Patients are told before surgery that after they remove their dressing they should palpate for lumps every few days. Any palpable lump should be squeezed firmly between thumb and forefinger and it usually will disperse. If they delay too long, or if the lump is not fat but tissue debris it will not dissipate. Most patients with an otherwise pleasing result are content even if a small lump exists. Others are devastated at even the tiniest nodule or contour irregularity and the surgeon should be prepared to remove it or to add fat to smooth out the contour. Other infrequent complications include hematoma beneath the flap and in the scrotum, fat extravasation, infection, necrosis of the tip of the flap, partial wound separation, pain lasting longer than 48 h, hypertrophic scar, urethral perforation and dysuria.

When patients are measured on the operating table after surgery, with few exceptions they have gained at least 2.5 cm and often up to 4.3 cm in length. Soon thereafter, unless the weight device is used, retraction will commence, with variable loss of length. As soon as the patient began to use the weight device as instructed, retraction ceases. Slowly, over the next few months the penis elongates as the weight device acts as a tissue expander. If patients wear the weight device intermittently as instructed for 4 months after surgery, the great majority will gain at least an inch in length. Many patients will wear their weight devices for months or even years, sometimes adding extra weight, and will continue to gain length.

Girth gains are more variable and less predictable. After 8 weeks about half the fat has already been reabsorbed and within the first year another 5%–10% may be lost. Most patients remain with a girth gain of between 2.5–5.0 cm. We have followed some patients as long four years. In general, what they have after a year is what they will retain.

Around 12% of patients undergo a second operation for
1. scar revision,
2. lump removal or contouring or
3. additional girth. Thin patients sometimes must gain weight before undergoing reoperation.

When we reported our first 162 patients in 1994, overall patient satisfaction averaged 5–6 on an ascending scale of 1–10. We now judge patient

Fig. 21, 22. Before and two months after length and girth enhancement

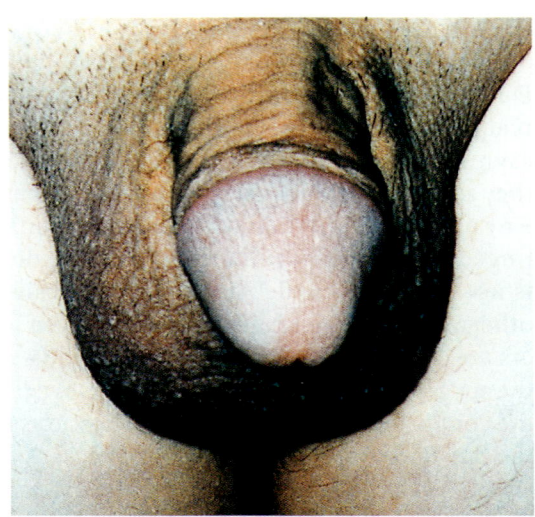

Fig. 22

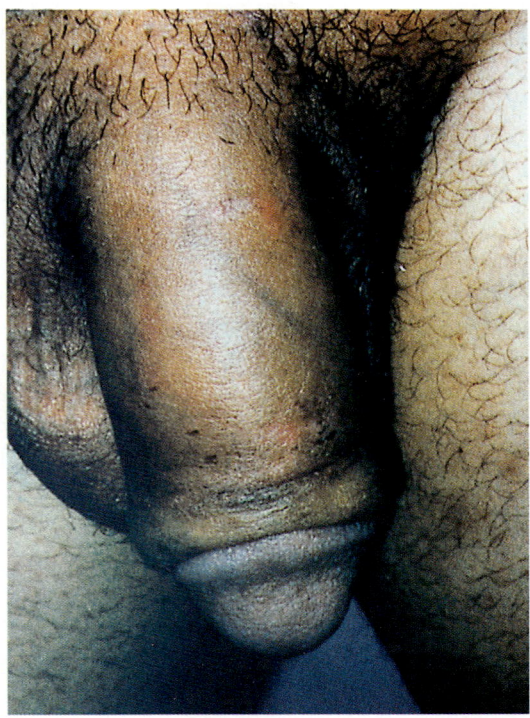

satisfaction to be around 7. Unlike our earlier series when detailed questionnaires were mailed and telephone calls placed to all patients by an independent research team, we have this time by necessity relied on information gathered at postoperative visits and telephone calls. Patients often live at a distance and don´t return or call unless they have a problem. Our information, therefore is anecdotal and probably skewed toward the less favorable. Our experience has shown that this is probably the best we can do.

When asked retrospectively if, knowing what he knows today would he chose to have his operation again, 10% said no (sometimes vehemently), 15% were undecided, and about 75% again said yes. As before, no patient reported erectile loss. No patient reported instability of the base (swiveling) or lower erectile angle. Subsequent weight loss did not seem to compromise girth gains.

As near as can be determined, our infection rate is probably around three percent, none within the last 12 months. Early reports of "pus leaking out," without other symptoms were probably attributable to seepage of excess fat. Infection in the new penile fat is a serious complication and is associated with significant psychological and physical morbidity. The infectious agents were staph. epidermidis and the enteric organisms. These have without exception cleared with Ciproflaxacin but before they subside much of the transplanted fat may be destroyed, requiring reoperation.

To these young healthy men even a small hematoma in their scrotum is alarming. But large or small these all clear with heat and rest and time, but instead of the patient returning to work in 2 or 3 days, he may return in 2 or 3 weeks.

Discussion

With experience we now insert much less fat then previously. We have come to believe that less is more. Fat that is sequestered in masses which cannot be penetrated by revascularization will not survive. If it is gently harvested, tenderly treated, transposed to an adequately prepared and vascularized recipient site, and properly immobilized, fat survival will very likely be adequate. The literature states that dermal fat grafts should not exceed 1.5 cm in thickness. Assuming that the graft is circumferential, this means that dermal fat grafts can add about 3 cm to the penis girth. In our experience about the same is true for autologous transplanted fat.

Enhancement phalloplasty is not a perfect operation and potential patients must be aware of its limitations. We agree with Alter that penis enhancement techniques continue to evolve and results are constantly being evaluated [1]. The same can be said for a great many common surgical procedures. Penis enhancement surgery can be performed with low morbidity and a high degree of patient satisfaction.

References

1. Alter GJ (1995) Augmentation Phalloplasty. Urol Clin of NA 22: 887
2. American Society of Plastic and Reconstructive Surgeons (1987) Report on Autologous Fat Transplantation by the ASPRS ad hoc committee on new procedures. Chicago, ASPRS
3. da Ros G, Teloken C et al. (1994) Caucasian penis: What is normal size. Presented at American Urological Association 89th Annual Meeting, San Francisco, May 16, 1994
4. Furlow W (1993) Presented at Los Angeles Urological Society, Los Angeles, CA
5. Subrini L (1984) Surgical treatment of Peyronie´s disease using penile implants; survey of 69 patients. J Urol 132: 47
6. Joshi PM, Kahn AG (1986) Augmentation phalloplasty. J Urol 135: Abstract 130
7. Burman SO, Kelly T (1994) Enhancement Phalloplasty. Poster presentation with discussion. VI World Meeting on Impotence, International Society for Impotence Research, Singapore Oct 1994
8. Roos H, Lissoos (1984) Penis lengthening. Int Aesthetic Restor Surg 2: 89
9. Reed HH (1994) Augmentation phalloplasty with girth enhancement employing autologous fat transplantation: a preliminary report. Amer J Cosm Surg 11: 85
10. Masters WH, Johnson V (1966) Human Sexual Response. Little, Brown and Co, Boston
11. Burman SO (1957) The effects of irradiation upon the revascularization and survival of skin autografts – I. Surg Forum 6: 575
12. Burman SO (1959) The effects of irradiation upon the revascularization and survival of skin autografts – II. Surg Gynec and Obstet 109: 683
13. Wessels H, Lue TF, McAninch JW (1996) Penile Length in the Flaccid and Erect States: Guidelines for Penile Augmentation. J Urol 156: 995
14. Ersek RR (1991) Transplantation of purified autologous fat: A 3-year follow-up is disappointing. Plast Reconstr Surg 87: 219
15. Lewis CH (1991) The current status of autologous fat grafting. Presented at the Ninth Annual Meeting, LSNA. Seattle, Sept 1991
16. Carraway JH, Mellow CG (1990) Syringe aspiration and fat concentration. A simple technique for autologous fat injection. Ann Plast Surg 24: 293
17. Ellenbogen R (see above) In: Carraway JH, Mellow CG (eds) Invited comment following paper

18. Agris J (1987) Autologous fat transposition: A 3-year study. Amer J Cosm Surg 4: 95
19. Bircoll M (1992) A nine-year experience with autologous fat transplantation: Amer J Cosm Surg 9: 55
20. Chajchir A, Benzaquen A (1986) Liposuction for grafts in face wrinkles and hemi-facial atrophy. Aesthetic Plast Surg 10: 115
21. Weber JR Jr (1986) Fat grafts: Do they work? Presented at the Annual Meeting of the Lipolysis Society of North America. Los Angeles, CA
22. Ellenbogen R (1986) Free autologous pearl fat grafts in the face. Amer Plastic Surg 16: 179
23. Peer LG (1956) The neglected free fat graft. Plast Reconstr Surg 18: 233
24. Fredericks S (1989) Fat grafting rejection for soft tissue augmentation (Discussion). Plast Reconstr Surg 84: 935
25. Illouz YG (1985) A surgical remodeling of the silhouette by aspiration lipolysis or selective lipectomy. Aesthetic Plast Surg 9: 7
26. Ibid (1984) Illouz´s technique of body contouring by lipolysis. Clin Plast Surg 11: 409
27. Ibid (1983) Body contouring by lipolysis: A 5-year experience with over 3000 cases. Plast Reconstr Surg 72: 591
28. Johnston JH (1974) Lengthening of the congenital or acquired short penis. Brit J Urol 46: 685
29. Kelly JH, Eraklis AJ (1971) A procedure for lengthening the phallus in boys with exstrophy (?) of the bladder. J Pediatr Surg 6: 645
30. Maizels M et al. (1968) Surgical correction of the buried penis. Description of a classi-fication system and a technique to correct this disorder. J Urol 136: 268
31. Horton CE et al. (1987) Hidden penis release. Adjunctive suprapubic lipectomy. Amer Plastic Surg 19: 131
32. Long DC (1990) Elongation of the Penis. Chung-Hua-Cheng-Hsing-Shoa-Shang-Wai-Ko-Tsa-Chih. Mar 6 (ii): 17-9,7 (Chinese)
33. Crawford DA (1977) Buried penis. Brit J Plast Surg 30: 96
34. Shapiro AR (1987) Surgical treatment of the "buried" penis. Urol 30: 554
35. Devine CJ, Jordan GH et al. (1984) Concealed penis. Soc for Ped Urol Newsletter 115: Nov. 14, 1984
36. Radhakrishnan J, Reyes HM (1984) Penoplasty for buried penis secondary to "radi-cal" circumcision. J Ped Surg 19: 629
37. Peer LG (1950) Loss of weight and volume in human fat grafts, with formation of a "cell survival theory." Plast Reconstr Surg 5: 217
38. Johnston JH (1977) Other penile abnormalities. In: Surgical Pediatric Urology. Saunders, Philadelphia, Chapt. 7.2, p 406
39. Johnston JH (1984) Concealed penis. Soc Ped Urol Newsletter, Dec 28, 1984, p 124

Penile Prostheses: Current Applications

William L. Furlow

Introduction

Alloplastic materials have been used by the medical profession for nearly half a century as a means of re-establishing erectile function in the impotent male. The chronological development of prosthetic devices is outlined in Table 1. The earliest alloplastic devices were single acrylic rigid rod devices implanted initially into the subcutaneous tissue of the penile shaft, followed a few years later by implantation into the cavernous tissue of the penis in order to better stabilize the device.

Proximal migration of single rod and paired devices was first addressed with the introduction of a bifurcate proximal attachment

Table 1. The history of alloplastic penile implants

1950:	Implantation of single acrylic rod prosthesis: (Scardino)
1952:	Implantation of single acrylic rod prosthesis: (Goodwin & Scott)
1956:	Implantation of single acrylic rod prosthesis: (Loeffler and Sayegh)
1960:	Implantation of paired polyethylene rod prosthesis: (Beheri)
1967:	Implantation of single silastic rod prosthesis: (Pearman)
1968:	Implantation of single silicone rod prosthesis: (Lash)
	Implantation of single silicone rod prosthesis with bifurcate crural attachment: (Lash-Maser)
1972:	Implantation of bifurcate teflon rod prosthesis: (Tudoriu)
1972:	Implantation of inflatable silicone penile prosthesis: (Scott et al.)
1973:	Implantation of paired silicone rod prosthesis: (Small-Carrion)
1973:	Implantation of single silicone rod prosthesis: (Gerow)
1973:	Implantation of paired malleable silver-wire prosthesis: (Jonas)
1977:	Implantation of paired flexible silicone rods: (Finney)
1983:	Implantation of paired malleable penile prosthesis: (AMS Study Group)
1983:	Implantation of inflatable silicone coated polyethylene Bioflex™ penile prosthesis: (Merrill)
1985:	Implantation of self-contained, single piece inflatable prosthesis: (AMS Study Group)
1987:	Implantation of two-piece inflatable penile prosthesis: (Mentor GFS™)
1994:	Implantation of two piece inflatable penile prosthesis: (AMS Ambicor™)

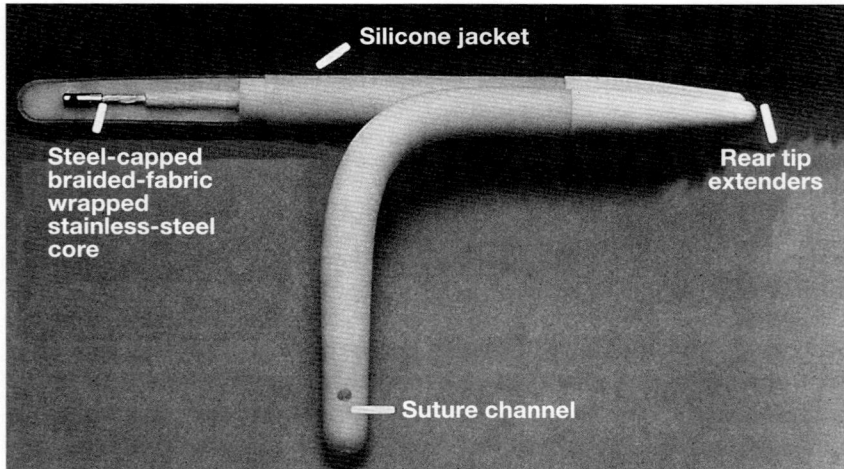

Fig. 1.   The AMS 600 malleable penile prosthesis

screwed into the proximal end of a solitary rod and seated, one limb in each crus [1]. Subsequently, paired rigid teflon and polyethylene devices used in the 1960s were replaced by devices made of silicone. These devices provided the patient with a permanent erection which was often difficult to conceal. A paired silver wire malleable prosthesis was successfully introduced by Jonas in 1973 in an effort to provide the patient with better concealment of the otherwise permanent erection [2]. This malleable concept was followed in subsequent years by the development of articulated malleable devices, braided stainless steel wire devices and paired hinged devices, all designed to improve and retain molding the erect penile shaft into a flexed position for better concealment (Fig. 1). Currently, these devices are primarily implanted using a subcoronal incision, and are usually implanted under local anesthesia.

In 1972 F. Brantley Scott introduced the first inflatable penile prosthesis [3]. The innovative design of this device provided the impotent patient and his physician with the option of selecting a prosthesis which would provide the patient with a controllable erection, fully erect and rigid when inflated and flaccid and easily concealable when deflated. The original three-piece inflatable device manufactured by American Medical Systems Inc. (Minnetonka, MN, USA) has been modified over the years through material changes in the properties of silicone to include controlled expansion cylinders and inflatable cylinders which expand both in diameter and length (Fig. 2). In 1983 the Mentor Corporation

Fig. 2. The three-piece
AMS 700 Ultrex Plus
inflatable penile prosthesis

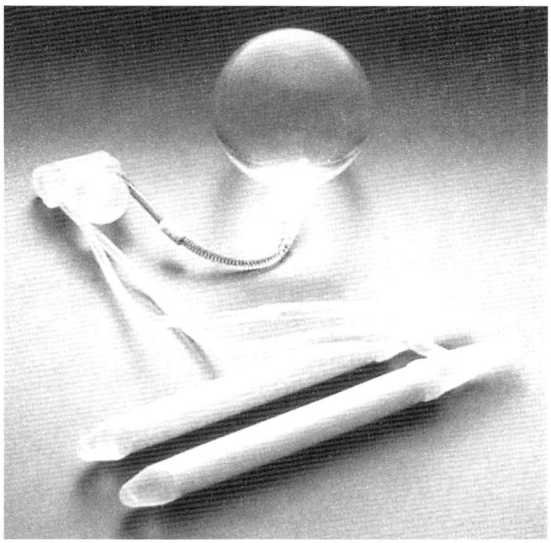

(Goleta, CA, USA) introduced a three-piece inflatable penile prosthesis utilizing a silicone coated polyethylene material [4]. These three-piece devices are currently implanted using either the AMS 700 CX or 700 Ultrex plus or the Mentor α1-inflatable prostheses, respectively. The recommended approaches for these devices are infra, suprapubic or penoscrotal.

Two-piece inflatable devices were first introduced in 1987 by the Mentor Corporation (Fig. 3), and subsequently in 1994 by American Medical Systems, Inc. (Fig. 4). These devices were designed to eliminate the reservoir component in an effort to simplify surgical implantation while preserving some of the desirable features of the three-piece devices. They consist of a scrotal pump with prefilled, pre-connected cylinders which can be implanted through either the suprapubic or infrapubic approach, or through a penoscrotal incision.

Self-contained inflatable devices were first introduced in the mid-1980s, consisting of paired inflatable cylinders with a self-contained fluid filled reservoir thus providing the patient with a controllable erection. Representative of these earlier devices is the currently available Dynaflex™ inflatable penile prosthesis (Fig. 5). This device is routinely implanted using a penoscrotal approach, and often employing local anesthesia as the anesthesia of choice.

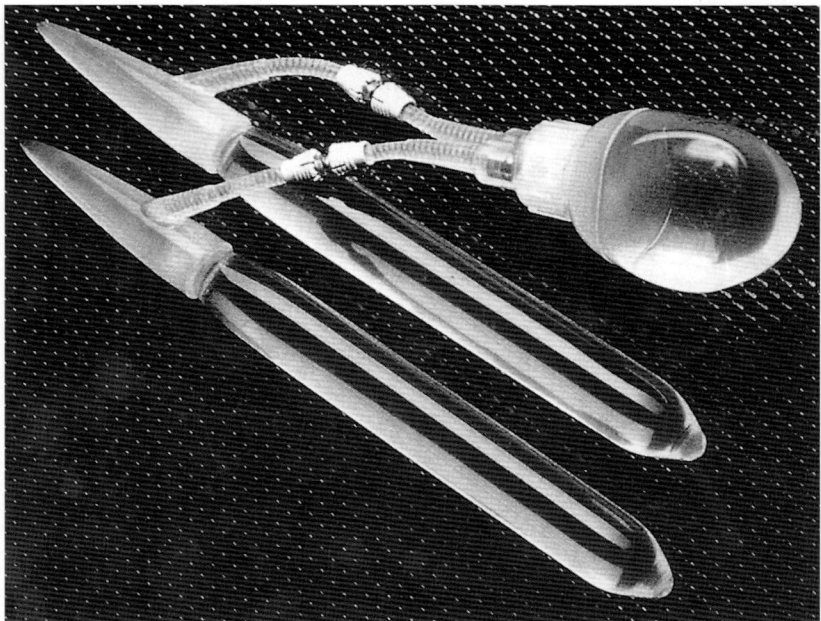

Fig. 3.   The Mentor two-piece GFS inflatable penile prosthesis

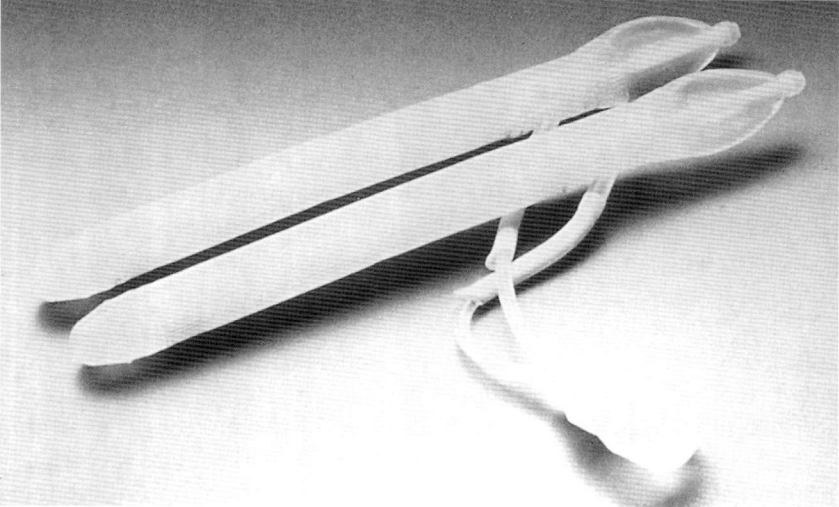

Fig. 4.   The AMS Ambicore two-piece inflatable penile prosthesis

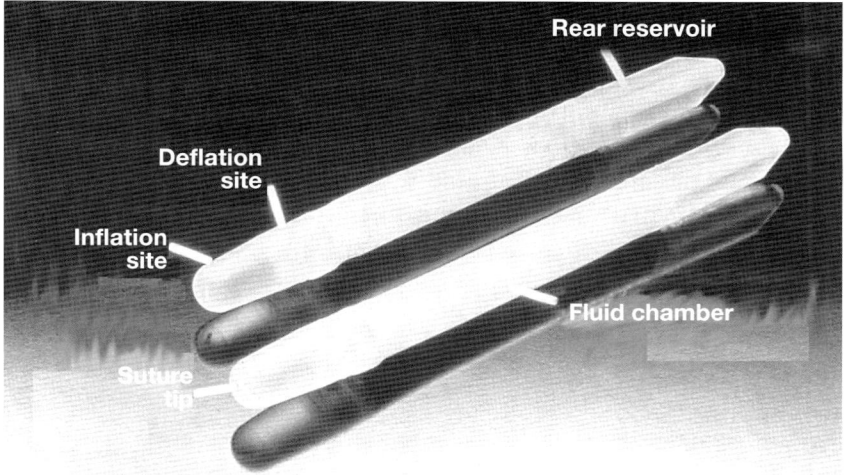

Fig. 5. The one-piece self-contained Dynaflex inflatable penile prosthesis by American Medical Systems, Inc.

The urologist´s decision as to which of the currently available devices should be implanted is based on a number of factors which include:
1. the physical and anatomical condition of the patient;
2. the patient´s habitus;
3. the urologist´s expectations as to the performance of the device, as well as the expectations of the patient´s partner; and
4. the training and preferences of the surgeon which may preclude selection of certain devices.

Penile Disorders and Penile Prosthetic Surgery

It is estimated that from January, 1985, through December, 1995, world-wide, more than 200 000 inflatable devices, and 75 000–85 000 semirigid rod devices have been implanted. In 1995 alone it is estimated that 20 000 inflatable devices and 4000 semirigid rod devices were implanted. Current estimates suggest that by the year 2000 A.D. nearly one-half million devices will have been implanted since figures became available in 1985 [5].

The majority of these implants have been performed on the organically impotent patient, patients that are best described as having irreversible erectile dysfunction due to a variety of well known causes. Arising out of this large pool of patients are three groups of implant patients that deserve our special attention today:

1. impotent patients with Peyronie´s disease;
2. patients with penile fibrosis requiring cavernosal reconstruction; and
3. patients who require penile lengthening. These groups are classified by the author as anomalous implants.

Peyronie´s Disease

Penile straightening can sometimes be achieved in the impotent patient with Peyronie´s disease by the implantation of a penile prosthesis. Some impotent patients with known Peyronie´s disease may have a perfectly straight penis after implantation, while others will demonstrate a severe curvature following implantation which will require surgical straightening (Fig. 6). In each case the implant should be inserted and the curvature clearly demonstrated before straightening is performed. The author´s standard practice when an inflatable device is implanted is to fully inflate the cylinders thus demonstrating the point of greatest curvatures. As an initial maneuver, there is some merit in attempting to manually straighten the penis by forcefully bending the erect penis in order to fracture the plaque material, thereby straightening the penis.

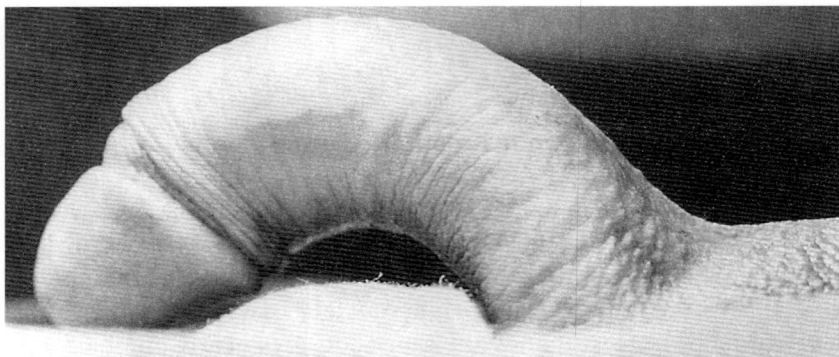

Fig. 6.   Severe dorsal curvature after inflatable device implantation in patient with Peyronie´s disease

This technique was first introduced by Wilson in 1994 and is currently used as the initial step prior to surgical straightening in the impotent patient with Peyronie´s disease receiving a penile implant.

If forceful bending fails to straighten the erect penis, the point of greatest curvature is then marked on the shaft of the penis after carrying out the usual degloving procedure to expose Buck´s fascia and the tunica albuginea. If required, the neurovascular bundle is then skeletonized at the point of greatest curvature on the concave surface. It is at this point that a transverse incision is made into the tunica using the cutting current of the electrocautery (Fig. 7). As the penis straightens, the resulting defect may or may not expose the underlying cavernosal tissue and the implant. Use of the cautery protects the underlying device from damage since silicone will generally not be injured by the cutting current of the cautery. The defect should not be covered with native or artificial graft material. Experience has taught us that the defect will fill in over the cylinder in about 4–6 weeks. In this way, one more step that might increase the patient´s chances of developing an infection has been eliminated. When an inflatable device is used, it is left partially inflated for

Fig. 7. Penile straightening with transverse incision of the tunica albuginea using the cutting current of the electrocautery

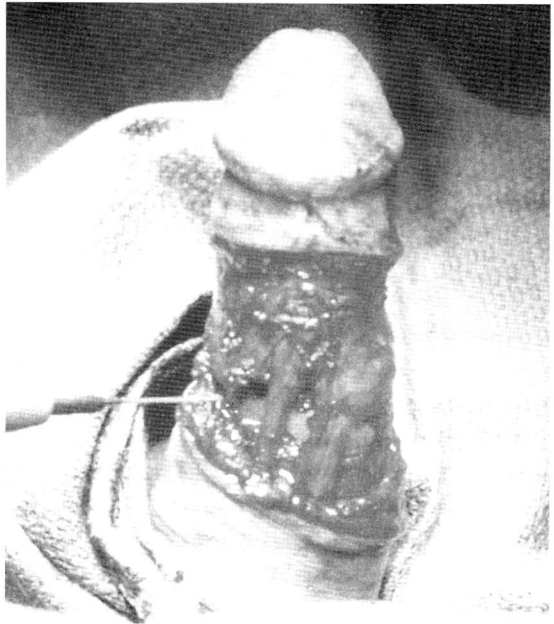

Fig. 8. Penis with device inflated following penile straightening and subcoronal skin closure

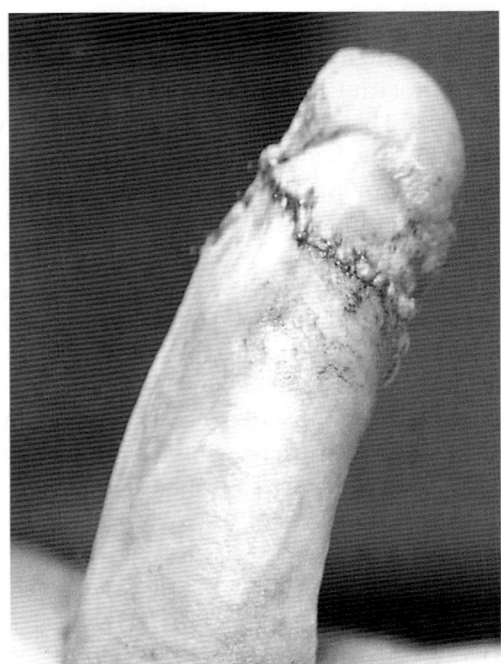

three days post-operatively, and then deflated fully as with a standard implant (Fig. 8). As a rule of thumb, defects larger than 2 cm in longitudinal width should be covered with a graft, preferably of Goretex (Fig. 9). With this technique the patient´s penis will be fully functional in from 4 to 6 weeks.

Penile Fibrosis and Cavernosal Reconstruction

The patient who is to be considered for the implantation of a penile prosthesis should be made aware of the potential of encountering penile fibrosis of varying degrees that may preclude routine insertion of the device, and that cavernosal reconstruction may be a possible alternative. However, the risk of encountering penile fibrosis requiring a reconstructive procedure in an otherwise normal male with no previous history of penile disease, trauma, or previous penile surgery is extremely small. On the other hand, extensive cavernosal scarring should

Fig. 9. Use of polyfluorotetraethylene
(Goretex) graft to cover the defect in the
tunica albuginea. Note preservation of
the neurovascular bundle

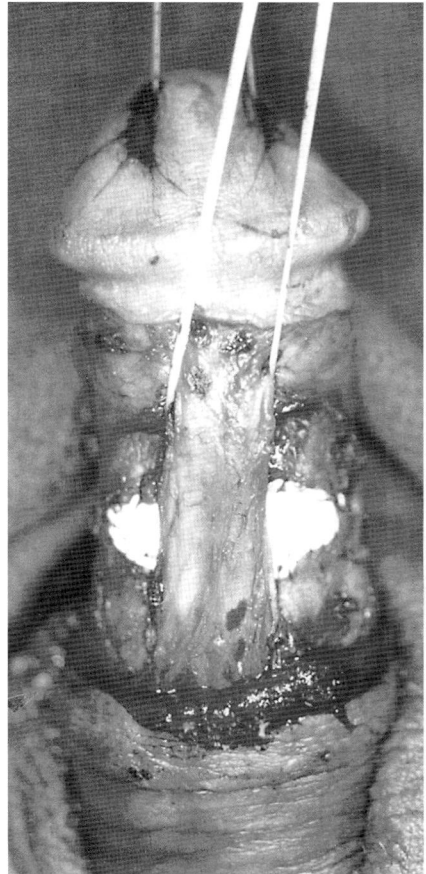

be anticipated in those patients with a prior history of cavernosal infection following prosthesis implantation and explantation, post-
priapism impotence, previous prosthetic explantation, penile straightening procedures, penile trauma, and Peyronie´s disease treatment, both
medical and surgical. It is within this group of patients that cavernosal
reconstruction may be required.

Cavernosal reconstruction implies the surgeon´s intention to recon-
figure a part or all of the fibrotic cavernous body into a hollow cylindrical tube which bridges the scarred portion, in order to implant a
penile prosthesis. This procedure was first introduced by the author at

the annual meeting of the American Urological Association in Las Vegas, Nevada in 1984. The basic principle is to bivalve the scarred portion of the cavernosal body and to then reconstruct the cylindrical shape of the normal erectile body using Goretex (Fig. 10a, b). While initially this bivalve technique utilized this synthetic material, additional techniques to enlarge the cavernous body diameter to accommodate penile device implantation have been introduced. One alternative method to correct the problem has been to dissect and remove the segment of fibrotic cavernous tissue from the overlying relatively normal tunica albuginea in order to create a space adequate to accommodate the prosthetic cylinder.

The technique has been most useful in cases of minimal to moderate fibrosis where cylinder dilation could not be achieved to an adequate caliber for the available cylinder. It is the author´s experience that patients with extensive fibrosis are best treated by the bi-valving technique with cavernosal reconstruction using Goretex, and in some

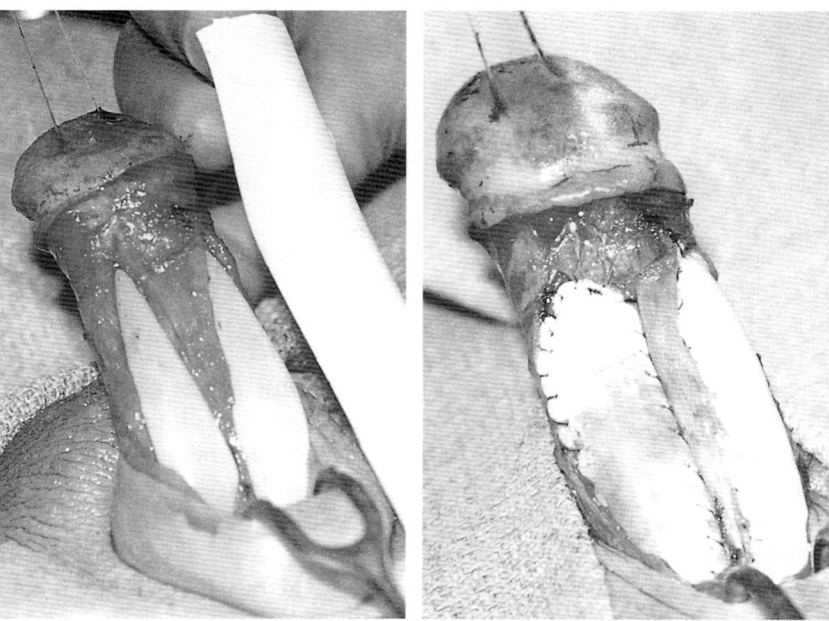

Fig. 10   a Segmental bivalving of the fibrotic cavernous bodies and implantation of the inflatable cylinders. Preparation of Goretex. **b** Goretex sutured in place to cover the exposed cylinders and completing the reconstruction

instances combining Goretex reconstruction with dissection and removal of fibrotic tissue where possible and safe to do so. In these patients, use of the inflatable penile prosthesis, AMS 700CX, manufactured by American Medical Systems, Inc., has been the prosthesis of choice [6, 7].

Over the past 10 years our group at the Center for Urological Treatment and Research has encountered more than 60 patients in whom it was not feasible to excise fibrotic cavernous tissue or dilate the cavernous body to accommodate an implantable cylinder. In one evaluation of 57 patients who underwent cavernosal reconstruction using Goretex and the implantation of an inflatable penile prosthesis, long term follow-up demonstrated that 70% of these patients maintained a functional device. In the remaining 30% removal of the implant and the graft was necessary as the result of infection [8, 9]. Further evaluation of these patients and the disappointing results led my group to conclude that if we could eliminate the necessity for dilating the fibrotic cavernous body up to the no.12 Hegar, the size required to insert the standard CX inflatable cylinder, by making available a downsized inflatable cylinder, we could reduce the inherent risks associated with reconstructive procedures and the use of artificial graft materials.

The downsized inflatable penile prosthesis(AMS 700CXM) manufactured by American Medical Systems, Inc. measures 9.5 mm in diameter and requires cavernosal dilation to only no. 10 Hegar distally and proximally. In the initial series, the downsized device was used in 20 patients with severe cavernous fibrosis [11]. Eighteen of these patients had undergone previous penile implantation and had their devices removed because of infection. Two patients had experienced severe priapism and had not undergone prior implantation. All 20 patients underwent surgery through a suprapubic incision and, in every case, severe cavernous fibrosis was encountered and the cavernous body could only be dilated to no. 10 Hegar. Use of the standard sized 12.0 mm diameter inflatable cylinder was not possible without extensive cavernosal reconstruction and foreign body grafting. Use of the downsized AMS 700CXM inflatable cylinder totally eliminated the need for the use of the polytetrafluoroethylene graft, and only native tissue reconstruction in seven patients. Only one patient (5%) experienced problems with postoperative infection. Follow-up over a period of 9–36 months demonstrated that 19 of 20 patients had a functional device and were experiencing satisfactory intercourse.

Clearly, use of the downsized inflatable cylinders in the patient whose fibrotic cavernous bodies cannot be dilated above no. 10 Hegar allows the implant surgeon to offer the patient a multi-component inflatable device without the need to bivalve the fibrotic segment and the necessity to use a polytetrafluoroethylene graft. This downsized device should be included in the implant armamentarium of every implanting urologist.

Penile Prostheses: Penile Fibrosis and Penile Lengthening

Successful penile prosthesis implantation in patients with penile fibrosis does not always provide the patient with sufficient length for satisfactory sexual intercourse. For this reason, it is important that the urologist thoroughly discuss the potential limitations of prosthetic implantation, and in particular, any unrealistic expectations regarding penile length. Penile prostheses do not increase the length of the penis. With this firmly in mind, there will still be those patients with severe cavernosal fibrosis who have undergone prosthesis implantation who will experience insufficient length and who may be suitable candidates for penile lengthening with flap advancement and tissue debulking [12].

The average adult penis in the flaccid state varies in length between 7.5 cm and 10.5 cm, and between 12 cm and 18 cm erect with a mean of 13 cm [11, 12, 13]. A penile size found to be below two standard deviations (10 cm in erect length) is considered to be a true micropenis [13, 14, 15].

A recent publication in the *Journal of Urology* by Knoll et al. chronicles the author´s experience with a new technique for penile lengthening in eleven patients who demonstrated no more than 10 cm of functional penile length after the implantation of a penile prosthesis and releasing of the suspensory ligament [12]. Nine of the eleven patients had undergone previous penile implantation with an inflatable device and had required removal secondary to infection without associated erosion. Two patients had severe priapism and had had no previous surgery. Clinically, all eleven patients demonstrated severe cavernosal fibrosis. In 10 patients, dilatation could be carried out to no. 12 Hegar and a AMS 700CX inflatable penile prosthesis was implanted. In two patients, the AMS 700CXM was used due to the inability to dilate to a size greater than no. 10 Hegar. Reconstructive procedures were not employed in any of the eleven patients.

The penile lengthening technique is as follows. Using the suprapubic approach, a U-shaped flap, based inferiorly, is designed, and the flap elevated and isolated to allow exposure of the dorsum of the penis and implantation of the prosthetic device. Following this, the suspensory ligament is exposed and carefully severed while protecting the neurovascular bundle. The cylinders are then fully inflated and the penis measured from the symphysis to the end of the penis. In all eleven patients penile length after inflation did not exceed 10 cm. Then, with the distal end of the flap oriented superiorly, one to two cm of the distal portion of the flap is de-epithelialized and the distal end sutured to the anterior portion of the pubis. After identifying areas in the lower abdomen from which excess fat should be removed, the adipose tissue is removed either by electrocautery or use of the liposuction cannula. When evaluated eight weeks post operatively all 11 patients in this series had a functioning device and were experiencing satisfactory intercourse. Of equal importance is the fact that all eleven patients demonstrated an increase in length from 3.5 cm to 6.5 cm after initial prosthetic implantation.

It is author´s contention that the above procedure can offer the impotent patient with a clinically foreshortened penis the opportunity to resume a normal sex life, rather than the premature termination of their sex life. The author, however, does not advocate this technique in the sexually active nonimpotent patient whose erect penis meets the published criteria for penile length set forth earlier in the text.

Conclusion

Implantation of the penile prosthesis for the treatment of irreversible male erectile dysfunction remains the gold standard by which all other methods of treatment must be measured. Under no circumstances should this form of treatment be considered the "treatment of last resort." The implantation of the inflatable penile prosthesis in more than 3000 patients over the past 25 years leads me to conclude that penile prostheses will always be a viable option in patient management throughout the world. An awareness of these special conditions in which the inflatable penile prosthesis has been particularly effective in the salvage of the patient´s sex life can be especially rewarding to both the patient and the urologist.

References

1. Lash H, Zimmerman DC, Loeffler RA (1964) Silicone implantation inlay method. Plast Reconstr Surg 34: 75–80
2. Krane RJ, Freedberg PS, Siroky MB (1981) Jonas silicone-silver prosthesis: initial experience in America. J Urol 126: 475
3. Scott FB, Bradley WE, Timm GW (1973) Management of erectile impotence: use of implantable inflatable prosthesis. Urology 2: 80
4. Merrill DC (1983) Mentor Inflatable Penile Prosthesis. Urology 22 (5): 504–505
5. Poston M Personal communication
6. Knoll LD, Furlow WL, Benson RC (1990) Management of Peyronie´s disease by implantation of inflatable penile prosthesis. Urology 36: 406–409
7. Wilson SK (1994) Non-surgical treatment of penile curvature. Presented at the International Society for Impotence Research, Singapore
8. Furlow WL (1983) Cavernosal reconstruction and implantation of the inflatable penile prosthesis. Presented at the 1983 Annual Meeting of the American Urological Association, Las Vegas
9. Knoll LD, Furlow WL (1992) Corporeal reconstruction and prosthetic implantation for impotence associated with non dilatable corporeal cavernosal fibrosis. ACTA Urologica Belgica 60(1): 15
10. Furlow WL, Knoll LD (1989) Clinical experience with controlled expansion cylinders: The AMS 700CX inflatable penile prosthesis. Urol Cl No Am 16 (1): 67
11. Knoll LD, Furlow WL, Benson RC, Bilhartz DL (1995) Management of non-dilatable cavernous fibrosis with the use of a downsized inflatable penile prosthesis. J Urol 153: 366–367
12. Knoll LD, Fisher J, Benson RC, Minich PJ, Furlow WL (1996) Managing penile fibrosis with prosthetic implantation and flap advancement with tissue debulking. J Urol 156: 394–397
13. Green R (1975) Human Sexuality. Williams and Wilkens, Baltimore, vol 1, pp 22
14. Winter JSD, Fraiman C (1972) Pituitary-gonadal relations in male children and adolesence. Pediatr Res 6: 126
15. Teague JL, Gonzales ET (1993) The many difficulties in managing micropenis. Contemp Urol 5: 15

Subject Index

Springer-Verlag
and the Environment

We at Springer-Verlag firmly believe that an international science publisher has a special obligation to the environment, and our corporate policies consistently reflect this conviction.

We also expect our business partners – paper mills, printers, packaging manufacturers, etc. – to commit themselves to using environmentally friendly materials and production processes.

The paper in this book is made from low- or no-chlorine pulp and is acid free, in conformance with international standards for paper permanency.